You'r_ _____, You're Full of "IT"

A Body, Mind, & Soul Cleansing Diet inspired by God

By David Ryals, Advanced MSc P.T., M.T.C.

Acknowledgements

As I feel "called by God" to write this book to help people, I acknowledge God first & foremost. I have been encouraged by thousands of my patients – as well as many nurses, therapists, and physicians (& other "friends & family" members) – to write this book for the past 18 years! I am grateful to them.   However, it was the Lord who convinced me to get over my fears and made it very clear I was to write this book to **reveal the truth about nutrition, diets, & the health of our bodies, minds, & souls** (whether I wanted to or not)!   *"For He has NOT given us a spirit of fear – but one of: **power**, love, & understanding!"* (2Timothy 1:7)   In 1990, God used me (someone who previous to this did not know the difference between a Phillips head or flat head screw driver!) as a vessel to invent a prosthetic robotic arm (in one week) & an android (in 10 weeks) to help people with disabilities!   In 2014, God used/inspired/convinced me to write this book to help people maximally cleanse (& optimize the health of) their bodies, minds, & souls!   Unless otherwise noted, all Scriptures quotations are from the *New American Standard Bible* (Copyright 2000 by: The Zondervan Publishing House).

     I also thank God for the many pioneers in the field of nutrition. Jordan Rubin, ND, C.N.C. is the author of *"The Maker's Diet."*[i] This fantastic book combines Scripture & nutritional science.   Phyllis Balch, CNC is the author of *"Prescription for Nutritional Healing."*[ii]   This thorough book (most recent edition) is an excellent resource on disorders – as well as giving advice on how to achieve optimal health.   Dr. Sherry Rogers (in her book *Detoxify or Die*) & Dr. Linda Greenfield (in her online self-instructional program for healthcare professionals entitled *"Over the Edge: Biological Stress & Chronic Conditions"*) illustrate how everyone in the world is *"**FULL OF**"* more direct body toxins (AKA: toxic heavy metals, industrial chemicals, pesticides, etc.) than ever before.   Dr. Rogers & Dr. Greenfield are referenced throughout chapter 3.

     I am also grateful to www.naturalsociety.com – a fantastic nutrition & health-based website – whose articles I reference throughout this book.

     I also thank God for "Moody's Radio" (a National radio station) & "Trinity Broadcast Network" (TBN = a National television station) that uses wonderful teachers to bring millions of people closer to God & God's love (one of the major goals of this book).   These wonderful teachers include, but are NOT limited to:

- Bishop T.D. Jakes, Charles F. Stanley, Dr. David Jeremiah, Clarence McClendon, Joyce Meyers, John Hagee, etc.

While they all have extremely different styles, their message is the same (*God LOVES you: He always has & He ALWAYS will* – this is actually the title of one of Dr. Jeremiah's books).

     I also thank God for all the times I was humbled in life:

- Having the physicians who delivered me tell my parents I would have cerebral palsy – or "be mentally challenged" the rest of my life.
- Having a child-prodigy older sister (who spoke fluently at age 6 months & wrote novels at age 4), brilliant cousins (who played piano in front of Carnegie Hall @ age 7), & family members who looked at me as "the good, but slow child."
- Having all the so-called "Christian" kids hate me from age 8-13 when they found out I was the only Jewish boy in the school. God used me & instructed me to do one more push-up every day until I could do over 1,000 consecutive push-ups. Every time a boy attacked me physically (due to their hatred of me being Jewish): they miraculously tripped over their feet & fell to the ground (God protected me so that I would not be physically harmed –nor would I physically hurt those who attacked me)! Every time a boy or girl threw coins, rocks, or snow balls at me (due to their hatred of me being Jewish): God protected me so that I was never physically harmed. I look back & believe God was using me to send the anti-Semitic children a message: "*I, God, will be your shield.*"
- Having extremely difficult university courses & being surrounded by all "geniuses" in college making me consider dropping out in my first week of college (By the second semester, God used me to tutor these "geniuses." These "geniuses" –who initially intimidated me with their superior intelligence, were later paying me to teach/tutor them in the courses we were taking!).
- Having all 3 physical therapy schools reject me in 1990 despite studying 100 hours/week & having close to a perfect GPA & score on the AHPAT test (similar to the "MCATs" for medical schools).

Every time life humbled me (every time life/"the world" knocked me down), I asked God with ALL my heart (& **tears in my eyes**) to help/USE me (& He "lifted me up"). Every time, God USED me to do miracles in my life that I would have never been able to (or even conceive to be able to) accomplish on my own accord if I was not first humbled. *Every time God has done wonderful miracles in your life (as well as mine & probably everyone in the bible), you were probably first humbled - & then worshipped God more than ever & then asked God to help you!* Perhaps we should ALWAYS be humble & ALWAYS praise & be thankful to God & then we can receive ALL the blessings God has for us!

I also thank God for giving me an earthly Dad who always gave me love –the greatest gift an earthly Dad can give to their children. I also thank God for an earthly Mom who gave me love & worked 3 jobs (as a single Mom) to support me when I was growing up. I am also thankful to God for having my loving Grandparents & the rest of my Jewish family recognize the dramatic change in my life when *God USED me* to go from the "weakest brain" of the family (as a child) to the "top 20 college students (in 1990 – at age 20) in the U.S."[iii,iv,v]

Preface

God has inspired me to write this book to help everyone (you, our nation, & hopefully the entire world) become closer to God & to maximally cleanse (& optimize the health of) their bodies, minds, & souls.   Authority figures (such as corporate, governmental, &/or religious leaders) have "**failed to disclose the truth**" to us in order to gain or maintain money &/or power.   This has led our nation to become misled & more "***FULL OF IT***" in the following areas: The word of God, Jesus Christ, our nation's anti-Godly tax & government policies, Diseases, Obesity, Chronic Pain, Disability, & especially Nutrition. This has led to Americans currently being "***FULL OF***" more body, mind, & soul toxins than ever before!

*"For the time will come when they will not endure sound doctrine; but wanting to have their **ears tickled**, they will accumulate for themselves teachers in accordance to their **OWN desires**, and will **turn away their ears from the truth** & will turn aside to **myths**."* 2Timothy 4:3-4
    If you don't want to hear **the truth** of how to maximally cleanse (& optimize the health of) your body, mind, & soul, don't read this book!   If you want to have *your ears tickled* & turn away from the truth (& stay "***FULL OF***" toxins in your body, mind, &/or soul), don't read this book!   If you are not concerned about the growing level of our body, mind, & soul toxicity: then do not read this book!   If you do not want to learn how the toxins (including **pain) in your mind & soul** are connected to the toxins (& **pain) in your body**, then don't read this book!
    Society's "irrational apathy & acceptance" regarding the rising *flood* of body, mind, & soul toxins we are bombarded with (&, unfortunately, "***FULL OF***") is very analogous to those who drowned in the flood during the days of Noah!   As this "*flood*" continues to grow on a yearly basis, my goal is that everyone jumps on the "***arc of salvation***" to cleanse (& optimize the health of) their bodies, minds, & souls!

My personal journey on writing this book came in 1/1/1997 when I became (what society labels) a "Messianic Jew."   Later that year (not a coincidence – but a "God-incidence") – after researching tons of articles, research studies, & reading many diet-books on colon cleansing (like Robert Grey's *Colon Health Hygiene Handbook*) & food-combining (like Mr. & Mrs. Diamond's *Fit For Life*) – I "created" a diet (a one-page handout of dietary rules) for myself (as well as over 1,000 of my ADULT friends & family).
    Since 1997 I have updated & improved this "diet" to create (what I strongly believe) are the 10 best <u>dietary</u> rules/commandments in the world to create optimal health!   This "diet" now includes "**super-cleansing foods/supplements.**"   By simply following these "**10 Dietary Commandments,**" I & over 1,000 of my "friends & family" (Patients, coworkers, etc.) have received dramatic, life changing improvements in

weight loss &/or body fat percentage (if needed), digestion/absorption, elimination, & overall health (& appearance).

As a physical therapist, I see patients (daily) suffering from the consequences of being "*FULL OF*" **physiological, intellectual, & spiritual Toxins**. These toxins are destroying their bodies – causing/contributing to chronic pain, obesity, musculoskeletal, neurological, cardiovascular, & immune diseases (as well as other, if not ALL diseases)! Being "*FULL OF*" toxins in their intestines leads to a whole host of postural dysfunctions (which leads to more chronic pain, weight gain, &/or diseases – which leads to more dysfunctions/diseases). These toxins are also being stored in their neurological system, cardiovascular system, &/or possibly every cell in their bodies.

It is God's desire that we maximally cleanse (& have optimal health of) our bodies, minds, & souls. God does not want you to be "*FULL OF IT*!" ☺ However, like my Jewish ancestors whom God freed from Egypt, most of us do not know (& therefore break: every day – sometimes 3 times per day!) these "10 Dietary Commandments!" As the people of "this world" have gone so far away from God & God's 10 Commandments, we have strayed farther away from (not ironically) these "10 Dietary Commandments." Haven't we wandered through the wilderness long enough?!

This is not your typical "diet book." This is the only diet book I know of that incorporates: ALL "**10** (of what I strongly believe are scientifically – as well as scripturally based) **Dietary Commandments.**" This book also includes the "**10 best non-dietary cleansing methods.**" This is the only diet book I know of that connects the body, mind, & soul in such a scientific, scriptural, academic, & intellectual (&, hopefully, educational, entertaining, & helpful) manner.

Thousands of my "friends & family" (which I include as nurses, therapists, physicians, patients, & their family members) have encouraged me write this book to help millions maximally cleanse (& optimize the health of) their bodies, minds, & souls! No more excuses. This book NEEDS to be read by *all the peoples of all the nations*!

So let it be written, so let it be done!

Table of Contents

Introduction

The title & sub-title of this book are better understood if these terms are defined.

Definition of a "**Toxic Body**" (AKA "**Physiological Constipation**") =
- Being "***FULL OF***" intestinal putrefaction ("***IT***") stored in your intestines.
- &/or Being "***FULL OF***" (storing) anti-Godly "**direct body" toxins** (AKA: "biological, material, &/or environmental toxins" – or "***IT***") in your intestines &/or anywhere else in your bodies -including, but not limited to your cardiovascular, neurological, musculoskeletal, & immune systems.   I use the term "**direct body toxins**" as these are toxins (like those from toxic heavy metals, industrial pollutants, harmful microorganisms, drugs, cigarettes, etc.) that **directly** attack the body.   Due to the strong body, mind, & soul connection: there are mind & soul toxins that indirectly attack the body.   In addition, this "Physiological Constipation": can destroy the health of your entire body (as well as your mind & soul)!

Definition of a "**Toxic Mind**" (AKA "**Intellectual Constipation**") =
- Being "***FULL OF***" anti-Godly Intellectual ignorance, Incorrectness, & sinful thoughts (also "***IT***") that destroys your mind (as well as your body & soul).

"My people are destroyed for lack of knowledge." (Hosea 4:6)

Governmental, Corporate, & Religious leaders have "**failed to disclose *the truth***" to us often for financial gain.   This has led us to become more misled & "***FULL OF***" ignorance in the following areas: The living word of God; Jesus Christ; Our nation's anti-Godly tax & government Politics; Diseases; Obesity; Chronic Pain; Disability; & especially Nutrition!   I am not attempting to judge or offend.   For example, I have no problem or issue with anyone eating "junk food."   However, when makers (& often political leaders who are financially supported by these makers) of this "junk food" lie to us & tell us that this junk food is part of a healthful, nutritious meal: That is my issue!   When this "junk food" breaks all of my "10 Dietary Commandments" (chapter 5), should we tell the consumer that it is healthful?   I think not.   ***The truth shall set you free***!

Definition of a "**Toxic Soul**" (AKA "**Spiritual Constipation**") =
- Being "***FULL OF***" anti-Godly Spiritual Toxins (SIN, ignorance &/or incorrectness - also "***IT***") that destroys your soul (as well as your body & mind).

Definition of "*IT*" = therefore, body, mind, &/or soul **Toxins**!   "***IT***" can be considered "***direct body***" **toxins** that <u>directly attack our bodies</u> (& indirectly harm our minds & souls).   "***IT***" can also be "***indirect body toxins***" (like greed, fear, hatred of others, etc.) that directly attack our minds & souls (& <u>indirectly harm our bodies</u>).

1

Definition of "***FULL OF IT*** Level of Disease, Obesity &/or Chronic Pain" is the level at which the accumulation & compounding of the combination of all the body, mind, & soul toxins cause or exacerbate diseases, chronic pain, &/or obesity!   This is analyzed in chapter 4.

Realize the term "***FULL OF IT***" is similar to the concept of "absorption &/or storing" toxins in our body, mind, &/or soul.   Intestinal waste matter is not truly absorbed "in" the body (it is "stored" in the intestines).   Jesus Christ was bombarded with mind & soul toxins – but never sinned (or had any sin "in" Him).   One may say that Jesus Christ never became "***FULL OF IT***!"

Before I discuss the "Goals of this book," let me preface by informing everyone what my intent is not! My intent is NOT (& NEVER has been) to offend anyone! My intent is NOT to offend:
-   Believers or Non-Believers in Christ
-   The obese or the emaciated
-   &/or the diseased or those who want to optimize their health!

Remember, Americans (whether thin or overweight) - as well as possibly everyone else across God's planet - are currently "***FULL OF***" more toxins ("***IT***") in their body, mind, & soul than ever before.   The question is: at what level does the **accumulation & compounding of these body, mind, & soul toxins** cause or exacerbate **diseases, obesity, &/or chronic pain** – in you?   I term this "level" the "***FULL OF IT*** Level of Disease, Obesity, &/or Chronic Pain."   This increased level of toxicity is the largest health care crisis of the 21st century as it is destroying the health of the bodies, minds, & souls of everyone on God's planet!

If this book improves or saves the life/lives of you &/or anyone else you know, then the book has served its' purpose!   I feel very strong that the number one goal of any health care PROVIDER (whether you are a Home Health Aide or the Wealthiest Physician) is **to HELP PEOPLE**!   There is nothing wrong with enjoying the financial fruits of your labor.   However, money should not be the number one reason why any health care provider works!   *No carpenter on this earth has ever built anything better than what my carpenter in Heaven has built for us!*

Thus, the major goals of this book are to help you:
- o   Share/disclose **the truth *(to set you free)*** in the following areas: **The living word of God; Jesus Christ; Our nation's anti-Godly Tax & Government Policies; Diseases; Obesity; Chronic Pain; Disability; Health of your body, mind, & soul; & especially Diets & Nutrition**
- o   **Become closer to God (& God's Love)**
- o   **Maximally CLEANSE (& optimize the health of) your body, mind, & soul.**

o **& prevent from becoming _"FULL OF IT"_ again** – _or possibly_ in the first place!   Our environment is more toxic (**_"FULL OF"_** an enormous, & growing, amount of direct body toxins – as well as mind & soul toxins) than ever before in the history of God's earth.   However, we don't have to become **_"FULL OF IT_**!"

This book teaches us how to do this via **dietary AND non-dietary methods** (**natural AND super-natural means**). To achieve these major goals, smaller below-mentioned goals should be achieved.

Goals of this book – **Read this book if you want to learn the** following:

- 1. **We are _"FULL OF"_ more mind & soul toxins (_"IT"_) than ever before (Chapters 1 & 2).**

Being _"**FULL OF**"_ these sins is a major reason why we are _"**FULL OF**"_ more disease, chronic pain, & obesity than ever before.   We are being exposed to/bombarded with more mind & soul toxins than ever before from the internet, television, radio, strangers, co-workers, even friends, family, etc.!   What's worse is that we are "holding on"/storing/accumulating (becoming "**FULL OF**") these mind & soul toxins – which indirectly (if not directly) hurt your body.

- 2. **We are _"FULL OF"_ more "direct body toxins" (_"IT"_) than ever before (Chapter 3).**

Being _"**FULL OF**"_ these "direct body toxins" (toxic heavy metals, industrial chemicals, pesticides, harmful microorganisms, etc.) is a major contributing factor to why we are _"**FULL OF**"_ more disease, chronic pain, & obesity than ever before.   We are being exposed to/bombarded with more "direct body toxins" than ever before from the food we eat, air we breathe, water we drink & bathe in, etc.!   What's worse is that we are storing/accumulating (becoming "**FULL OF**") these direct body toxins (in our intestines, brains, cardiovascular system, &/or every cell in our body) – which indirectly (if not directly) hurt your mind & soul.   Remember: treating your _body (the temple of the Holy Spirit)_ like a sewer is also a sin!

- 3. **We should "blame" our being _"FULL OF"_ more diseases, obesity, & chronic body pain than ever before on the increased exposure to - & accumulation & compounding effect of - the COMBINATION of the increased body, mind, & soul toxins reaching our _"FULL OF IT_ Level of Disease, Obesity, &/or Chronic Pain."**

WHY/HOW we become diseased, obese, &/or in chronic pain is best explained (in my strong opinion) by this "**FULL OF IT** Level" concept.   Although we are **living** longer, we are **NOT thriving** longer.   We are living longer – with a lower level of health & fitness.   More Americans are at or above this "**_FULL OF IT_** Level" than ever before.   Therefore: We are "**_FULL OF_**" more diseases (especially chronic diseases), obesity, &/or disability – with chronic pain than ever before.

Our being "_FULL OF_" "direct body toxins" ("_IT_") is strongly related to the Mind & Soul Toxins ("_IT_") we are "_FULL OF!_"   Said differently: Our "**Physiological Constipation**" (toxic build up stored in our intestines & the rest of our bodies) is strongly related to our Toxic Minds & Souls!

        The strong similarity amongst all 3 abovementioned definitions is by no mistake or accident. The mind-body-soul connection has been studied & written about before –but is still extremely under-recognized.   In addition, no other book has ever come even close (in my strong opinion) to connect all 3 in such an educational (&, hopefully, entertaining) manner!   One may say that: if you do _NOT_ believe there is a strong connection between the health of your body, mind, & soul – then "**_YOU'RE FULL OF IT!_**"   This book will help the reader decide the answer to the following questions (pertaining to the body-mind-soul connections):

    o   **Have our "Toxic Bodies" <u>caused</u> our minds (including our personalities) & souls to become toxic!?**

         ▪ Asked differently: Has our "Physiological Constipation" (Being "**_FULL OF_**" direct body toxins) <u>caused</u> our minds & souls to become "**_FULL OF IT_**!?" Additionally: Can our chronic body pain cause "pain" in our minds & souls?

    o   **Have our "Toxic Minds & Souls" <u>caused</u> our bodies to become toxic!?**

         ▪ Asked differently: Has our "Intellectual & Spiritual Constipation" caused our bodies to become "**_FULL OF IT_**!?" Additionally: Can the "pain" in our minds & souls cause our chronic body pain?

    o   **Should we blame diseases (including obesity & chronic pain) on <u>just one</u> body, mind, or soul toxin?**

         ▪ **Should we blame diseases (including obesity & chronic pain) on <u>just one type</u> (body, mind, or soul) of toxin?**

    o   **What is causing us to be more "_FULL OF_" of diseases, obesity & chronic pain than ever before?** Is it our increased exposure to - & becoming "**_FULL OF_**" – more "direct body toxins" ("IT") than ever before? Or is it our exposure to - & becoming "**_FULL OF_**" – more mind & soul toxins than ever before?   **Our being "_FULL OF_" more diseases, obesity, & chronic pain (as well as disability) than ever before should be blamed on our increased exposure to - & <u>accumulation & compounding</u> of - the <u>combination</u> of the increased <u>body, mind, & soul</u> toxins reaching our "_FULL OF IT_ Level of**

Disease, Obesity, &/or Chronic pain!" It is not wise (in my humble opinion) to believe that diseases, obesity, &/or chronic pain are caused by just one (or even one type/category of) body, mind, or soul toxin. There are thousands of peer-reviewed scientific studies showing how being "***FULL OF***" one specific direct body toxin (a certain pesticide, toxic heavy metal, industrial pollutant, etc.) can *increase the risk* of one or more diseases. **However, I strongly believe (& hope to prove) that our increased exposure to - & accumulation & compounding of - the COMBINATION of increased multiple body, mind, & soul toxins to the "*FULL OF IT* level of disease, obesity, &/or chronic pain" is the #1 reason why we are "*FULL OF*" more diseases, obesity, & chronic pain than ever before! This concept of combining & multiplicity is important to understand when attempting to optimize the health ("*CLEANSING*") of your body, mind, & soul.**

○ **At what level does the accumulation & compounding of "IT" (these body, mind, & soul toxins) cause or exacerbate diseases, obesity, &/or chronic pain - in YOU?** You may be "***FULL OF***" a level of toxicity just below the amount that would trigger diseases (including obesity &/or chronic pain). If you become "***FULL OF***" more toxins, then you become so "***FULL OF IT***" that you cause or exacerbate diseases (including obesity &/or chronic pain). You may pray, get a colonic, go to a sauna, go on a raw organic vegetable juice fast, etc. - to reduce the amount of toxins (in your body, mind, &/or soul) "***YOU'RE FULL OF***" so that you no longer have the disease (or an inflammation/exacerbation of the disease). But because of our ignorance of nutrition, diet, & health (of our bodies, minds, & souls): we soon become "***FULL OF***" more toxins which bring us back into this diseased &/or inflamed state (I call the "***FULL OF IT*** Level of Diseases, Obesity, &/or Chronic Pain**" – analyzed in chapter 4). Chapters 1-4 basically explain how/why we raise our "***FULL OF IT*** Level.**" Chapters 5-7 show how/why we can lower our "***FULL OF IT*** Level.**"

This book can change your life - & hopefully change the world for the better. This is not just some diet book. It is a way of life. It is a cleansing of the body, mind, & soul! Should we ignore the truth that most of our "media," "Hollywood," our anti-Godly tax & governmental policies (as well as our so-called governmental "representatives"), & the rest of "society" are poisoning our minds & souls?

We should not ignore the truth that our nation has become "***FULL OF IT***" in the following areas:

- **Health & Nutrition** (including our <u>diets, exercise –or lack of exercise, posture, obesity, diseases, disability, chronic pain, & our overall health</u>);
- **Intellectually** (in the above areas –as well as other areas like **tax policies, politically, & socio- economically** that are hurting ourselves & our nation);
- & **spiritually** (including **morally, socially, & attitudinally**)!

Should we ignore the connection between the satanic poisoning ("**_IT_**") of our minds & souls & the poisoning of our bodies! We have ALL gone astray so far away (& so often) away from God? Is our wandering in the intellectual & spiritual wilderness NOT destroying our bodies - as well as our minds & souls!? Is our wandering in the wilderness of health & nutrition NOT destroying our minds & souls – as well as our bodies!?

- **4. <u>To recognize the strong connections between all of our nation's largest deficits in the following areas:</u>**
  - **God deficit**. This is indubitably a mind & soul toxin – but (as seen in chapter one) an extremely under-recognized body toxin. For **non-believers**: this is a **direct** body toxin (see chapter 1). However – even for believers: This is an indirect body toxin our "God-deficient" society puts on us. We are more deficient in God as a country than ever before. More Americans consider themselves "**convinced atheists**" than ever before (this is mentioned & referenced in Chapter 2). As our country has strayed farther away from God than ever before, the financial debt of our country has skyrocketed. We have seen an increase in divorce rates, & the amount of money we spend on health care. We have an increased number of working aged Americans on disability benefits. We are "**_FULL OF_**" more diseases, obesity, & chronic body pains than ever before. These are NOT coincidences. As our "God-deficit" has grown in our nation, we have become (as a nation): less healthy, more in debt, less intelligent, & more immoral.
  - **Health Deficit**. We are "**_FULL OF_**" more disease(s), obesity, & chronic pain (as well as disability) than ever before! We often treat our toxic bodies - "**_FULL OF_**" diseases - with more toxins ("**_IT_**")! As our health deficit has grown in our nation, we have become (as a nation): more "God-deficient," more in debt, less intelligent, & more immoral.
  - **Financial Deficit**. Our nation is in more financial debt than ever in our history! Our society ("the world") wants to remove the words: "in GOD we trust" from our currency. If we don't trust God, who do we trust? Our country was built

& blessed "under God." As we remove God from our country, we become less blessed & more cursed. It is easy to see how our health & moral deficits have also contributed to our financial debt. This financial debt is a mind & soul toxin – as well as an indirect body toxin. As our nation's financial debt hits record highs, we have become (as a nation): more "God-deficient," less healthy, less intelligent, & more immoral.

- **Intellectual Deficit**. This is a mind & soul toxin – as well as an indirect body toxin. We have more access (via T.V., radio, internet, cell phones, books, etc.) to the Living Word of God. However, we have replaced the Living Word of God with immoral sinful food for our brains? It is simply a coincidence that our country has become more ignorant in health, nutrition, diets, exercise (or lack of exercise), posture, chronic pain, obesity, diseases, economics/tax-policies, & of God's Living word than ever before? Have we become lazier than ever before –physically & mentally? Is it a coincidence that our elementary schools (K through 12) have become similar in quality to some 3rd world nations?! We can't teach children "creationism" – but are forced to teach them "Darwinism!" Have we removed God from our schools? We have removed praying - & "I pledge allegiance UNDER GOD**!**" **If you believe in the bible, you are considered "arrogant!?"** If you are 100% convinced that God does NOT exist, you are considered "open-minded," a "free spirit!?" Do we really have to wonder why we have fallen so low intellectually!? As our nation's "intellectual deficit" has grown, we have become (as a nation): more "God-deficient," less healthy, more in debt, & more immoral.

- **Moral Deficit**. This is a mind & soul toxin – as well as indirect body toxin. Despite the **difficulty in objectively** measuring our country's over-all immorality being greater than ever before, this book will attempt to prove just that. We have removed God from our culture & have become more sinful. Are we surprised at how low we have fallen? If morality was listed on the stock exchange, we would be at an all-time low! ☺ As our nation's immorality hits record highs, our nation has become: more "God-deficient," less healthy, more in debt, & less intelligent.

We have failed to recognize how GOD, our morals, finances, & health (of our bodies, minds, & souls) are ALL strongly connected to each other!

Our nation's largest God, Financial, Intellectual, & Moral Deficits are toxic to your mind & soul – as well as your body. As these deficits are larger than ever before (&, unfortunately, growing), we are more "***FULL OF IT***" than ever before.   Thus: we have become ***FULL OF**" more diseases, obesity, disability, & chronic pain – than ever before in our nation's history!

Society's "*irrational apathy*" to the **_flood_** of body, mind, & soul toxins (including the abovementioned "deficits") we are "***FULL OF***" is very analogous to those who drowned in the **flood** during the days of Noah! How much more time or warning do we need?

- 5. **The "10 Dietary Commandments" illustrated in Chapter 5 may be the best "diet" in the world to cleanse (& optimize the health of) our bodies –as well as our minds & souls.**

If you believe simply avoiding physical laziness & gluttony (both part of "Dietary Commandment #1") are the only 2 factors responsible for achieving optimal health of your body, mind, &/or soul – then "***YOU'RE FULL OF IT***!"

Is the field of **nutrition** a science or an art?   I consider it a **scientific ART** because every human is different & ever changing.   Every human has their own genetic predispositions for diseases.   In addition, every human has their own individual preferences (which can change during their lifetime) for food: Tolerances; Allergies; Taste preferences or dislikes; Positive & negative reactions.

Even the "super-cleansing foods &/or supplements" (mentioned in chapter 6) may have a negative reaction on certain individuals.   However, every human adult (& most teenagers) will benefit from reading (& **absorbing** the information) in this book.   Every human adult (& most teenagers) may benefit from following ALL of these "10 Dietary Commandments" (which are based on scientific & scriptural principles) to "cleanse" (& optimize the health of) their bodies (as well as their minds & souls).   This is because we are "***FULL OF***" more direct body (as well as intellectual & spiritual) toxins than ever before in our world's history.   Considering the growing level of toxicity we are "***FULL OF***" in our bodies (as well as our minds & souls), every adult may benefit from reading this book & following these "10 Dietary Commandments."

Despite the body of knowledge in nutrition doubling every 7 years, we have become "lost" wandering through the wilderness of diet & nutrition. We have become slaves to our "physiological constipation" we intentionally & ignorantly put our bodies through –mostly via breaking these "10 Dietary Commandments!"   ***Most adults are breaking ALL of these "10 Dietary Commandments" – often a few times per day! Is it any wonder why we are more diseased, obese, & in chronic pain than ever before!***   Imagine if you broke ALL *10* of *God's Commandments* every day – three times per day! How healthy would your body, mind, or soul be? ☺   As society has strayed farther away from God's *10 Commandments*, we have (by no coincidence) strayed farther away from these "10 Dietary Commandments."

GOD'S COMMANDMENTS = HIS "*EMPOWER-MENTS*"

When God **commands** you to do something: *He always enables/helps/**empowers** you to accomplish it.* (Isaiah 41:10)

By simply following these "dietary rules/commandments," thousands of my "friends & family" have received/reported dramatic, life- changing ***empowered*** improvements in the following areas:

- Achieved optimal health & appearance (as per themselves others. However, beauty is in the eye of the beholder.);
- Lost intestinal putrefaction – created optimal elimination;
- Lost hip &/or waist size, weight & body fat (if needed, to an optimum weight & body fat percentage);
- Improved mental functioning, energy, & vitality (reported);
- Felt "cleaner," "more spiritual," &/or "closer to God;"
- Reduced or eliminated allergy symptoms;
- Improved their immune function & reported a "decongesting" of their nasal sinuses – with reports of improved air flow &, therefore, sense of smell & cardiopulmonary functioning;
- Detoxed from the bombardment of toxins we are "***FULL OF***!"
- Reduced or eliminated colitis, heartburn, &/or other acid-reflux symptoms.
- & improved digestion/**ABSORPTION** of the healthful foods they consumed!

What I've said for years: *Just because you break these "10 Dietary Commandments" – does NOT mean you will be diseased!   Nor am I* promising *to reverse your disease process.   However, you will never achieve your own personal optimal health by breaking "My 10 Dietary Commandments" (on a daily basis)!   How well did my ancestors do when they broke God's 10 Commandments?   Haven't we wandered through the nutritional/dietary wilderness long enough?*

As Americans have been **increasingly breaking** these "10 Dietary Commandments" since the 1970s (if not longer), we have become: **more diseased, obese, disabled, & in more chronic pain** – than ever before in our nation's history.

Some "Diet books" mention part of 1 or even a few of these commandments in their Diets. However, this is the 1st "Diet Book" (that I am aware of) to include ALL 10!

Thus, one of this books goals is to "set you free" from the nutritional & dietary "bondage" (or ignorance/misconceptions/"con jobs") that we have believed. We have believed that many healthful foods are harmful & many harmful foods are healthful. Even when we get it right – we get it wrong! We believe certain foods have "no value" – when they actually should be considered "super-foods!"

This concept of optimal absorption benefit can be applied to what we "feed & absorb" in our bodies – as well as our minds & souls. *Your mind & soul becomes what you feed it & **ABSORB**!* If an atheist reads the entire bible & remains an atheist, they did NOT ABSORB it! If a believer in Christ reads & listens to God's word in the bible - but does not have love (for all humans) & forgiveness in their heart, they did NOT ABSORB His message!

Said otherwise, when you feed & **ABSORB** satanic violence & pornography in the movies, video games, televisions, & the internet: you become ***FULL OF IT!***   In fact, we have become "desensitized" to this - & other forms of anti-Godly toxicity – that we have polluted our minds & souls with them!   Our minds & souls have strayed so far away from God.   We have accepted this - & other forms of "Intellectual & Spiritual Constipation" as the norm.   Murderers, terrorists, vampires, & other satanic creatures have become "famous," popular, & accepted as "normal" parts of our culture.   Believers in God & God's word are considered "radical!?"

When you read &/or listen (**& ABSORB**) God's word in the Bible: you become alive, full of peace, love, & joy!   God wants us to *renew like Eagles*. Eagles only "eat" living things!   God wants our minds & souls to eat & ABSORB the **living** word of God!   God also wants His creation to have optimal physical health –as well!

In summary, goal # 5 of this book is to illustrate how following all 10 of these "10 Dietary Commandments" on a daily basis is a **major dietary method to achieve OPTIMAL:**

- **Digestion & ABSORPTION of the healthful nutrients you consume**
- **Elimination of the toxins in your intestines – as well as the rest of your body**
- **& health ("***CLEANSING***") of your body (as well as your mind & soul).** However, it is NOT the only method.   There are Non-Dietary – as well as other dietary (such as certain "Super–Cleansing Foods & Supplements") methods needed to follow to truly achieve **optimal health (&** "***CLEANSING***"**) of your body, mind, & soul.**

6. **To achieve optimal health (&** "***CLEANSING***"**) of your *body, mind, & soul* by using a COMBINATION** of: Dietary & Non-Dietary Methods.   This includes "Natural" –as well as - "Super-Natural" Methods.   This is the major goal of this book.   Too many of us believe the lie that simply consuming one "**Super-Cleansing Food or Supplement**" (listed in Chapter 6) or performing one non-dietary cleansing method (chapter 5) or following one "Dietary Commandment" will create the optimal health of our body (or our mind or soul)!   Therefore, **optimal health (& maximal "***CLEANSING***") of your body, mind, & soul** may be achieved by following ALL of the below mentioned methods:

-        Trying your best to avoid all spiritual & intellectual toxins you're bombarded with (chapters 1 & 2)
-        Trying you best to avoid all direct body toxins you're bombarded with (chapter 3)

-        Following most, if not ALL, of the "10 Non-Dietary Cleansing Methods" (chapter 5)
-        Following ALL of the "10 Dietary Commandments" (chapter 5)
-        & consuming many of my "Super-Cleansing Foods & Supplements" (chapter 6).

Remember: God wants you to have optimal health of your body, mind, & soul.   God wants you to have a perfectly "clean" body, mind, & soul.   These goals can only be achieved by lowering your "**_FULL OF IT_** Level" to zero – or as close to zero as possible (God does not want you to be "**_FULL OF IT_**)!"   I believe this book shows you "the way."

"LIFE IS BUT A SCHOOL. SOMETIMES YOU ARE THE TEACHER - & SOMETIMES YOU ARE THE STUDENT."   I have been stating this since 1988 when I began my college studies.   This favorite quote of mine is derived from the famous theater quote: "Life is but a stage -."   However, I believe my quote is more appropriate here.   Time to go to school! ☺   Hope this book achieves its' primary goal of bringing **you** (the **student** when you first read it &, then, the **teacher** when you teach others) **closer to God & cleanse (& optimize the health of) your body, mind, & soul!**

11

CHAPTER 1: *"YOU'RE FULL OF"* SIN - causing More Diseases, Obesity, & Chronic Pain in our world's history

This chapter's primary goal (as well as the primary goal of this entire book) is to bring you closer to God (& God's Love) & maximally cleanse (optimize the health of your) body, mind, & soul.

This chapter should demonstrate the following facts:

- Every human (whether obese or not) is "*FULL OF*" SIN (a type of "*IT*"). Said differently, "*YOU'RE FULL OF IT*" – whether *YOU'RE obese or not!*
- Sins are directly toxic to the mind & soul - & indirectly toxic to the body. Said differently, *YOU'RE overweight*, in chronic pain, &/or **DISEASED**: because "*YOU'RE FULL OF IT*" (body, mind, & soul toxins). Said differently: the "pain" (sins) in our mind & soul can exacerbate or even cause our body pains (as well as obesity, diseases, & even death)!
- The **accumulation of these sins** (added to the direct body toxins – AKA "biological," "material," "environmental" toxins –discussed in chapter 3) can reach your own "*FULL OF IT* Level of Disease, Chronic Pain, &/or Obesity!"

This chapter may also help the reader answer the following question:

- Does being "*FULL OF*" SIN cause diseases (including obesity) & even death – **DIRECTLY or INDIRECTLY**? This is similar to the chicken or egg question (of which my answer has always been = eat chicken & eggs - in the "Lifestyle Phase" of this diet book – illustrated in chapters 5 & 6). ☺

Consider the following 2 examples:

- Example #1: "*YOU'RE FULL OF*" laziness & gluttony (under-recognized sins illustrated later) on a regular, prolonged basis. According to God's living word, these sins (like all sins) can **DIRECTLY** cause diseases (including obesity) & even death. Being "*FULL OF*" these 2 sins may **directly** cause the following **immediate** physiological stress: Weight gain & obesity; Abdominal/gastrointestinal discomfort; Bloating, gas, acid reflux, indigestion, poor absorption of food, & constipation. Thus being "*FULL OF*" these sins can make you "*FULL OF*" intestinal putrefaction (one type of "*IT*" for this book)! This way the body, mind, & soul toxins truly begin to compound destroying your entire body, mind, & soul!

According to the living word of God, being "*FULL OF*" these sins (like all sins) causes **psychological stress** because only God can give you optimal peace. The prolonged physiological (mentioned above) & psychological **stress** of being "*FULL OF*" these 2 sins can (**indirectly**) **eventually** lead a cascade of "**physiological stress reactions**." The sympathetic nervous system (the "flight or fight" response) dominates over the parasympathetic ("relaxation" response) nervous system.

This can lead to prolonged elevated cortisol (a **stress** hormone released by the adrenal cortex in response to **stress**) levels which may predispose you to the following **long-term** physiological reactions (illustrated further in chapter 3):

- Atherosclerosis (due to constricting of blood vessels, increased heart rate & blood pressure); Insomnia, chronic fatigue syndrome; Thyroid disorders (which can make you "***FULL OF***" intestinal waste matter); Dementia, Alzheimer's, learning difficulties, ADD, ADHD, & OCD; Depression, **panic attacks, & anxiety**;*** Erectile & fertility dysfunctions (which can make you "***FULL OF***" more psychological stress reinforcing the cycle); Immune system suppression (which can predispose you to cancers, autoimmune diseases –as well as the cold & flu); Diabetes; **Chronic pain** (which can lead to physical inactivity – an under-recognized killer); & (as mentioned above) weight gain, obesity, mal-absorption, acid reflux, indigestion, & constipation! It is obvious to see how all of the abovementioned "stress reactions" can lead to more physiological & psychological stressors & diseases. Thus, the <u>cycle of SIN causing diseases</u> **directly & indirectly** continues.
- Example #2: "***YOU'RE FULL OF***" fear (an under-recognized SIN discussed later). You may be fearful of losing your finances, health, &/or relationships.   According to God's living word this sin (like all sin) can **DIRECTLY** cause diseases (including obesity & chronic pain) & even death.   In addition, being "***FULL OF***" this sin (like all sin) for a prolonged period of time can **directly** create tremendous psychological stress (as you are not trusting God with your problems in life & only God can give you optimal peace) – leading (**indirectly**) to the abovementioned physiological reactions.

Thus, being "FULL OF***" **fear** for a prolonged period of time can actually cause your body to create more anxiety, panic attacks, & fear. This way the cycle of SIN causing diseases **directly & indirectly** continues! "***YOU'RE FULL OF***" SIN - & this **directly & indirectly** leads to becoming "***FULL OF***" diseases (including obesity, chronic pain, & even death)!

I.   ***"YOU'RE FULL OF"* SIN = an under-recognized & *Modifiable* cause/risk factor of ALL Diseases - including Obesity, Chronic Pain - & even Death**

Asked differently: Is our "Intellectual & Spiritual Constipation" the #1 **modifiable** cause of: ALL diseases & even death? Additionally: Is the "pain" in our minds & souls causing the pain (as well as obesity &/or diseases) in our bodies?

Most diet books usually put a "spiritual" aspect of their diet towards the end of the book. However, I believe this is part of the problem we have in society. We turn to God for help -*AFTER* we have tried things every other

13

way. After "the world" has failed us, then & only then, we (hopefully) turn to God to help us.   No matter what, He always has time to listen & help us! There is no better Physician in the world than God.   You don't need health insurance or have to make an appointment (waiting days or weeks) to see Him! ☺

Is a "Toxic Mind & Soul" _modifiable_?

God's word defines the word "repentance" as a change of your mind/attitude resulting in a turning away from wickedness & towards belief & acceptance in a relationship with God. (Jeremiah 8:6; 31:19, 20)   If you "**feed**" your mind/soul **(& ABSORB)** wicked sins of the flesh (Galatians 5:19-21), you will become wicked!   If you "**feed**" your mind/soul **(& ABSORB)** the word of God, you will bear the _fruits of the Holy Spirit = love, joy, peace, patience, kindness, goodness, faithfulness, gentleness, & self-control._ (Galatians 5:22-23)

This foundation of this entire "diet" book is based on the law of **ABSORPTION**!   Your body, mind, & soul are what you feed it & ABSORB!   If you feed your body the most healthful foods & supplements, but do not ABSORB them, you did not receive any benefit from them!   If you feed your mind & soul the word of God, but do not ABSORB His word, then you did not receive the benefit!   If you feed your mind & soul the word of God, but are still "**_FULL OF_**" hatred, un-forgiveness, jealousy, greed, laziness, gluttony, &/or other SINS – then you did not ABSORB His message!

The relationship between a toxic body & a toxic mind/soul is currently under-recognized in society.

Most diet books would include ancient Greek philosophers (like Socrates or Aristotle) or Roman philosophers (like Senaca) to illustrate the mind-body-soul connection.   Many of their philosophies may (or may not be) based on God's living word.   However (like everything in life), God's living word has the best answer to demonstrate this relationship.   These philosophers are _dead_!   God's word _lives_ forever.   The reader should notice that the word "modifiable" is underlined.   This is because we –as humans (God's creation) has been given _free will_!

The following relationship is NOT a coincidence (it is a "God-incidence"):

- As our nation has become more sinful ("**_FULL OF_**" Mind & Soul Toxins) than ever before, we have also become "**_FULL OF_**" more pain meds (& pain med overdosing), obesity & diseased ("**_FULL OF_**" Direct Body Toxins) than ever before!   It is no coincidence that our "deficit in GOD" has led to the deficit in our health (as well as our financial, moral, & intellectual deficit).

The following biblical verses may be seen as scriptural evidence that:

- o SIN (a major mind & soul toxin) may be a major cause (if not the #1 cause) of Disease (including Chronic Pain & Obesity) - & even Death!

14

- God's will is for you (His creation) to have optimal health: a clean body, mind, & soul!

1 Corinthians 15:56 – *"The sting of **death is sin**."*

Romans 7:9-11 - *"When the commandment came, sin became alive & I died...for **sin** deceived me & through it **killed me**."*

Romans 8:6-7 - *"For the **mind** set on the **flesh [fleshly SINS]** is **death**, but the mind set on the **Spirit** [of God] is **life** & **peace**. The mind set on the flesh [fleshly SINS] is hostile toward God."*

Romans 8:13 -*"For If you are living according to the flesh [fleshly **SINS**], you must die. But if by the Spirit [of God] you are putting to death the deeds of the body, you will live."*

1 Corinthians 3:17 – *"If anyone destroys God's temple: God will destroy him. For God's temple is holy and **you are that temple**."*

1 Corinthians 6:18-20 – *"**Flee immortality**. The **immoral man [with a "TOXIC SOUL"] sins** against his own **BODY**. Or do you not know that <u>your body is a temple of the Holy Spirit</u> who is in you, whom you have from God, and that you are not your own? You have been bought with a price. Therefore: <u>**glorify God in your body**</u>."*

Romans 12:1-2 – *"Present your <u>**bodies**</u> a living & holy sacrifice, acceptable to God, which is your spiritual service of worship. Do not be conformed of this world. Be transformed by the renewing of your <u>**mind**</u>, so that you may prove that the will of God is that which is good & acceptable & perfect."*

Proverbs 3:7-8 – *"Fear the Lord & turn away from evil. It will be **healing to your body** & refreshment to your **bones**."*

Proverbs 4:20-22 – *"For <u>**My words**</u> are **LIFE** unto those who find them, - and **health** to ALL their **whole body**."*

Proverbs 14:30 – *"A tranquil [AKA peaceful] heart is **life to the body**."*

Proverbs 17:22 – *"A **joyful heart** is **good medicine**. But a **broken spirit** dries up **the bones**."*

Psalm 103:2-5 – *"Bless the Lord, O my soul, & forget NONE of his benefits: Who pardons all your iniquities; **who heals all your diseases**; Who redeems your life from the pit; who crowns you with loving-kindness & tender mercies; Who satisfies your years with good things; so that your **youth is renewed <u>like the eagle's</u>**."*

Psalm 107:20 – *"He sent His word, and **healed them**, & delivered them from their destructions."*

Isaiah 53:4-6 – *"Surely our grief [AKA sickness/diseases] He Himself bore, and our <u>**diseases**</u> [AKA sorrows &/or pains] <u>**He carried away**</u>. Yet we ourselves esteemed Him stricken, Smitten of God, and afflicted. But He was pierced through for OUR transgressions. He was crushed for OUR iniquities [SINs]. The chastisement for our well-being fell upon Him. And **by His scourging [stripes of blood] we are healed**. All of us like sheep have gone astray. Each of us has turned to his [or her] own way. But the LORD has caused the iniquity of us all to fall on Him."*

Matthew 8:16-17 – *"He healed all who were ill. "HE HIMSELF TOOK <u>OUR INFIRMITIES & CARRIED AWAY OUR DISEASES</u>" (Isaiah 53:4-6).*

1 Peter 2:24 – *"By **His stripes we are healed**"* (Isaiah 53:4-6).

Isaiah 40:29 & 31 – *"He gives strength to the weary. He increases power to him who lacks might. – Those who wait for the Lord will **gain new strength**. They will mount up with wings <u>**like eagles**</u>. They will run & not get tired. They will walk & **not become weary**."*

Jeremiah 30:17 – *"I will **restore your health**. I will **heal your wounds**, declares the LORD."*

Mark 5:34 & Luke 8:48 – *"He said to her, 'Daughter, your <u>**faith has made you well**</u>; go in **peace** and be <u>**healed of your affliction**</u>."*

Matthew 4:23 & 9:35 – *"Jesus was healing **every** kind of **disease & sickness**."*

Matthew 10:1 – *"Jesus summoned His twelve disciples & gave them authority over <u>**UNCLEAN**</u> spirits, to cast them out, & to **heal every kind of disease & every kind of sickness**."*

John 14: 12-14 – *"Truly I [Jesus] say to you, he who believes in me, the works that I do **[such as healing ALL diseases]**, he will also do; and greater works than these he will do; because I go to the Father. Whatever you ask in my name, I will do, so that the Father may be glorified in the Son. If you ask Me anything in My name, I will do it."*

3 John 1:2 – *"I pray that in all respects you may prosper and be in **good health**, just as your **soul prospers**."*
2 Corinthians 7:1 – *"Let us **CLEANSE** ourselves from all defilement of **flesh** & spirit."*
1 John 1:9 – *"If we confess our sins, He is faithful & righteous to forgive us our sins & to **CLEANSE us** from all unrighteousness."*

This "**cleansing**" may be seen as a cleansing of our soul – as well as our mind & body (which includes our intestines & the rest of our body).

The above scriptures support the concepts that:

- Sin is toxic to our souls, minds, & bodies.
- God's will is for you (His creation) to have optimal health of your body, mind, & soul! Said differently: His pain = your gain!

At the last supper: <u>AFTER supper</u> (The Old Covenant is over) Jesus said: *"Take this cup & drink. This is my NEW covenant."* (Jeremiah 31:31-34; & Luke 22:19-20). If you are a believer in Christ, & believe the Devil has authority over you, you are "***FULL OF IT.***" Jesus said, *"It IS FINISHED."* In other words, Jesus has won & fulfilled the prophecies to bring the new covenant. Now all believers in Christ have authority over Satan & Satan's desires (disease, stress, poverty, fear, unfaithfulness, rejection of Jesus, & all other SINS Satan wants us to commit). It is the will of God for you not to be burdened. *"I have set you free."* Before Jesus said *"it is finished"* (John 19:30), He said *"I am thirsty"* (John 19:28). The abovementioned statement Jesus made represents: *"I am thirsty"* for:

- You to be whole – to have 100% peace (AKA *shalom*) in your body, mind, & soul; & for you to have optimal health of your body, mind, & soul.

Satan's punishment (mentioned In Genesis) is that he must eat dust forever. Our FLESH is made of dust! When you let your sinful flesh dominate you, Satan grows in power in your life! Jesus cleans away your sins (they are forgiven & forgotten)! Don't let your past hold back your present & future what God called you to do! Cleanse your mind & soul so you can cleanse your body of intestinal putrefaction, excess body fat, & toxins stored in your entire body!

II.   "*YOU'RE FULL OF*" 10 Under-Recognized SINS that increases the risk of Diseases - Including Obesity &/or Chronic Pain

Keep in mind, ***EVERY un-repented SIN*** (soul & mind toxin) can, therefore, be seen as a modifiable risk factor/cause of any & all diseases. Society is somewhat aware that the "direct body" toxins (being stored in our <u>bodies</u>) have an **accumulative** damaging effect on our health. However (as society has strayed so far away from God's word), our nation has forgotten the biblical truth that:

- The **accumulative** effect of **ANY &/or ALL un-repented SIN(s)** - can cause all diseases (including obesity & chronic pain)! Remember,

EVERYONE SINS!   Like all of you, I have fallen short of the glory of God. I am still a work in progress. The SINS I am tempted by, may not be the SINS you are tempted by. Only the Messiah was & is without SIN! If you believe you never sinned: "**YOU'RE FULL OF IT**!"

The question many of us must ask ourselves is: "What are *the bondwomen in our lives?*" (Genesis 21:10 & Gal 4:30 – 5:1) What SINS are enslaving us? What SINS: - fear, anxiety, depression, hatred (of ourselves & others), un-forgiveness (of ourselves & others), greed, idolatry, gluttony, laziness, addiction, &/or any other Sin - haven't you "*released yet?*"   What SINS are holding us back from all the gifts & blessings that we are promised.   "*For Christ has set us free!*"

If SIN(S) can exacerbate or even cause diseases (including obesity & chronic pain), how do I stop sinning?

The answer may be in Romans 6:14 where it is written: "*For SIN shall NOT be master over you* [those that are "in Christ" –believers in Jesus Christ as their personal Lord & savior], *for you are NOT under LAW but under GRACE.*"

We should spend less time focusing on SIN (the breaking of the LAW of GOD). When you focus (or even become obsessed with) SIN, it becomes your master. This is like telling yourself - 100 times a day: "Don't think of a purple cow!" This is why many diets fail. We should not focus on the junk foods we should not eat. We should focus on God & cleansing (& optimizing the health of) our bodies (the temple of the Holy Spirit), minds, & souls.

We should focus on God's **GRACE - & LOVE of us.**

We should NOT focus on the SINS - & their contribution to diseases.

We should focus on Jesus Christ who <u>forgives & cleanses us from ALL SINS - & heals ALL diseases</u>!   For He has set us free!

However, our country has strayed so far away from God – that so many disease-causing SINS have become severely under-recognized (& mostly "acceptable" behaviors in our culture)!

I do not mention these SINS to judge or condemn anyone – but to make us more cognizant of how these under-recognized SINS may be contributing factors in all diseases (including obesity & chronic pain). Again, my goal is to bring everyone closer to God (& God's Grace - & LOVE) & to cleanse (optimize the health of) our bodies, minds, & souls.

1. **Polluting your body (the temple of the Holy Spirit) with direct body toxins**. We do this by:
   - Bombarding our bodies with direct body toxins – mentioned in Chapter 3.
   - & Breaking (on a daily basis –if not multiple times per day) the "10 Dietary Commandments" mentioned in Chapter 5.

Many believers of Christ ignorantly believe that they do not need to be concerned with the food they eat. They will ignorantly claim: "Dietary Rules were part of the 'Old' Covenant. We are part of the new covenant –so we can eat whatever we want & not concern ourselves with whether the food is

17

healthful or harmful. We can get as obese & diseased as we want – as it is not a sin to treat your body like a sewer!" I guess these people need to be reminded that *"your body is the temple of the holy spirit!"*   Many Christians will also ignorantly believe that God never uses the natural to heal us – only the super-natural.   God can heal people in any way He chooses. There are examples in the bible of how God healed people via super-natural methods – as well as natural methods.

We are polluting our bodies with toxins from foods, beverages, cigarettes (including passive or "second-hand" cigarette smoke from "friends & family"), drugs, alcohol, medications; the water we drink & bathe in; & even the air we breathe inside & outside our own homes! These "stored" direct body toxins - causing obesity, chronic pain, & diseases - are discussed further in Chapters 3 & 4.

2. **Choosing to "store" (become *"FULL OF"*) these toxins in our bodies (the temple of the Holy Spirit).**   We choose NOT to detoxify/cleanse our bodies (the temple of the Holy Spirit) by:
- Breaking (on a daily basis – if not multiple times per day) the "10 Dietary Commandments" mentioned in Chapter 5.
- Avoiding ALL 10 of the "10 Non-Dietary Cleansing Methods" – mentioned in chapter 5.
- & avoiding ALL "Super-Cleansing Foods/Supplements" mentioned in Chapter 6.

The accumulative effect of these "stored" toxins may cause all diseases (including obesity & chronic pain).   By storing these toxins in our bodies (the temple of the Holy Spirit), we are polluting our minds & souls.   By polluting our minds & souls we cause our bodies to become toxic.   We must choose to break that cycle!

These 1st 2 abovementioned "SINS" are truly "direct body toxins" that have an accumulative detrimental effect on our health (& possibly our weight)!   One storage area for these toxins is our intestines.   Intestinal putrefaction can be a breeding ground for a whole host of harmful viruses, fungi, yeast, bacteria, other harmful microorganisms, & other toxins.   Some adults may be *"**FULL OF**"* over 40 pounds of intestinal putrefaction!   This can put excess stress on the low back area – predisposing those people to **chronic pain** anywhere from the low back to the toes (discussed further in chapter 3).   This may also mimic Obesity, slow down your metabolism, & therefore, lead to body fat storage.   **This results in a cycle of us being *"FULL OF"* chronic pain&/or excess body fat (as well as disease-causing toxins)!**

Other storage areas for direct body toxins include, but are not limited to, the brain, liver, muscles, arteries, or any other organ system or cell in the body!   Realize (due to the strong connection between the body, mind, & soul) we also store (become *"**FULL OF**"*) toxins in our bodies due to other sins (mind & soul toxins) we become *"**FULL OF**."*

18

3. **Being _"FULL OF"_ Greed, Jealousy, Fear [all fear except the "fear"/respect of God] or Any OTHER SIN that causes "STRESS" (the "Anti- PEACE") in your life**.

Realize society has falsely accepted certain so-called "innocent" SINS (such as conceit, lying, perjuring, greed, envy, & anxiety) to be "normal." Some may foolishly argue that they are not SINS at all! This would be a lie –which of course would be another SIN! These "less offensive" SINS (Phil 4:6-7; Prov 12:25; John 14:27; Is 26:3; Matt 6:27 &34) can reduce your peace [create a lot of emotional stress] in your life. This "stress" (the "anti-peace") can make your soul & mind toxic.

Stress is a risk factor for atherosclerosis, cancers, digestive disorders, obesity, & almost all other diseases! Stress stimulates the sympathetic nervous system (i.e. "flight or fight reaction") – which increases your heart rate, constricts your blood vessels, & takes blood supply away from your gut. Therefore, stress decreases your digestion & absorption of the foods you consume.

For example:
- Greed, jealousy, & fear [all fear except the fear of God] are 3 sins (not trusting in the Lord) that can destroy/dominate the health of your body, mind, & soul – as well as your Investments/finances! This of course becomes a viscous cycle of "stress" in many areas of your life. It should not amaze us that so many stock brokers & day traders have gastrointestinal, cardiovascular, & overall immune-system diseases.
- Jealousy is breaking one of the 10 Commandments (Ex 30:17). Be thankful for the blessings God has given to you – so you can continue to receive more blessings from Him in the future!

The greedy banks, buyers, mortgage & stock brokers have led to the real estate collapse. It is not a coincidence that these loans (debt) are considered **TOXIC!**

In addition, stress can increase cortisol production which forces your body to convert energy to FAT! Thus, stress can lead to **obesity**. This excess weight/load can predispose you to **chronic pain** (as well as a whole host of other problems discussed further in chapter 3). God wants you to have optimal peace. (Psalm 119:143; Gal 5:22; Matt 11:28-29) "Fear NOT" is mentioned 366 times in the Bible (once for every day of the year – including leap year)!

"For God has not given us a spirit of **fear** [also translated as "timidity" or "cowardice"], _but of power and love and discipline_ [also translated as "sound judgment" or "**sound mind**"]" (2 Tim 1:7) This scripture is additional evidence showing how God wants us to have a healthy mind & soul – even when faced with stressful events (including diseases – as well as other trials & tribulations) in our lives. God knows you can't achieve optimal health of your body – without optimal health of your mind & soul. God knows you can't have a perfectly "clean" body – without a perfectly "clean" mind & soul! No child is born without self-esteem. Many parents give their children a fear of failure: "why can't you be more like your siblings?" This fear becomes an encumbrance in their life. Jesus came to set you free from this & all SINS!

As a Physical Therapist, I see more patients currently <u>dominated</u> by anxiety than depression. Anxiety "cripples" them. Anxiety becomes their master! They become afraid of leaving the home, exercising, & receiving all the health care benefits they need! ***"And who of you by being worried can add a single hour to his life?"*** (Matt 6:27)

I believe **Mary Magdalene** was one of the greatest disciples of Jesus Christ. Jesus healed & fed thousands of people who witnessed His miracles (including raising people from the dead, healing the blind, deaf, lame, & all diseases).   Where were all those thousands of people when "the world" turned against Jesus? Who was there when they tried Him in the courts (with the Jewish high priests – as well as with Pontius Pilate)? Who was there when they tortured Him? Who was there when He dragged the cross? Who was there when He was crucified? Who was there when He said "It is finished?" Who was there to 1st see the empty tomb? Who did the resurrected Christ appear to 1st to bear witness to His other disciples? Who did Jesus choose to have bear witness to His resurrection? (Matt 28:1, 8-10; Matt 27:55, 56, 61; Luke 24:10, 11)

Jesus saved **Mary Magdalene's** life physically & spiritually.   Mary Magdalene (according to the scriptures) **never stopped loving Him & appreciating Him. Mary Magdalene never seemed to fear** what "the world" may do to her for being "with him" (AKA "In Christ")!   Yes, Jesus' mother Mary was there also. But Mary Magdalene was not related to Him. Mary Magdalene is one of the greatest role models for how Jesus forgives our sins & changes our life (makes us a "new creation in Christ")!   ***Mary Magdalene was not afraid to stay with Jesus Christ – despite "the world" being against Him***! So often (2,000 years ago – as well as currently) Jesus gives us an amazing blessing (heals our diseases; heals a loved one's diseases; performs some miracle in our lives; answers our prayers, etc.), & we soon forget (& stop appreciating) the One who <u>gave</u> us that blessing!   When "the world" turns against Jesus, are you afraid to be "with/in Him?"

When life seems to be falling to "pieces," you can find perfect "peace" if you keep your mind on God! (Isaiah 26:3)   I have often joked with my patients suffering with anxiety: "I, too, have the gene for worrying!" If you are a believer in Christ & believe you should be burdened with ANYTHING, you may be "***FULL OF IT***!"   Don't condemn yourself for the SINS you have done in the past. Jesus bore the SINS of all of us. Jesus has set us free (including a clean mind & soul).

"Rejoice in the LORD always! Be anxious for NOTHING! Pray about everything" (Phil 4:4-7)
"Come to Me - all who are weary & heavy-laden, & I will give you rest. (Matt 11:28) You will find rest for your <u>souls</u>." (Matt 11:28; Jer 6:16)

4., 5, & 6. Being "Full of" Laziness, Drunkenness &/or a "Gluttony"

(Titus 1:12; Prov 23:20-21; & Prov 20:1)

Eating excessively (to be a "Glutton"), drinking alcohol excessively, & Laziness (lack of exercising) are 3 under-recognized sins that may be **major causes of diseases (including obesity & chronic pain).**

Are people committing suicide with these sins?   Society does not view these sins (or any other sins for that fact) as suicide.   But we can't ignore the fact that *the wage of sin is death*!   Are we killing ourselves with alcoholism, gluttony, &/or laziness!?

Being "Full of" Laziness = "Lazy *Tushy* Syndrome" = lack of exercise "Lazy *Tushy* Syndrome ("LTS"):" lack of exercise has become a ***world-wide epidemic***.   33% of the world's adults may be considered "lazy" regarding exercise.   33% of adults across the globe (increased in "high income" countries like America) do NOT exercise (moderately) more than 150 minutes per week - & ***it's killing us***![1,2]   According to studies featured in the medical journal The Lancet, this physical inactivity (less than 150 minutes of moderate exercise a week) is a major contributor to life-threatening diseases like ***heart disease, Type 2 diabetes, & breast & colon cancer***.[1,2]   This lack of exercise (a form of laziness) was considered a ***major causative factor of 5.3 million deaths in 2008*** (more than smoking —considered the major cause of 5 million deaths in 2008).[1,2]   Realize "LTS" applies to almost everyone.   Even if you are unfortunately confined to bed or a wheelchair, there are exercises you can do!

Have the advancements in technology given us an excuse to be lazy?   My robotic inventions in 1990 did not make me rich.   In fact they ended up costing me lots of money to invent them.   The reason they did not make me rich is because I underestimated how lazy abled-bodied society would become.   I invented the prosthetic robotic arm & the android to help people with disabilities (not to help the abled become lazy)!   That is why I never patented them.   I never thought of patenting a "voice activation system" that typed out words without having to touch a keyboard (it was primitive in 1990).   I never thought of patenting a "robotic vacuum cleaner;" "robotic lawn mower;" an android that converted into a motorized wheelchair.   All of these technological advancements have helped disabled people become more independent —but have given excuses for the abled to become "lazy."   No one forces you to take the elevator!   Now you can't watch the television without a remote control!

"Whatever you do, do your work heartily (with ALL your might) as for the Lord" – Ecclesaistes 9:10 & Colossians 3:22-24.   This may apply to any occupation you have on this earth —working for your earthly "boss."   This may also apply to "working" for your "spiritual master (boss)"= God!   If God —the Holy Spirit - wants you to *Glorify Him in His temple* (your body):" being lazy (choosing not to exercise) may be seen as *"sin against God's temple (your body)*!"   Our laziness may be related to our employment problem as well.   You may be

"**_FULL OF IT_**" - if you think it is a good thing that there are many jobs that Americans either:
- Don't WANT to do (like home health aide, landscaping, etc.)
- Or aren't qualified to do (like those in the engineering or computer science fields).

So what's left for teenage Americans to become? Health Care Professionals, Politicians, Government workers, & Insurance salespeople!

Being "FULL OF" Drunkenness = Drinking Alcohol Excessively

Excessive alcohol consumption can destroy your liver, brain, & even increase the risk of bleeding!   This liver toxin may cause liver disease(s). The liver is the organ in the body considered most responsible for filtering the toxins in our bodies.   Damaging the liver, therefore, severely impairs one's ability to detoxify!   If the alcoholic beverages (like wine) one excessively consumes are high in sugar, they will also become at increased risk of type II Diabetes. If the alcoholic beverages one excessively consumes are high in calories, they will also gain weight - & possibly increase the risk of obesity.

It is NOT a coincidence that alcoholic beverages can be referred to as "**_spirits._**"   These alcoholic "spirits" can dominate the alcoholic's mind (including their personality), soul, & body.   You will often hear their loved ones' make excuses for their other sins by claiming: "It's the alcohol speaking! It's not them!"   The same could be said for other drug addictions! ***

***Just because I've never had an alcoholic drink (or taken any "recreational drugs") in my 44+ years of life on this earth, does NOT mean I have never been under the influence of any drug. In college, I developed a severe addiction to CAFFEINE!   Most of my classmates thought I was high on speed or some other drug.   Keep in mind, the "spirit" of caffeine can dominate your mind (including your personality), soul, & body – just like any other drug.   I was a "maniac" high on massive amounts of caffeine (in any & every form available) which made me very aggressive, short-tempered, & "hyper" (without peace). This was a sin-full way of living for me. I would excuse my sin-full behavior by telling people: "It's the caffeine speaking. It's NOT me!" Most people would laugh it off as society "accepts" this specific drug addiction!   After 3 years of this addiction, I had to have an "intervention" where the "girlfriend" I had at that time (threatened to end our relationship) - & my "boss" confronted me to let me know how concerned they were that my addiction to caffeine was hurting myself!   I went "cold turkey" off the caffeine & within weeks had "knocked it out."   I lost my aggressiveness & temper - & regained peace in my life!

Being "FULL OF" "Gluttony" = Eating Excessively

If you are not sure that God considers "Gluttony" a sin or not, consider where & how the word glutton is used in the bible.   The word "gluttony" (eating *excessively*) is usually accompanied (in the bible) with other sins like:

- **Heavy Drinking** – which (combined with gluttony) leads to poverty & drowsiness (Proverbs 23:21-22); Humiliating your father (Proverbs 28:7); Lying, deceiving, & being full of myths so that people turn away from the truth (Titus 1:10-14); Selfishness (Titus 1:14); Evilness (Titus 1:14); & **Laziness.** (Titus 1:14). **It is by no coincidence the word "gluttons" is so connected to the word "lazy" ("*Lazy Gluttons*")!** (Titus 1:14) America (& the rest of the world) has become "***FULL OF***" lazy gluttons!

Eating excessively puts a large amount of physical stress on your gastrointestinal, cardiovascular, endocrine, immune, & (eventually) our skeletal systems. Therefore, gluttony, drunkenness, & laziness may actually worsen or cause chronic pain. Realize a "Glutton" eats "excessively." Individuals that exercise regularly (like athletes) & "burn" the calories they consume are NOT Gluttons! However, most of us are NOT Olympians burning 5,000 calories per day!

Being a lazy, drunk (especially of high-calorie beverages), glutton are major risk factors of obesity, & therefore, obesity-related diseases such as: type II diabetes, hypertension, cardiovascular disease, & disability.[3] Some of the reasons why we have become lazy, drunk, gluttons are discussed below (& illustrated further in chapter 4).

There are physical, cultural, emotional, psychological, & spiritual reasons why we are "over-eating." These include:

- Poor **ABSORPTION** of the foods we are consuming because we **break the "10 Dietary Commandments" – mentioned in Chapter 5.** You are what you absorb –not what you necessarily eat. If the food/beverages you consume do not get digested/absorbed, they stay in your intestines (as intestinal putrefaction). Your brain tells your body to continue to eat – "over-eat" to absorb the nutrients your body needs.
- Our **portions** in restaurants **have quadrupled** since the 1950s.[4] This affects our culture & how we eat at home. This may be why American adults are consuming 20% more calories than 50 years ago![4] It has become acceptable behavior in America to "waddle" out of restaurants with our belts & pant buttons undone!
- Our brain's satiating sensors have a delayed reaction (20 minutes or so) & will not tell you that you're full immediately after swallowing your food! **If you become full *while* you are eating, you may have eaten too much!**
- Avoiding "Breaking-the-Fast" & **eating only 1 meal per day** causes us to store our fat, slow down our metabolism, & become "*starved*" (depriving your body of necessary food/nutrients). We should eat breakfast & small meals throughout the day. Many Americans eat a very small (or no) breakfast & then a huge dinner! I believe this is diametrically opposed to good healthful sense!

- Trying to *"fill a **VOID**"* in our lives. Many have replaced God with food! *We are all like sheep have gone astray.* When we have problems (sadness, anxiety, or any other kind of stress in our life), we will often over-eat as an "answer/solution." **Besides focusing on what, how, & when we are eating, we also need to ask ourselves: *"What's EATING YOU?!"***
- Lack of DISCIPLINE to NOT "over-eat." This can be seen as under-recognized SIN # 7 that can cause or worsen chronic pain, Obesity, & Diseases.

7. **Being *"FULL OF"* Disorder – Lacking Discipline, Self-Control, & Patience** (Gal 5:22) Lacking Discipline, Order, Self-Control, & Patience are SINS.   You must be disciplined to regularly exercise your body, mind, & soul to become closer to God (& farther away from sin & Satan)!   God wants us to have discipline & order in our diets - as well as every other part of our lives. Thus, this can apply to our lack of discipline to follow God's 10 Commandments –as well as the "10 Dietary Commandments" (mentioned in Chapter 5).   These "10 Dietary Commandments" (as well as the "10 non-Dietary Cleansing Methods" – mentioned in Chapter 5) include regular exercise.   Therefore, a lack of discipline to commit to an exercise regimen: may predispose you to chronic pain, obesity & diseases.   Most diets & exercise regimens fail because many lack order & discipline.   If Jesus & Moses fasted, why can't we avoid breaking these "10 Dietary Commandments?"

Discipline is part of Godliness. Do I choose to be led by my sinful flesh – or do I choose to be led by the Holy Spirit that dwells in me?   Are we led by our fleshly "YOLO" attitudes (You Only Live Once) which corrupts our bodies with sexual immorality as well as Obesity & disease?   Following the "YOLO" attitude nutritionally (eating sugar & other junk foods all day long) has led to obesity & disease.   Jesus & His disciples fasted (which took discipline). Doing the will of God, takes discipline to NOT do our fleshly sinful will –but that of God's. Treating your body like the temple of the Holy Spirit takes discipline!   The scriptural verse in 2 Timothy 1:7 often translates *"the spirit God gives us – as one of **discipline**."* (New American Standard Bible)

If you believe you will achieve optimal health without the discipline & commitment to regular exercise & following the "10 Dietary Commandments" (mentioned in Chapter 5), then: ***"YOU'RE FULL OF IT!"*** From age 8 to 11, I: did not curse or even belch (unlike all my classmates); consumed no sugar (unlike all my classmates); & did 1 more push-up every day.   By the time I was 11: I had tremendous strength (over 1,200 consecutive push-ups) & health (of my body, mind, & soul)!   I never would have received this blessing from God: if I lacked the **discipline & commitment** to do the above.

If you believe you can be the best student you can be without having the discipline to study = "*YOU ARE FULL OF IT*!"   In college, I studied 100 hours per week!   Most of my classmates started college far ahead of me. But no one worked harder than I did.   I did not go to parties. I did not socialize. I did not go on dates. I studied!   Yes, God answered my prayers & blessed me. He took me from a "slow child" & the worst student at age 18 (considered dropping out of college my 1st week) - to the "All U.S.A. Academic Team" nominee (at age 21).   He took me from someone intimidated by the "geniuses" I was surrounded by – to the top student whom these "geniuses" paid to tutor them (after only my 1st semester in college) in almost every math or science course I enrolled in!   But I never would have received these blessings if I didn't have the **discipline & commitment** to study harder than any other student I ever met.

As we have "strayed away" from God (& God's love), we have strayed away from our spouses! Have we become blind to the fact that falling out of love with your spouse may be directly correlated with the falling out of love with God!?   Is this why our nation is "*FULL OF*" divorce?!

You will never be the best athlete, spouse, parent, child, friend, employee, &/or employer: without **discipline & commitment**.   Most millionaires had the **discipline** to work & save for many years to become millionaires.   Many people want a success in their finances, careers, relationships, & health – but do not have the **discipline** to stay committed to achieve their goals.

Discipline is also related to financial success.   Our nation has been undisciplined (since 1997 –see chapter 2) with our debt which has grown tremendously.   Americans abuse their credit cards (the worst invention for most consumers as it gives them an income they often don't have) - causing their own personal debt to grow. The banks allowed our homes to be used like credit cards in the early to mid-2000s. The **lack of financial discipline** (an under-recognized sin) by our nation's government & tax policies, our banking/mortgage system, & our own personal debt creates a huge burden/toxin to our minds, souls, & (eventually) our bodies!   This is analyzed further in chapter 2.

We should all have goals in our life (a positive vision).   First & foremost goal= to love God 1st & foremost. We should stay committed to this.   We must praise the Lord when things are going great & even when "the world" turns against you.   Then: love one another (including family & friends –whether they are homosexuals, criminals, on drugs, or atheists)! Remember: are you bringing people closer to God? God loves you always. If you love someone ONLY when they are wealthy, healthy, & kind to you: how deep is your commitment to love them?   If you think a perfect relationship is when you TAKE everything without earning it (because you lack the discipline & commitment to earn it) & NEVER GIVE back = "*YOU ARE FULL OF IT*!"

*"All things must be done in an **orderly manner**."* (1Cor 14:40)

Before Jesus fed 4,000 people (with 7 loaves of bread & a few small fish) He had them "get" in order. (Matt 15:35)   Before Jesus healed large crowds (who were lame, crippled, blind, mute, & many others) He had them "get" in order. (Matt 15:30)

"All discipline for the moment seems not to be joyful, but sorrowful. Yet to those who have been trained by it, afterwards it YIELDS the peaceful fruit of righteousness." (Hebrews 12:11)   This can apply to our diet & exercise regimen.

It is discipline (not desire) that determines our success. I see this everyday with my patients. Many patients want to get better. However, they lack the discipline to follow 100% of their home exercise program. Most comply with about 20% of their home exercise program!   When I was 8 years old I started doing 1 more push-up every day. After 3 years, I could do over 1,200 consecutive push-ups without stopping. I had the discipline. For the last 30 years, I have performed 15 minutes of stretches every single day. It just becomes part of your disciplined routine (like teeth brushing). Have you missed brushing your teeth in the past 30 years?

Many people *want* to achieve optimal health & fitness.   Some people truly do not know how to. They do not know what foods to eat &/or how to achieve optimal health (these are the people I truly wrote the book for).   However, many people do not have the discipline or commitment to break away from their lazy gluttony – or other sins destroying the health of their body, mind, & soul!   What are you waiting for? Remember, *your body is the temple of the Holy Spirit*!

Wait on the Lord, & keep His way (Psalm 37:34). Patience & self-control are mentioned together as "fruits of the Holy Spirit." (Gal 5:22)   Patience is needed to achieve success in every area of our lives (from our relationships with friends, family, & even God – to finances/careers)!   Our society has become fast-paced & impatient.   We want "fast-foods" & instant love, money, success, & gratification!   We want to spend more than we make via the use of credit cards – versus buying items we desire when we have saved enough.   Then we wonder why we are not achieving success in these areas!

As a Physical Therapist, I see patients struggle with patience all the time.   I have patients that have suffered with excruciating pain from pinched nerves for decades - relieve their pain in one session & complain the session took too long! I have had patients reverse their so-called paralysis in one session & complain it took so long to find a therapist with a powerful enough electrical stimulation machine to reverse their "paralysis."   I have had patients become impatient when they don't receive a 100% cure in a couple of sessions.   Patients may become upset that they do not achieve their goals – despite the fact they are 100% non-compliant with all home recommendations.   If you don't floss or brush your teeth (& suck on sugary candy) for 90 days – do not become frustrated, impatient, shocked, or discouraged that you may get or worsen a dental cavity!   **Great patients** (as

26

well as parents, children, spouses, & other **followers of God**) *require great patience*.   Great health requires great patience.   If you avoid all "10 Non-Dietary Cleansing Methods" & continually break all "10 Dietary Commandments:" do not be impatient (or discouraged) that you haven't achieved optimal health!

8. **Being *"FULL OF"* Addiction**

This is very similar to the previously mentioned under-recognized SIN!   Any addiction that tries to "fill ourselves" with anything besides God, is a SIN! Most of society is aware that immoral SIN-full addictions are SINS.   However, even "good" behaviors can become addictive.   The following is a list of examples of certain addictions that are considered SINS (if we are trying to replace God with them) we are *"FULL OF"* addictions to:

-   Video games
-   Text messaging
-   Social media websites
-   Sexual addictions (including pornography)
-   Drugs, alcohol, cigarettes
-   **Over-eating** (includes "binge eating") – being a "glutton" (breaks part of "Dietary Commandment #1")
-   **Sugar** - have we become "**carb-addicts" or "sugar junkies?"**   This breaks part of "Dietary Commandment #9."   Many people believe they are addicted to chocolate. However, most people addicted to chocolate are probably addicted to the combination of cocoa with sugar!
-   Junk food = breaking most – if not all of the "10 Dietary Commandments" mentioned in Chapter 5 (as well as Chapter 6 – to understand what should be considered junk food)
-   Caffeine
-   Work (includes money. Remember, the love of money is a root of all sorts of evil. -1Tim 6:10)
-   Shopping

What are you trying to fill the void in your life with?   What are you trying to fill the God-deficit in your life with?   Remember: what do you think of when you wake up?   When you go to sleep?   What do you think of during the day? When the addiction becomes your master, where is God in your life?   Only God can truly fulfill us with all of our present & current needs.

Even gifts we receive from God, we can turn into addictions! Sometimes we get so enamored with our gifts (from God), we forget about the giver!

One of the best ways to cure addictions may be found via the biblical numbers "12" & "144." For example, most smokers know what time they have the 1st cigarette. If it is 7am, they can wait until 7:05am. The next day, they can wait until 7:10am. After 12 days, they have cleansed themselves of cigarettes for that 1st hour awake. After 144 days, they have "cleansed" themselves of cigarettes for the 1st 12 hours awake. Hopefully, by the end of your day - you will realize the absurdity of having your 1st cigarette at night. If not, continue this trend until you are "100% clean." This possible addiction cure may apply to many other forms of addiction. However, try not to focus on the addiction. Try to always focus on God. God does not see you as an addict. God Loves you & sees you as a believer in Christ or one that will be a believer in Christ (hopefully before your flesh dies)! (Psalm 22)

9. **Being *"FULL OF"* Hatred or Un-forgiveness of others or ourselves**! (Matt 6:14 & 18:21-22) & John 3:16)

"God is Love!" How can God forgive us of our SINS, if we do not forgive others of their trespasses against us!? God wants us to love & forgive everyone. If you claim to be a believer in Christ, but do NOT have Love & forgiveness of everyone, you may be *"FULL OF IT*!" You are not born a racist or an anti-Semite!

I admit, it can be extremely difficult for some of us to truly forgive (& love) others for some of the horrific acts they have done to us or our loved ones. Most of my Jewish family have not forgiven (& will probably never forgive) the Nazis for the satanic acts they did to our relatives. In my opinion, the hatred of non-believers (by some so-called believers) may be the #1 reason why they stay as non-believers! Unfortunately, most of my Jewish family will never read (or desire to hear) about the prophecies of the Jewish Messiah (found in Isaiah 7, 9:, 52-53, 61; Psalms 16 & 22; Jeremiah 31; Micah 5; Zech 9 & 11, etc.).

If you are truly a believer & follower of Jesus Christ, you will Love (& forgive) everyone. As an animal lover, I can truly see the beauty in all animals. As a believer in Christ, I can truly see the beauty in all humans! I had to work on forgiveness –as I held on to this for years with people who had "trespassed against me." How many blessings from God were being "returned to sender" by my un-forgiveness? I need all the blessings I can get!

To truly forgive someone of some horrific acts they have done to you &/or your family members can't be done without God. The world will say, "That kind of forgiveness is not possible. It is not human! It is supernatural!" The last part is correct! (Matt 6:14 & 18:21-22; John 3:16) When they mocked & taunted Him & pierced His hands (possibly the median nerve - causing "excruciating" pain), He told His Father (in Heaven): *"Father, forgive them; for they do not know what they are doing."* (Luke 23:34)

Believers must become more aware of how non-believers view us. So-called Christian kids hated me when I told them I was Jewish. They called me horrific names. They would throw pennies, rocks, & snowballs at me. I forgave them. However, from age 8 to about 22, I ignorantly believed "Christians hate Jews!" Do the Christians today love or hate non-believers (like the non-Messianic Jews, Islamists, Buddhists, Hindus, etc.)?   How do Islamists look at so-called Christians who don't act Christ-like!   How do any non-believers look at Believers ("The Body of Christ")?   **Hatred of non-Believers (felt, heard, & seen) from so-called "Christians" (who are obviously not acting "Christ-like" – in fact they are acting "Anti-Christ-Like"), may be the #1 reason why non-believers remain as non-believers! Are you Jewish?** How do you know? Anti-Semitism & Racism reveals historical & biblical ignorance. Many Jews in the 1st century believed in Jesus as the Messiah (as their Lord & savior). These Jews called themselves Christians & separated themselves from the "non-messianic" Jews (like my ancestors). However, these "Messianic Jews" still had the Jewish "nationality" (descendants of Jacob – AKA "Israel") in them.   These (messianic Jewish) Christians married & had children – who were told they were no longer Jewish (they were told they were "Christians").   Truly the Jewish nation became split, diversified, & diluted. Jesus said (in Matt 10:35 & 37), "*I came to set a man against his father, & a daughter against her mother, a daughter-in-law against her mother-in-law. (Micah 7:6) He who Loves their father or mother MORE than ME is NOT worthy of ME. He who loves their son or daughter more than ME is NOT worthy of ME.*" (Deut 33:9) Jews are the spiritual branches of Christians. (Romans 11:19)

    Two thousand years later, many anti-Semites are ignorant of the possibility that their ancestors may have come from these 1st century Messianic Jews! Many racists are ignorant of the possibility that their ancestors may have come from people whiter or blacker than they could have ever imagined! Consider the fact that my mother's Grandparents came from Latvia & my father's grandmother was Seminole Indian. I don't speak Latvian or "Seminole." I don't follow any Latvian or Seminole Indian customs. However, I can't deny the fact that I have Latvian & Seminole Indian "nationality" in my blood. Can you deny the possibility that your ancestors 2,000 years ago were definitely NOT Jewish (or Black, Red, Yellow, Brown, or White)?! Remember God does NOT identify us by our nationality or the color of our skin. There is no longer Gentile & Jew. There are only two identities under God: those who already believe in Jesus & those who have not YET believed in Him! (Psalm 22)

    Believers must ask themselves (on perhaps a daily basis): "Was I a shining light of God helping to - bring others closer to Christ – or bring people further away?! Shining the bright light of the Holy Spirit &/or God's Living Word into the face of a non-believer may turn them away. However, letting the Holy Spirit lead us/"shine on us" will attract non-believers to us (& hopefully Jesus Christ). If we can LOVE them (as we have been commanded to), they will feel the LOVE (of our Commander)!   The above is discussed further in section III of this chapter.

10. Being *"FULL OF"* Ourselves – with Egocentric Arrogance & Conceitedness (Rom 11:25 & 12:16; & James 4:16)

We should boast that the Truth of Christ is in us, & it should not be stopped by "the world." (2Cor 11:10)   No one should boast of any good works they do as *we have been saved **by grace through faith**, & that **NOT of ourselves**. It is the **Gift of God**!* (Eph 2:8-9)   Therefore, we should NOT be selfishly ambitious. (Roman 2:8)   We should work hard to glorify God!

Non-Believers also have the capacity to do good deeds. You are created in God's image whether you believe it or not. You can be tremendously blessed by God –whether you acknowledge where your blessings come from!

*"God is opposed to the **proud**, but gives grace to the **humble**."* (James 4:6; Psalm 138:6; Proverbs 3:34; Matt 23:12; 1 Peter 5:5)   *"**Humble** yourself in the presence of the Lord, & **He will exalt you**."* (James 4:10)

When life knocks you down – you can either:
-   Look down & punch the ground you are on;
-   Or look up & pray to God to help you!

What I've always said is: "**If God can use a Jackass, He can surely use you & me**!"   When life humbles you, God can use you (& raise you up) to do greater things than you ever imagined! Think of David. He started as a shepherd boy, was looked down upon by his earthly father, had multiple murder threats by Saul (but God, the Father loved him because David's heart was with God), & he became a king!   Almost every person mentioned in the Bible that God used to do amazing things was humbled before that.

Did not Paul become blind before God used him to be one of the best Disciples of Christ (to bring people "into Jesus Christ")?   Was not Mary Magdalene once a prostitute & shunned by most in society before God used her to be (in my humble opinion) one of the greatest Disciples of Christ?

Was Jesus not born in a manger?

Was Jesus not despised?

Did Jesus not wash the feet of His disciples?

Was Jesus not beaten, whipped, & crucified (one of the most humiliating & "excruciating" ways to have your flesh die) for the SIN of all humankind?

Perhaps this is why He told us to *Love your enemies*. Perhaps this is why He told us to *love those who curse you*. These things can humble you & God can then use you even more.*

*Personal Journey to being humbled. This is not about me. However, this story may help others become closer to God. I was born with the umbilical cord strangling my neck depriving my brain of oxygen. The obstetrician told my parents I "would have either cerebral palsy, mental retardation, or be *on the slow side*." I did not talk until almost age 3 (& I haven't shut up since!). I could only drink out of a "baby bottle" until age 7 (beverages taste better out of a nipple!). I had a speech impediment until age 9. I was a bed-wetter until age 13. I was surrounded by a genius sister & genius cousins. I was told I was "slow & stupid." I thank God for this was a blessing to be humbled.

At age 8, I lost all my friends when the "anti-Semites" (so called "Christian kids") found out I was Jewish. They would throw pennies & rocks & snow balls at me (ironically –I was never injured by them). Many of the anti-Semitic kids attacked me physically (but God always protected me –these kids seemed to miraculously fall/trip when they physically confronted me!). After 3 years of this, I was able to do over 1,000 consecutive push –ups (what doesn't kill you makes you stronger). I always forgave these kids for their hatred of me for being Jewish - as this was a blessing.

In my first week of college, I was humbled once again by how many geniuses I was surrounded by. I prayed to God to help me. I studied over 100 hours per week (*whatever you do – do with ALL your heart & might*). After 1 year of college, I was tutoring all the courses I was taking to the fellow classmates that I was originally intimidated of!

After 2 years of college, I became "*FULL OF*" myself. I had become enamored with the blessing God had given me –but forgot about He who gave me the blessing! I failed to achieve my dream in life & was rejected by 3 Physical Therapy Schools. I had hit rock bottom again. I went from sadness to anger to forgiveness to complete humility. I cried out for God to help me once again. He USED me to invent (in 9 days straight without sleep) a prosthetic robotic arm for people with above-elbow amputations. Then He USED me to invent (in July/August of 1990) an android to help people with disabilities to: mow the lawn, type (with a voice activation system), vacuum clean their homes, ride with as a motorized wheelchair, & walk with as a motorized walker. I was then chosen to represent my University as one of the top 20 college students in the U.S.A! This never would have happened if I hadn't hit rock bottom - & humbled myself & asked the LORD to help me.

Life may knock you down – but you have to become humble & ask God to help you when this happens. Many people get knocked down & never get humble & never ask God to help them!

Even if "the world" (which may even include family members, co-workers, etc.) REJECTS (or even hates) you: Jesus loves & ACCEPTS you! Even if "the world" considers you cursed & worthless, Jesus considers you blessed & gifted!   We are ALL His creation.   He did not create any human soul without a purpose or a gift(s)!

III.   "*YOU'RE FULL OF*" Repelling people AWAY from Christ - versus leading people towards Him

Put yourself in the shoes of an atheist, homosexual, or Muslim. If all you know about Jesus Christ is that His so-called disciples/followers ignorantly hate you or your parents – then you may ignorantly believe that Jesus does as well! From age 8 to 13, all the "so-called" Christian kids hated me because I was Jewish. How was I supposed to perceive their leader? Christians are **SUPPOSED TO love everyone** (including the atheist, homosexual, non-believer, etc.) – just as Jesus LOVES EVERYONE! Are you so perfect that you are without sin? If you believe you're perfect, then "*YOU'RE FULL OF IT*!"

Mentioning or showing the Old Testament Messianic Prophecies (that Jesus fulfilled in the New Testament) to non-believers IS ONE of the best ways God may use you to bring non-believers "to Christ." Mentioning or showing non-believers the love & gospel of Jesus may be another way God may use you to bring them "to Christ." Healing their diseases &/or their loved one's diseases may be another great way God may use us to bring non-believers closer to Christ. Giving a book like this one to a non-believer may

31

also hopefully bring a non-believer closer to Christ.   Praying for non-believers may be another great way God may use us to bring them closer to Christ.

However, the best way may be to:
- LOVE them. To let the Holy Spirit shine on you. If you shine a light in someone's eyes, they will turn away. Think about that.
- & to be the best representatives of Christ we can be spiritually, intellectually, & **physically**! Living "the Christian Life" is an under-recognized way God may use you to bring non-believers closer to Christ.

Remember: *we have NOT been saved BY good works*. We have been saved *TO DO* good works. We must Love everyone. God forgives & forgets all your repented sins. But God remembers ALL your good works of LOVE!
Thus, we **should be "FULL OF":**
- *"Love, joy, peace, patience, kindness, goodness, faithfulness, gentleness, & self –control (Galatians 5:22-23)."*

We should also treat our bodies like the temples of the Holy Spirit!   Thus, we should eat healthful foods, exercise regularly, not smoke, not get drunk, & not be lazy gluttons, etc.!

What message are we giving to non-believers (as well as believers "in Christ") when they see Christians treat their bodies (the temples of the Holy Spirit) like an "over-sized sewer!?"

Consider the following parable. A 10 year old boy has lost his father & has 2 uncles as his 2 male role models in his life. "Uncle Sam" is a Christian that goes to church every Sunday. However, "Uncle Sam" is an obese glutton (eats excessively regularly), gets drunk, smokes, is lazy (never exercises), complains of chronic body pains, & seems full of hatred (as well as fear, greed, & depression).   "Uncle Bruce" is currently an atheist. "Uncle Bruce" is thin, healthy, exercises regularly, eats healthful foods, & seems full of love (as well as joy).   Which uncle is this 10 year old boy more attracted to? Which uncle are non-believers more attracted to?   Which uncle are believers more attracted to?

Consider a similar parable. Remember: *your body is the temple of the Holy Spirit.* Consider 2 "temples."   One "temple" is filthy & "*FULL OF*:"
- Toxic garbage; cigarette smoke; hatred; high-stress; depression; drunks; & lazy sinful gluttons.

The other "temple" is clean & filled with:
- Happiness; peace; love; joy; hard-working, healthy, & fit righteous people.

Which "temple" are you more attracted to?   Which temple are others more attracted to?

What kind of role models are we to our friends & family? If we are "*FULL OF*" toxins, what kind of spouse, parent, child, or friend will we be?

What did Jesus do before He started His ministry? He fasted 40 days & 40 nights. (Matt 4:2)

What did His disciples do before they began their 1st missionary journey? They fasted. (Acts 13:2-3) They sacrificed the fleshly pleasures of earthly food for spiritual food. Are we not His disciples?

I am NOT suggesting that we HAVE to (or should) eliminate all food for 40 days & 40 nights BEFORE God can use us to bring people "into Christ." However, are we not capable of sacrificing the fleshly pleasures of earthly JUNK food for spiritual food?

I AM suggesting that we would be better vessels (better representatives) for Christ (better "equipped" to be used by God to bring people "into Christ") by:
-    Trying your best to AVOID direct body toxins (chapter 3)
-    Following the "10 Dietary Commandments" (chapter 5)
-    Following some –if not all of the "10 Non-Dietary Cleansing Methods" (chapter 5)
-    & consuming certain "Super-Cleansing Foods/Supplements" (Chapter 6).

BY avoiding toxins & "detoxing" – we will have a "cleaner"/healthier body. By optimizing our physical health, we can better optimize the health of our minds & souls. We will also "look" more attractive to others.   By ***cleansing*** all the toxins out of your ***body, mind, & soul*** - it will be <u>easier</u> to be filled with *Love, joy, peace, patience, kindness, goodness, faithfulness, gentleness, & self-control*!

In Luke 24:5, it is written: *"Why do you seek the LIVING ONE among the dead?"*

When we read or preach the word of God, we should (therefore) keep in mind that "The Word" of God is ALIVE! He IS the Living Word of God. He has risen!   "The world" (including most believers) looks at you & judges you by how you look. They will judge you by how tall you are. They will judge you by the color of your skin, eyes, & hair. They will judge you by the sound (or accent) of your voice. They may or may not like how you look or talk.

But how does God see us?   God has called all believers to preach the gospel to all the nations. If someone does not like the way you look or the sound/accent of your voice –tell them not to look or listen to you that way. Tell them to "feel the love" God has for them. Tell them to receive/"feel" the Love you have for them. Do not look at me like that Jewish, 6'1", blue eyed, brown haired, white (12.5% Seminole Indian), Floridian with a New York accent!   Don't look at the vessel – listen, hear, & read the Living Word of God.   Don't look at the vessel - receive the Love that God has for you (which is greater than any Love you will ever receive)!   If God can use a jackass to get His message across to man, He can certainly use me!

CHAPTER 2: Why "_YOU'RE FULL OF_" more _Mind & Soul_ toxins than ever before

I hope to demonstrate in this chapter the answer to the following question:

- What are the 4 major reasons why Americans (as well as the rest of the world's people – in general) are "_**FULL OF**_" more SIN than ever before? This is at least part of the reason why we are "_**FULL OF**_" more diseases, obesity, &/or chronic pain than ever before!   Remember: it is the **accumulation & compounding effect** of all these SINS (added to the "direct body toxins") that cause or exacerbate diseases (including obesity, chronic pain, & even death)!   Additionally: the "spiritual pain" (sins) in our minds & souls can exacerbate or even cause the pain in our bodies (as well as obesity, diseases, & even death).

As mentioned in chapter 1, the following under-recognized relationship is NOT a coincidence (it is a "God-incidence"):

- Our nation's **God- deficit** (straying farther from GOD) is related to our health, moral, intellectual, & financial **deficits**. **As our nation has become more sinful** ("_**FULL OF**_" intellectual & spiritual toxins), **we have become "_FULL OF_" more diseases, obesity, disability, & chronic pain**!   As society has strayed farther away from God's 10 Commandments, we have (not ironically) strayed farther away from the "10 Dietary Commandments" (mentioned in chapter 5).

The strong relationships/connections between God, your health, finances, & morality are severely under-recognized. Our nation's largest **God deficit** has led to our largest: **Health, financial, & moral deficit**. Our nation's largest **Health deficit** has led to our largest: God, financial, & moral deficits.   Our nation's largest **financial deficit** has led to our largest: God, health, & moral deficits. Our nation's largest **moral deficit** has led to our largest: God, health, & financial deficits.

Do you see the connections/relationships?   If you believe these body-mind-soul connections are simply "coincidences" (versus "God-incidences"): then "_**YOU ARE FULL OF IT**_!"   As we have removed (or "pushed" away) God from our lives/nation/world, we have become: More broke economically/financially; More immoral; More obese, diseased, & dead from prescription painkiller overdoses; & less intelligent!

There are many reasons why the minds & souls of our nation have become more sinful than ever before.   I will list (what I believe) are the **4 major reasons** why &/or how the minds & souls of our nation have become more sinful than ever before.   My goal of writing these reasons is not to condemn our nation. It is for our nation to wake up & rise up.   I write these reasons so that our nation (& the entire world) can get closer to God (& God's Love) & cleanse (optimize the health of) our bodies, minds, & souls! If we can get back to God (& God's love): we can become, once again, the greatest nation in the world.

I. *"YOU'RE FULL OF"* More Direct Body Toxins - & society *"Irrationally Accepts"* this as "normal"

Society currently has an *"Irrational Apathy & Acceptance"* regarding the increased level of direct body (as well as mind & soul) toxins we are bombarded with (&, therefore *"**FULL OF**"*). I believe society's apathetic view of the *flood* of direct body (as well as mind, & soul) toxins we are bombarded with &, unfortunately, *"**FULL OF**"* is extremely analogous to those who eventually drowned during the days of Noah! God warned the people of this **flood**. This book warns our society of the abovementioned "flood." How much more warning do we need? Should we be so apathetic & accepting of this *flood* that it continues to grow larger & larger by the day?! *"YOU'RE FULL OF IT"* – but you can change this!

The bombardment & "storing" of toxins in the intestines & the rest of our body is destroying the health of our *bodies (the temple of the Holy Spirit)* – as well as our minds & souls. We have achieved this by:

- Breaking (ignorantly &/or volitionally) most – if not all - of "10 Dietary Commandments" on a daily or even multiple times per day basis! These are mentioned in Chapter 5.
- Avoiding ALL of the "10 Non-Dietary Cleansing Methods" (mentioned in chapter 5).
- Avoiding ALL the "Super-Cleansing Foods/Supplements" mentioned in Chapter 6.
- Being bombarded with & storing direct body (dietary & non-dietary) toxins from the environment, our posture, etc. (chapter 3).

We have "chosen" (either ignorantly or volitionally) to do the above. By choosing to do the above, we are storing these direct body toxins (as well as mind & soul toxins that indirectly destroy our bodies). Therefore, we have chosen to become *"**FULL OF IT**"* – which destroys our bodies = *the temple of the Holy Spirit* in infinite ways/examples. Some of these examples include (discussed further in chapter 3):

- o We have created an intestinal breeding ground for harmful virus & microorganisms. This is why it is so difficult to reverse many virus-based diseases (like Hepatitis, etc.)
- o We end up storing nicotine & other addictive drugs in our intestines. This may be why many drug addictions become so difficult to cure (the addictive substance can still be stored in their intestines or other body part for years after their last cigarette)!
- o We end up storing mercury, pesticides, & other toxins in our intestines, brain, & any other body part the toxins want to be stored in! This may be why mental disorders (like OCD, ADHD, Depression, Anxiety, etc.) & neurological diseases (like Parkinson's, Multiple Sclerosis, Alzheimer's, & ALS) have become so difficult to reverse (the blood-brain barrier is a difficult barrier to cross).

35

- We end up storing industrial chemical toxins & toxic heavy metals damaging our brains (as well as our entire nervous system), cardiovascular systems, endocrine systems, the rest of our body, including every living cell in our body. This can predispose us to cancer – which we often treat with more carcinogenic toxins!

We have <u>accepted</u> or chosen NOT to do everything in our power to prevent or reverse diseases! We have <u>chosen</u> NOT to do everything to optimize our health. Perhaps many people simply do not know (where the word "Ignorant" comes from). *"Forgive them for they do not know."* This might sound harsh. However, consider the following examples:
- If you do not know that having intercourse with your neighbor's wife is a SIN: is it still a SIN?
- If you do not know that smoking cigarettes is harmful to your health (like perhaps in the early 1900s) &, therefore, a SIN: is it still a SIN?
- If you do not know that spraying toxic perfumes on your body or spraying toxic pesticides in your homes is harmful to your health &, therefore, a SIN: is it still considered a SIN?
- If you do not know that being "stressed-out" (lacking peace), lazy, undisciplined, drunk, or a glutton is harmful to your health &, therefore, a SIN: is it still a SIN?
- If you do not know that storing/being "***FULL OF***" toxins in your body is harmful to your health &, therefore, a SIN: is it still considered a SIN?

Is America's Health Care "Culture" Backwards - & DO WE HAVE IRRATIONAL ACCEPTANCE & APATHY REGARDING THIS?

We have become a **disease-based (versus health-based) society**. We have replaced health with diseases. In America's health care system: **when you are "positive" = this is negative** (or bad news that you do have "a disease")! **When you are "negative" = this is positive** (or good news that you do NOT have "a disease")! Our health care system is NOT HOLISTIC. It has become so specialized. Our focus has gone from looking at the patient as a "whole" ("Holistic") to looking at their 1 body part or organ system. We have believed the myth that absence of disease (which we often use direct body toxins to evaluate & treat) is optimal health! Optimal health is the optimal functioning of every cell in your body! We are "***FULL OF***" **certain health-care myths – like good health care is** (analyzed further in Chapter 3 & 4):
- Treating most chronic diseases & chronic pain - caused by being "***FULL OF***" body, mind, & soul **toxins** ("***IT***") - with more direct body **toxins (like pharmaceuticals, radiation, etc.)**!
- Treating the symptoms of chronic diseases (including chronic pain) with direct body toxins versus treating all the causes (being "***FULL OF IT***")!
- Treating cancer & autoimmune diseases with carcinogenic, immune destroying direct body toxins!

- Treating acid reflux with ant-acids (often bound with toxic artificial flavors, colors, & even toxic heavy metals) on a daily basis. There are patients of mine who take prescription (&/or over the counter) ant-acids every day for years! Taking these ant-acids on a daily basis may block the absorption of necessary nutrients (like calcium) & interfere with the digestion of your food. Thus, you may truly end up: "**_FULL OF_**" intestinal putrefaction (which slows down intestinal motility) – which may predispose you to <u>more gastrointestinal reflux</u>! This can create a habit harmful to your body - as well as your wallet!
- Treating all influenzas with antibiotics!
- Treating all diseases with toxic medication, surgery, &/or other toxic methods (radiation, chemotherapy, etc.).
- Prescribing/Recommending the same dosage of medications (or dietary supplements) for a 300 pound 30 year old & an 80 pound 80 year old!
- Treating all degenerative joint diseases with "Total Joint Replacement" Surgeries!
- Treating all herniated discs with discectomy surgeries! For over 25 years we have known of the "False Positive" findings of disc protrusions by radiologists. Using CT scans: it has been proven that many people with herniated discs have no pain/symptoms.[1,2]
- Treating/Preventing Blood Clots with Anticoagulants - & Neglecting the risk of Bleeding &/or Anemia from the anticoagulants (both pharmaceutical & "natural")! This is illustrated again & in greater detail (with a hopeful solution) in "Dietary Commandment #6" (in Chapter 5).

We believe **other health-care myths like optimal health is achieved by**:
- Taking some "super-medication(s)."
- Taking some "super-supplement(s)." If you do not follow the "10 Dietary Commandments" (in Chapter 5), you may not optimally ABSORB the supplements & foods you consume. In addition, certain supplements absorb better than others. Also, many supplements have serious side effects – especially when taken with: Pharmaceuticals; Each other or in excess; Someone already having a disorder/disease in which the side effects of the supplement increase those side effect risks; &/or someone who is near surgery &/or trauma.

We have believed the following **myths about dietary supplements** (analyzed further in Chapter 6):
- They will heal all our diseases, create optimal health, eliminate our obesity, make us look great, & cure world peace!
- All dietary supplements are 100% safe, natural, & organic (they usually aren't).
- Dietary supplements won't interact with medications (they might)!

Again, if we break the "10 Dietary Commandments" (illustrated in Chapter 5) even the most healthful supplements will not get absorbed!

We have believed (become "**FULL OF**") some of the following myths **about nutrition & obesity** (these - & many more of these myths will be these will be discussed again in further detail in chapters 4, 5, & 6):

- All **FOOD** is equally healthful regardless of whether it is:
  - Organic versus sprayed heavily with pesticides &/or genetically modified;
  - Alive & Raw versus dead (vegan "Raw" usually does = alive. However non-vegan "Raw" – like raw eggs, fish, meats, etc. = dead!);
  - Alive & Raw versus fried with hydrogenated oils & trans-fats;
  - Alive & Raw versus sugar & salt added;
  - & combined correctly to assure optimal absorption versus combined incorrectly!
- All **FIBER** sources are equally healthful. The fiber found in raw vegetables, fruits, seeds, & nuts is "super-cleansing fiber." The fiber found in most cereals, breads, & pastas is not.
- All **Soy** is equally healthful. There are "super-cleansing soy" food sources like natto, doenjang, sprouted soybeans, & tempeh. However, most Americans are consuming the "junk-food," processed soy sources (like soymilk, soy cheese, soy burgers, soy ice cream).
- All **Fats** are equally healthful. There are "super-fat" food sources (mentioned in chapter 6). However, Americans (since the 1950s) have been consuming a lot of extremely harmful (possibly satanic) trans-fats & hydrogenated oils! As explained in chapter 6, this is why some **Meats** are harmful (as they are injected with hormones, antibiotics, & raised on non-organic feed high in grains – as well as cooked/fried in hydrogenated oils)! There are "super-meats" discussed in chapter 6.
- All **Carbs** are equally healthful. Americans have become "carb-addicted." Americans have also been consuming a lot of sugary sodas & grains. Remember the USDA "food pyramid" of the 1970s recommended we consume grains as the largest category of our diet.[3] Even recently, the "MY Plate" endorsed by the USDA recommends 25% of "our plate" be grains.[3]
- All **Dairy** is equally healthful. Some milk (like organically raised goat's milk) is healthful. However, most milk we consume in America may be harmful to our health & our waistlines!

Some of the reasons our bodies are more toxic/ "**FULL OF IT**" than ever before is because millions have believed (&/or followed the advice of) the abovementioned myths. I will demonstrate (in greater detail) that the above (& many more nutritional fallacies) are myths in chapters 4, 5, & 6.

It seems like our nation is almost proud of being a bunch of sinful, "stressed-out," addicted, greedy, ignorant, jealous, anxiety-filled, hateful, impatient, unfaithful, undisciplined, lazy, drunk, "drugged-out" (especially on pain killers), gluttons!   We seem almost proud of being the most obese nation in the world!   We seem apathetic to avoid the bombardment of direct body toxins. We seem apathetic to detox from the toxins stored in our bodies. We seem apathetic to stop all the other sinful causes of obesity, chronic pain, & diseases!

In addition **we "reward" people for being diseased &/or disabled**! This may offend some people – but it is NOT my intent to offend anyone. I remember as a child my Jewish mother giving me delicious chicken soup every time I got a cold. She would also give me more attention & love! Her attitude changed when I hit approximately 15. She told me she hated when I was sick. The chicken soup & extra love & attention stopped. I stopped getting so many colds!

Our Society Rewards Disease!

We have to realize as health care providers & healers (who may use the power of the Holy Spirit & the name of Jesus Christ to heal diseases), NOT everyone wants to be healed!

- **Many people "hold onto" (identify themselves) their diseases**. They identify themselves with their diseases (whether or not they have been correctly diagnosed or not with that disease). If you dare tell them they have been diagnosed incorrectly for the past 5 years (like with "lymphedema" versus "edema"), some of them may get upset. They tell their friends & family they "have" such & such disease(s). They "doctor shop" to find physicians to prescribe the drugs (like pain killers) that they are addicted to.
- **Many people are psychologically rewarded for their chronic pain &/or disease(s).** They get more sympathy from friends, family, strangers, & even health care providers (who are supposed to be empathetic versus sympathetic).
- **Many people are rewarded financially - & with better (& more attentive) health care for their chronic pain, disease(s) &/or disability.**   If you are disabled for 2 years or more, you qualify for Medicare.   If you are "injured" at work, you may receive 60-80% of your salary for 2 years (or for life if injured as a government employee) tax free! They may receive financial benefits from the government – as well as disability insurance. They may receive better (& more affordable) health care from the government.   Many patients "doctor shop" to get prescription pain medicines to sell to friends, family, strangers, etc. Unfortunately, the tremendous percentage increase (analyzed further in chapter 3) in deaths from prescription painkiller overdosing may have something to do with these "rewards." **These "socio-economic rewards" for disease(s)/disabilities (as well as the tax "punishment" for working since 1997) may be major reasons why the number of Americans receiving more disability benefits has been skyrocketing since approximately 1997** (no coincidence!).   The

tremendous increase in the number of Americans receiving disability benefits in the past 20 years will be dissected & referenced further - later in this chapter.

The fact that the abovementioned bombardment & storing of body, mind, & soul toxins causes diseases – including obesity & chronic pain - will be discussed further in Chapters 3 & 4.

Our anti-Godly society is imprisoning our health care providers from providing the health care their patients deserve!

Since certain patients want to *sue our neighbors* (including health care providers) versus *LOVE our neighbors,* health care providers spend an excess of time doing legalistic paperwork to "CYA" (Cover Your Assets) from being sued!   Since our insurance companies & their representatives do **NOT** *love thy neighbor,* health care providers spend an excess of time doing legalistic paperwork to CYA from being denied payment for their services!   Health care *providers* are supposed to *provide* health care (versus write about it)!

As medicine has become more specialized, we have become more distant & "cold" as health care providers. Health care providers have to protect themselves from negligence, malpractice, insurance denials, & even sexual harassment!   Have we forgotten the fact that our "neighbors" (***love thy neighbor***) include patients – as well as health care providers?   Have we gone so far astray from God that we have forgotten one of his greatest commandments: *"To Love EVERYONE*!?"

We have accepted cold distant apathy as the norm for how health care providers treat us. Health care providers (like myself) who love &/or care too much about their patients are criticized & even mocked! I have been told by coworkers, patient's family members, & even patients: "You're not Jesus you know. Stop caring so much about your patients!"   Health care providers need to have a professional distance. However, the norm has become a different area code!

How would our current anti-Godly society view some of the actions Jesus Christ did?

These days our society would arrest &/or sue Jesus Christ for:
-    Disturbing the peace; Vandalism of the temple; & healing ALL disease without a license to practice medicine!

Today's society would criticize Jesus for:
-    Raising Lazarus & the little girl from the dead – but not making them wealthy; Healing all diseases – but not making those people rich; Healing all diseases – but not submitting the proper paperwork to their insurance companies; Giving the masses fish & bread – but not money, wine, chicken, or filet mignon!

Money has become society's master today.   Society's obsession with money replaces God (& God's love) with riches.   Society's obsession with money is an under-recognized toxin/sin that destroys the health of our bodies, minds, & souls.

<u>**Our Attitude = "Irrational Acceptance/Apathy" of Diseases & Obesity**</u>! We have **accepted** & chosen to:

- Be bombarded with - & become "***FULL OF***" mind & soul toxins (Chapters 1 & 2) – as well as non-Dietary direct body toxins (chapter 3);
- Break all of the "10 Dietary Commandments" multiple times per day (Chapter 5);
- Avoid all of the "10 non-dietary cleansing methods" (Chapter 5);
- & avoid all of the "Super-Cleansing foods/supplements" (chapter 6)!

<u>**So, what should our attitude be towards health care: Adam's, the Atheistic Existentialist's, or God's?**</u>

<u>**Adam's view**</u>: Currently, <u>**our nation**</u> has the attitude towards health care of Adam = <u>**Irresponsibility**</u>.   When Adam 1st sinned he blamed Eve, the devil, & even God!   When something goes wrong with our health, we look to blame (even sue) others – including the well-intentioned health care providers. Are we much different from Adam in our sense of personal irresponsibility? Do we *love thy neighbor*? A "good" year for a physician is when no one attempts to sue them! We blame our physicians for prescribing all these toxic medications, radiological tests, & surgeries. We also blame our physicians when they **don't** prescribe toxic meds, radiological tests, &/or surgeries!

I must confess - existentialism has its place in health care. We need to increase the level of responsibility towards our health.   Pure <u>**Existentialists**</u> believe you are 100% responsible for your own health care!   I believe this part of existentialism is correct.   The person most responsible for your health care is YOU!

It is mostly <u>**our fault that we choose to store**</u> (become "***FULL OF***"- & choose not to detoxify from) these toxins. <u>**We can choose to:**</u>

- Avoid – as best as possible - mind & soul toxins (chapters 1 & 2) – as well as many direct body toxins (chapter 3); Follow all "10 Dietary Commandments" (Chapter 5); Follow most (if not all) "10 Non-Dietary Cleansing Methods" (chapter 5); & consume some "super-cleansing foods/supplements" (Chapter 6).

The above can help us avoid & detoxify from body, mind, & soul toxins!

However, an <u>**atheistic existentialism**</u> is not a healthy philosophy for all aspects of your life. Atheistic existentialism may teach that you are 100% responsible for the famine & wars in the world (as you are not doing everything possible to stop them)!   If you follow existentialism as a life philosophy, you may be promised 3 things in your life: *forlornness, despair, & unhappiness*! One of Jean-Paul Sartre's (a famous author of existentialistic books, plays, etc.) plays is appropriately entitled: "*NO EXIT!*"

Atheistic existentialism is diametrically opposed to what Jesus promised.   Jesus said, "*You are never alone. I am with you always.*" Some of "*the fruits of the Holy Spirit are peace & joy."* Not despair or unhappiness. *"Rejoice in the LORD always!"*

In summary: **it's not *100%* your fault that** *"YOU ARE FULL OF IT!"* Society's **acceptance** of our bodies being bombarded &, therefore, *"FULL OF"* toxins in our food, water, homes, the air we breathe, etc. – has leeched into our brains as being **acceptable**. Similar to the way we *accept* that our non-organic foods are *"FULL OF"* neurotoxins, carcinogens, etc. – we also accept brutal violence, blasphemy, theft, pornography, adultery, etc. (on our televisions, radios, etc.). It's just part of our culture! Other countries ban GMO foods or force food companies to label when a food contains Genetically Modified Organisms. However, the United Secrets of America is that ALL of our food is Genetically Modified or contains pesticides/herbicides, etc. –UNLESS it is labeled: "non-GMO" or "100% Certified U.S.D.A. Organic" (which usually implies non-GMO – as well as no pesticides or herbicides sprayed on the food).

II.   *"YOU'RE FULL OF"* more Sin than ever before because "SIN is IN" – "Intellectual & Spiritual Constipation" are the norm

I believe this is still the best nation in the world. However, we are no longer the "envy" (or the role-model) of the world we once were. There are many reasons for this! "Right" has become wrong in our nation! Wrong has become "politically correct." ***Our society needs a colonic!*** Has America become like "the world" during the time of Noah!? Genesis 6:5-6 – *"Then the LORD saw that the wickedness of man [mankind] was great on the earth, & that **every intent** of the **thoughts** of his **heart** was **only evil continually**. The LORD was sorry that He had made man on the earth."*

America has forgotten that we are founded on a Judaic-Christian (Godly) foundation. Believers & real-followers of Christ are ***supposed to be*** ***"FULL OF"*** *"fruits of the Holy Spirit: Love, joy, peace, patience, kindness, goodness, faithfulness, gentleness, & self-control."* (Gal 5:22) However, those who proclaim to believe God's word are considered by our nation to be: "radical, extreme, narrow-minded, politically incorrect, & even ignorant!" God's 10 Commandments have been removed from the U.S. courtrooms & schools! Our nation doesn't want to watch a movie or television program about some beautiful God-loving people who dedicate their lives to helping others in need out of the good-ness of their heart. Our society finds these stories: "BORING!"

"Sin is IN" & "*YOU'RE FULL OF*" Atheism! Are we *still* considered "One Nation under God?"
From 2005 to 2012, the percentage of Americans that believe in God has shrunk – while the percentage of "convinced Atheists" has increased 500%![4] The percentage of Americans who identify themselves to be "***convinced***

atheists" has skyrocketed five-fold from 1% in 2005 to 5% in 2012![4] Consider where we are spiritually in America: "convinced Christians" are considered arrogant & close minded; whereas "convinced atheists" are considered open-minded!?   Unfortunately, this percentage of Americans that consider themselves "**_convinced atheists_**" will most likely grow far above 5% by the time you read this book.

As mentioned in chapter one, there are many atheists who act more like Jesus Christ/God-like than many devout believers in God!   However, we can't deny the fact that as Atheism has grown –so has our level of immorality as a whole nation!   In addition, this "Atheistic movement/growth" is becoming stronger & more widespread (like a cancer) infiltrating every aspect of our society!   The atheists in our country are actually starting to attempt to sue their local governments for emotional pain & suffering due to public statues of Jesus, the 10 Commandments, etc.!   How low have we fallen?   We must still Love these atheists – even if they may be "**_FULL OF IT_**!"

SIN & Satanic symbols are accepted & even rewarded in our country. I remember when my beautiful niece was 14 years old (in 2009), she asked me: "What are you: a vampire or a werewolf?! Everyone in our school is either one or the other!" Have these 2 satanic symbols become the role models of our children?   Our media makes murderers, terrorists, pedophiles, kidnappers, rapists, thieves, blasphemers, & other sin-full, satanic symbols famous!   Would we ever have known of these murderers –if it wasn't broadcasted for weeks & weeks on every media venue?

Falling out of love with God (& God's love & God's word) is the "IN" thing in our nation.   As our nation has become "**_FULL OF_**" more atheism & sin (than ever in our history), we have also become "**_FULL OF_**" more obesity, chronic pain, disease, disability, divorce, debt, immorality, etc.   Have we become blind to the concept that falling out of love with God may cause you to fall out of love with yourself, spouse, neighbor, &/or country?!   Perhaps this is too deep!   These days we think of abortion & divorce as something we order at a restaurant!   "Yeah –I'll have the chicken & we'll have a Divorce with that!"

"SIN is IN" & "_YOU'RE FULL OF_" **Intellectual Constipation & Emotional Instability!**   _"My people are destroyed for lack of knowledge."_ (Hosea 4:6)

As our connection to God has declined - so has our intelligence levels!   The fact that we are "**_FULL OF_**" "Intellectual Constipation" (& its' relationship to our toxic bodies & souls) has been illustrated previously in this book. I am not the only scientist that believes humans are becoming intellectually weaker & emotionally more unstable![5]   This may be due to:

- The direct body toxins that we are bombarded with (& become "_FULL OF_") from the:
  - Food we eat – breaking all of the "10 Dietary Commandments" (chapter 5) on a daily basis – & often multiple times per day;

43

- o Water we drink (filled with toxins like chlorine, antibiotics – as well as lead, & Fluoride which may lower your I.Q.);[5]
- o Air we breathe – containing pollution, pesticides, etc.;
- o & other toxins our bodies are bombarded with (see Chapter 3).
- The Intellectual **laziness** "*allowance*" of advanced technology. As technology has advanced to *allow* physically & mentally challenged people to "rise up," it also allows the "un-challenged" to stop challenging themselves & "fall down!" We force students at an early age to use a calculator & wonder why they need one to multiply 55 x 65 (it's 3,575 -& no, I didn't need a calculator. It is called "the difference between two squares." Thus, 60x60 = 3600 – 25 = 3575)! ☺ There are children in 3rd world countries who know this. However, most American adults need a calculator!
- The spiritual satanic toxins that we are bombarded with - & become "*FULL OF*" Remember, there is no coincidence that our nation's largest God deficit has led to our nation's largest intellectual (as well as health, financial, & moral) deficit!
- &/or that Charles Darwin was wrong or right!? Geneticists have explained that "*Darwin's theory of 'survival of the fittest' is less applicable in today's society as people with adverse genetic mutations are more likely than ever to survive & live amongst the strong.*"[5]

Our "Intellectual Constipation" will be discussed again throughout this book – especially later in this chapter when it is illustrated why we have <u>accepted</u> our Anti-Godly tax policies!

SIN sells in "Hollywood"! I do not blame "Hollywood" (movie, television, & video game producers) for "pushing" SIN – because SIN sells! Movies, television programs, & video games don't "sell" unless they contain the following SINS:

- Brutal violence, murder, sexual immorality, greed/swindlers (con-men & con-women), sorcery, idolatry, outbursts of anger, lying, abusive language, blasphemy, laziness, gluttony, drunkenness, conceited-ness, &/or jealousy!

Our culture seems to "demand" these SINS (& sin-full "role models") from "Hollywood." When real people of our society "copy" these sin-full "role models," we claim "they're sick!" HELLO?! We have become a sin-full nation - which has *made us* "sick!"

If you look hard enough through the pollution on the television, you can find "Godly" programs showing real people helping the needy, preaching the word of God, etc. Remember: your mind & soul is what you feed it (**if it gets "absorbed")!**

What we call a "dysfunctional home" "*FULL OF*" violence & abuse – God may consider a "Generational curse!" Remember: Jesus **ended all generational curses**! (Jeremiah 31:29-31 & John 19:28-30)

Before Jesus said "*It is finished*" (John 19:30), He said "*I am thirsty*" (John 19:28) – to **END ALL generational curses** (Jeremiah 31:29-31; John 19:28-30).

What we call "pigging out," or "getting drunk or wasted," or a "couch potato" - God calls SINs ("gluttony," "drunkenness," & "laziness") - & causes of diseases –including obesity &/or chronic pain!

What we call "being stressed out" or "undisciplined" – God calls a SIN (& a major cause for diseases – including obesity & chronic pain)!

What we call "pest-control" – God calls a SIN (destroying the temple of the Holy Spirit = our bodies)!   If you believe pesticides are harmless because they may be odorless, then "**_YOU'RE FULL OF IT_**!"   My Jewish ancestors were killed in the Holocaust with odorless gas.

What we call "having a cigarette break," or "getting high on drugs" – God calls a SIN!

We have become a society of "TAKERS" without "GIVING."   If you believe a successful relationship (this includes relationships with: your spouse, parents, children, friends, employer, employee, & even your country) is one where you TAKE everything you can from them - & NEVER GIVE back anything = "**_YOU ARE FULL OF IT_**!"   Many people <u>want to</u> lose excess body fat &/or waste matter, reduce or eliminate their body pains, optimize their health & appearance: but don't want to "GIVE" a commitment to doing so. We are committed to our laziness, gluttony, & lack of discipline. However, we tell everyone how much we want to get healthy (lose excess body fat, waste matter, reduce our body pains, optimize health & appearance).

America is "**_FULL OF_**" more SIN than ever in our nations' history! It is no coincidence that we have become "**_FULL OF_**" more obesity, chronic pain, & diseases than ever before!   This relationship is severely under-recognized & under-appreciated!

God does not refer to us as sheep because sheep are highly intelligent. Most sheep herders will tell you they are not. God refers to us as sheep because sheep <u>NEED a GOOD SHEPHERD</u> to live/thrive for their _entire life_! We were a "nation under God" (God is the greatest most powerful shepherd in the world) for decades. However, now we have become a nation that is _like sheep that has gone astray_. This growing "God deficit" has led to America's growing: health, economic/financial, intellectual & moral deficits!

Where are the "Noahs" of our nation?!   Don't "drown" in society's flood of SINS.   Jump into the _arc of Jesus_ & He will lift you up & give you peace & joy & LOVE during the storm.   Now, more than ever –God needs His believers to rise up & be the "salt of the earth."   He needs us to be lights in a darkened world!   I pray this nation -& our entire world – become closer to God!

III.   "_YOU'RE FULL OF_" Deficiencies, Mal-absorptions, & Misconceptions of God's Living Word

<u>Deficiency of God's Living Word</u>

As mentioned above, our nation has strayed far from God. God wants us *renew like eagles*. Eagles (unless they are held in captivity) eat things that are **ALIVE**! Chickens, crows, & buzzards eat dead things. God doesn't want you to be a chicken! He wants you to read the *living word of God*. If we develop a deficiency in the living word of God, we may become deficient in all other areas in our lives! If we want optimal health of our bodies, minds, & souls —we should feed our minds & souls the Living word of God. This can include choosing to listen & watching the word of God on the radio, television, -& of course reading the living word of God on a daily (if not multiple times per day or for those who are tempted like myself —all day long) basis. "LORD: *Give us our daily bread.*"

God does not want us to feed our souls & minds with "dead" anti-Godly things. This includes what we hear & see on the internet, television, radio, cell phones, etc. It may also include what our friends, family, & even co-workers "feed us."

Friedrich **Nietzsche** (famous author of books such as *Thus Spoke Zarathrustra*) was considered a strong supporter of **atheism**. Nietzsche was also considered the greatest influence on **Mussolini, Stalin, & Hitler**. Need I say more?! Jesus Christ was considered the greatest influence on Mother Teresa & international missionaries (who sacrificed their time, money, & lives to help the poor, needy, hungry, & sick to come closer to the Love of Christ). Who influences you, your family, & your country?

The minds of our nation have become so polluted, we don't even know when life begins (or ends)! My Jewish Grandmother (in the 1980s) used to tell me the following joke: "Did you hear the new Jewish philosophy on abortion? You're a fetus until you graduate college!"

We have failed to recognize the connection between America's growing "GOD-DEFICIT" & our growing:

- Health Deficit. As our nation has become more sinful than ever before, we have become "*FULL OF*" more diseases, obesity, & chronic pain.
- Financial Deficit. As our nation has become more sinful than ever before, we have become "*FULL OF*" more financial debt than ever in our history. We have failed to connect our spiritual deficit with our financial deficit! Society wants to remove the words: "*In GOD we trust*" from our currency. Our country was founded "under GOD." As we remove Him from our country, we become less blessed (& more cursed)!
- Moral Deficit. As we have removed God from our culture (& replaced Him with SINS), we have become "*FULL OF*" more immorality! Society's morality has fallen to record lows. If morality was sold on the stock exchange, it would be hitting record lows!
- Intellectual Deficit. As we have removed God from our schools & our society, we have become "*FULL OF*" more ignorance (less intelligence). We have more access (via the T.V., radio, internet, cell phones, etc.) to God's Living word. However, we have chosen "to feed" our brains with SINFUL toxins! We wonder why our schools (K through 12) have fallen to that of 3rd world countries! Teachers are forced to teach children "Darwinism" &

__forbidden__ to teach them "Creationism!"   They want to prevent children from praying in schools!   They want to eliminate the words: "_One nation UNDER GOD_."

All of the abovementioned deficits become toxic to our bodies, minds, & souls!   What are you trying to fill the "God-deficit" (void) in your life?   Only God can truly fulfill us with ALL of our present & eternal needs!

Mal-absorption of God's Living Word

Your mind & soul is NOT (necessarily) what you __feed__ it.   Your mind & soul IS what it "eats __& absorbs__!"   This is very similar to our bodies.   You are not what you eat.   You are what you absorb!   Some people refer to this as "passive listeners."   If an atheist reads the entire Bible, & still remained an atheist: they obviously did NOT absorb God's living word. ***

***Personal comment/story

My 1st week in college, It took me 8 hours to read the 1st 5 pages of a Biology text book.   However, I had no clue of what I had just read – as I did NOT absorb it!   I prayed to God to make me "the best student in the world!"   This sounds arrogant.   However, God said "_Ask & you shall to receive._" In addition my prayer was God-based so I could eventually get into physical therapy school to help people.   I worked harder (_with all my heart & might_) than any other college student I knew by studying 100 hours per week. This only left 38 hours per week for sleeping (as I was in class 20 hours per week & commuted 10 hours per week).   I had no social life.   After 3 years I was chosen by my University to represent them as one of the top 20 undergraduate college students in the U.S.A.!   After 4 years of this __disciplined__ studying regimen, I was able to "speed-read," memorize, & __absorb__ an entire text book in 1 hour (cover to cover).   However, there is one book I have never been able to (& should not try to) "speed read."   That is the living word of God!   God's word is alive! Living "food" for the mind, soul, & body!   __I believe God's living word –like our food- needs to be "chewed on" thoroughly & slowly to be __optimally absorbed__.   There is not a more powerful book in the world!

Plant God's "seed" (like God's most healthful foods) on __good soil__ to have optimal __absorption & become "FULL OF" God's word/love__.   This concept is repeated many times in the Bible to get it through our stubborn, fleshly minds! (Mark 4:4-20)

If God's living word [seed] is read or heard by someone with a mind, soul, &/or "_heart that is __beside the road__ where the word is sown:_" they will __not absorb__ the word of God.   When they hear the word of God, immediately _Satan comes & takes away the word which has been sown in them!_   Therefore, these people never __absorb__ God's living word.

If God's living word [seed] is read or heard by one with a mind, soul, &/or "_heart_" that is __on rocky places__, they will have a short-lived __absorption__ of the word of God.   "_When they hear the word, they immediately receive it with joy. However, they have no firm root in themselves, but are only temporary. When persecution arises because of the word, __immediately they fall away__._"   Therefore, these people only have a temporary (short-lived) __absorption__ of God's living word.

If God's living word [seed] is read or heard by one with a mind, soul, &/or "heart" that is __among the thorns__, their "thorns" will interfere ("choke")

47

the word of God. *"These are the ones who have heard the word [of God], but the worries of the world, & the deceitfulness of riches, and the desires for other things enter in and __choke the word, & it becomes unfruitful__."* No further explanation needed in my opinion!

If God's living word [seed] is read or heard by one with a mind, soul, & heart that is on **good soil**, *they hear the word & accept it (__optimally absorb it__) & __bear fruit thirty, sixty, & a hundredfold__!"* *"To you (true believers - followers in Christ whom hearts, minds, & souls are like "good soil") has been given the mystery of the kingdom of God."*

However, those who are outside get everything in parables, so that *"__THEY MAY SEE & NOT PERCEIVE, AND THEY MAY HEAR & NOT UNDERSTAND__."* (Is 6:9-10 & 43:8; Jer 5:21; Ezek 12:2; Matt 13:14; Luke 8:10John 12:40; Rom 11:8) Those who read the old covenant – but do NOT believe in Jesus Christ – have a *"**veil**"* over their __hardened minds & hearts__. (Isaiah 6:10; John 12:37-41; 2 Corinth 3:14-16) *"But when a person turns to the Lord, the __veil__ is taken away!"* (2 Corinth 3:14-16)

"Life & Death is in the tongue." Therefore, be careful what you say! Your life (including your words & actions) should be like the *"fruits of the Holy Spirit: love, joy, peace, patience, kindness, goodness, faithfulness, gentleness, & self-control."* (Gal 5:22)

If you have a "hard" (or "rocky") soul/mind, you will do what your sin-full "flesh" desires. If you have a "good" (or clean) soul/mind, you will NOT do what your sin-full "flesh" desires. As Jesus (our best role model) said: *"I do the will of my Father!"*

Jesus is the best Shepherd & the best Farmer! He can remove (*"**cleanse**"*) the stones, rocks, thorns, & weeds in your heart & mind. **Jesus cleanses us to give our mind & soul – as well as our body: "GOOD SOIL!"** This way you will optimally "absorb" the word of God to bear the *"fruits of the Holy Spirit!"*

This concept of mal-absorption also applies to our diets

If you break any of the "10 Dietary Commandments" (in chapter 5), you will NOT optimally **absorb** the food (or supplements) you eat! In other words, you will become "***FULL OF IT***!" If you do not absorb the food you eat, your body becomes deficient in the nutrients it needs/demands. Therefore, your body tells you to continue to eat (over-eat). Since your intestines are so "***FULL OF***" waste matter ("rocky or thorny soil"), the **absorption** of the food (even the most healthful foods in the world) will not be optimal!

If you eat healthful foods & do NOT **absorb** them (due to breaking the "10 Dietary Commandments"), they served no benefit to your health. In fact, if the foods you eat can create more intestinal putrefaction – which can:
- Slow down your metabolism; Create a breeding ground for toxins (such as harmful microorganisms, metals, drugs, etc.); & make you become more at risk for diseases (including obesity & chronic pain).

If you consume healthful foods on **"good soil"** (a clean colon –as well as the rest of your body; & a clean mind & soul), you can achieve the optimal benefit from these foods.

Misconceptions of God's Living Word

The "under-recognized Sins" mentioned in Chapter 1 represent some of the many misconceptions about God's Living Word.

These misconceptions (among non-believers - & even believers) have brought many of us away from God. In fact, many believers even divide themselves amongst each other due to these misconceptions. Satan wants to *divide & conquer*. Believers must be cognizant of how non-believers view us. Again, I mention these misconceptions as a way to:
- Bring our nation closer to God & God's Love.
- Optimize the health of our minds, souls, & bodies.
- Use The Living Word of God to UNITE & bring everyone closer to the love & power of God. Despite using the Bible to answer these misconceptions, they are still **my answers**. Only God knows the entire 100% truth. Only God is *THE TRUTH*! *"I am the way, & **the truth**, & the life; no one comes to the Father but through Me."* (John 14:6)

Some of these misconceptions may be controversial subjects amongst believers. Remember, only Jesus **IS THE TRUTH**! (John 14:6) Too often, Christians become "close-minded" on certain issues. Too often Christians have the opportunity to "open the minds" of non-believers & bring them closer to Christ (& His Love). We are not God & only God knows everything! If they want to know "The Truth" –show them. If they want to know the answer, they can ask Him! Jesus loves **everyone**. He died for everyone! He did *not* say – we should seek Him AFTER we have cleansed our bodies, minds, & souls! He said *"Come to ME!"*

In the 1st letter of Paul to Timothy (1 Timothy 1), the 1st chapter is devoted towards "Misconceptions in Doctrine & Living." *"The goal of our instruction is **LOVE** from a **pure heart** & a **good conscience & a sincere faith**."* Society's misconceptions of God's Living Word have caused our nation to stray so far away from God that many (if not most) Americans currently do not know the answers to the following questions:

1. **Can Jesus & His "Disciples" (In the name & power of Jesus Christ) Still Heal ALL Diseases?** **My bible-based answer = YES!**

Two thousand years ago, no one doubted Jesus' ability to Heal ALL diseases (or perform ALL miracles). Jesus was known as a healer (& miracle worker) before He was known as the Messiah! As mentioned in chapter 1, Jesus gave His disciples the authority to heal ALL diseases. People believed in His disciples to Heal ALL diseases. There were even people who did not believe in Jesus as LORD, yet used His name, to heal diseases! The question two thousand years ago was: Is Jesus the Messiah!?

Today, everyone who reads the Messianic prophecies in the Old Testament (AKA "Old Covenant"), believes He is the Messiah. The questions many people (including believers) have are:
- Is Jesus Still able to Heal ALL Diseases?!
- & Are His Disciples Still able to Heal ALL Diseases?!

Jesus never told His disciples to Heal some diseases. Jesus never told His disciples to stop healing ALL diseases. What has happened to our faith?!

Two people in the New Testament that had "great faith" were actually gentiles (a centurion & a Canaanite mother of a diseased child). They probably knew nothing of the LAW of God or God's word. However, they had great faith in God's Love & in Jesus Christ to heal all diseases.

As mentioned in Chapter 1, we must NOT focus on our SINS (the breaking of the law of God). We must focus on the GRACE - & Love of God. We must focus on Jesus who cleanses us from all sins.

We should not focus on the diseases.

We should focus on the healer of ALL diseases & for our optimal health!

Do we still have the faith to believe & ask God for 100% healing of ALL diseases (as well as miracles & other things we desire)? God can do anything! There is no limit to His power. We should not ask for a slight improvement of our diseases! If we need to lose 30% of our body fat to achieve optimal health, we should ASK for a 30% reduction in our body fat! Do you believe God can only help you lose 10% of the body fat you need to lose to achieve optimal health? How strong is your faith? We should ask & believe in God to give us 100% healing of our diseases (as well as our body pains). We should ask & believe in God to give us optimal health! In John 14:12-14, Jesus told His disciples: *"he who **BELIEVES in Me**, the works that I do, he will also do; & **greater works** than these he will do! If you **ASK for anything in My name**, I WILL DO IT."*

It reminds me of when I owned a tutoring company in 1988-1991. Many students would tell me "All I want is a 'C' or a 'D.'" Today, many of my patients will tell me "I just want to be able to walk around the house (versus around the supermarket). I just want to decrease my pain (versus eliminate their pain)." Some of them have already given up – stating: "I don't think I'll ever walk again. I don't think I'll ever get off the pain medication." *We have not because we ask not!*

When the blind man asked Jesus to help him, he could have asked for food or clothing or shelter. Instead, he had **strong faith** & **boldly** asked Jesus to heal his blindness! There are many stories where faith in Jesus to heal themselves, their friends, & family members of all diseases = caused their diseases to be healed. Where has our faith gone? God is not limited by anything! He created the universe. There is no limit to His power.

Remember, Jesus did NOT heal everyone! I believe this had (& has) to do with 3 major reasons:

- One, many people don't want to be healed. This may sound harsh – but there is a lot of truth to it that we must acknowledge. As mentioned in section 1 of this chapter, society rewards diseases (with money, more attention from friends, family, strangers, & health care providers). People also identify themselves with the diseases (as well as their chronic pain &/or obesity). You may "have" Parkinson's disease. But you ARE NOT "Parkinson's!" You may have an amputation. But you are not an "amputee!" This may sound like semantics –but it's deeper than that!
- Two, many people don't believe Jesus or His disciples can heal their disease(s).

- Three, many of His Disciples don't 100% believe they can heal diseases. They may say the right words, but if they don't believe it - . By the way, the words (I believe the Bible tells us to use) are: "Dear God the Father, in the name of Jesus Christ our Lord & savior - & the power of the Holy Spirit, we ask -- (Person's name) to be 100% healed of --- (fill in the disease(s)."

Remember, there are no "power shortages" in heaven. There is no "love shortage" either! Why do you spend 99% of your time worrying about your earthly problems - & only 1% focused on God? Is not God more powerful than your problems? He said: *"I am the alpha & the omega! ... I am THE way. I am the truth. I am the life. ... I created everything. Before Me: Nothing existed! I, therefore, can heal your diseases, optimize your health, & maximally cleanse your body, mind, & soul. I, therefore, can heal all your diseases & burdens."*

2. **How many Religions or Identities can we have? My bible-based answer = Two.** According to God's Living Word, there are only two:
- Those who already have accepted Jesus Christ as their own personal LORD (& Savior)
- & those who have not done so YET! (Gal 3:28) *"**All** will bow down before Him, even those who cannot keep their soul alive!"* (Psalm 22:29)

"The world" identifies humans in so many different ways/categories. However, God defines us by our heart. According to God's word [regarding who lives eternally with Jesus] there are **currently no**:
- Blacks, whites, browns, yellows, or reds. Thus, there should be no racists.
- *Jews or Gentiles.* For that matter there are no Buddhists, Atheists, Lutherans, Catholics, or 4,000 other Christian denominations! Thus, there should be no anti-Semites.
- Homosexuals or Heterosexuals.
- Republicans or Democrats.
- Socialists, liberals, communists, or conservatives.
- Wealthy or poor.
- Slaves or free men.
- Males or females.
- Short people or tall people.
- Blondes, brunettes, redheads, or even those who are bald.
- Ectomorphs, mesomorphs, or endomorphs.
- Single, married, or widowed.
- Smokers or non-smokers.
- Lawyers, physicians, teachers, politicians, bankers, bakers, or candlestick makers.
- NY Yankee fans or Boston Red Sox fans.
- Vegans or meat-eaters.

All children who (tragically) pass away - go to Heaven. It doesn't matter if they were baptized or not. It doesn't matter if the parents were believers in Christ or not! God said: *"ALL CHILDREN are MINE!"* (Ezekiel 16:20-21 & 18:20; Matt 19:14) This includes (in my opinion) those whose minds stay like a child's (AKA "mentally challenged"). You can NOT truly reject the Messiah unless you are of the mental age (possibly 13 for many as the "Bar- & Bas-Mitzvahs" are performed at age 13?).   No one (except God) knows what that "intellectual age of responsibility" is.

ALL *(except the Messiah) have sinned & fallen short of the GLORY of GOD.* (Romans 3:23) We are ALL sinners who need God's grace.   You can choose to accept God's love & grace - & accept/believe in His only begotten Son. You can, therefore, choose not to perish (Psalm 22:29 & Psalm 89:48; 1 Cor 15:25-27; Rev 20:14-15 & 21:8), but have eternal life. (John 3:16)   I pray everyone becomes "in Christ" (AKA "Children of God" or "Believer of Christ" as the Messiah & personal Lord & savior). This is the will of God!

3.   Who are Believers in Christ supposed to <u>LOVE</u>? Answer = God the most - & then **ALL** Humans.

"You shall LOVE the LORD your God with all your <u>heart</u>, & with all your <u>soul</u>, & with your <u>mind</u>. This is the great & <u>foremost commandment</u>." (Deut 6:5 & Matt 22:37-38)   *"The second (greatest commandment) is like it, 'YOU SHALL LOVE YOUR NEIGHBOR AS YOURSELF."* (Lev 19:18 & Matt 22:39)   Your neighbors include enemies who curse & trespass against you. Your neighbors include **EVERYONE** – including non-believers. If you are a believer in Christ **& do NOT love** your enemies, homosexuals, Islamists, Hindus, Buddhists, & Atheists: **"*YOU'RE FULL OF IT*!"**   I know many atheists who are more Christ-like than most Christians. I also know many "Homosexuals" that are Christians.

The English language does not perfectly translate from the original Biblical languages (ancient Hebrew, Aramaic, & Greek).   This is most true with the word "LOVE."   Surely, we can recognize the following "loves" are different:
-    The Love you should have for your "neighbors" (including fellow believers & non-believers; including friends & enemies).
-    The Love you should have for your Mom or Dad.
-    The Love you should have for your children (& your pets. I know there is no mention of this in the scriptures. However, God did create every living creature. If a pet can give us so much love. I believe we can love our pets & actually bring us closer to God. Just remember to LOVE God foremost! Also remember, to Love Humans!).
-    The Love you should have for your spouse or "significant other."
-    The Love you should have for God (*with ALL your heart, mind, & soul*)! As mentioned above, this is the most important commandment. If you deny Jesus to please your parents or children or in-laws, you are not worthy of Jesus! I believe this is why Jesus said (in Matt 10:35 & 10:37) "*He who loves [their parents or children] more than ME is NOT worthy of ME*." This is why you should Love Jesus more than anyone. You should *honor your mother & father*. However: if a friend, spouse, parent, or other family member tell you to reject Jesus or love them more than Jesus: they are asking you to break God's *greatest & foremost commandment*.
-    The Love that God has for YOU!

This last love is the *greatest LOVE of ALL!* (Rom 3:5, 4:25, 5:6, 8:32, 8:39; John 3:16, 15:13; Gal 2:20; Eph 5:2)   It is a LOVE you will never understand without accepting Jesus as your Lord & savior! *"God is LOVE."* (John 3:16)   **Without LOVE**, you have nothing! (1Cor:13)   God loves you greater than anyone else in the world (even greater than the love your parents, grandparents, spouse, etc. –have for you). Because GOD **IS** LOVE, God LOVES us 100% of the time!   As Dr. David Jeremiah stated (in his book *God Loves You: He Always Has & He Always*

Will): *"You can't say that about anyone else in your life – your spouse, your parents, or your favorite uncle. For God to fail in His love for you – even for a second - would mean God would stop being God because: God IS love."*

As Dr. David Jeremiah stated (in his book *God loves you: He always has & He always will*): God loves you: Before you were born; Even when you don't love or appreciate or even recognize Him; While you sin; & while you treat your body (the temple of the Holy Spirit) like an undersized sewer!

Jesus said, *"Who is my brother, sister, mother?"* If you are a health care provider, treat your patients like your family (assuming you love your family). If you are a financial advisor or in any other business, treat them like your family (assuming you love your family).

IN THE "GAME" OF LIFE: I BELIEVE SUCCESS SHOULD BE MEASURED BY HOW MUCH LOVE YOU HAVE GIVEN & RECEIVED TO/FROM GOD &, THEN, OTHER PEOPLE. AT THE END OF ONE'S LIFE, WE SHOULD CONCLUDE THAT A PERSON WAS A "WINNER" IF THEY GAVE & RECEIVED AN ABUNDANT AMOUNT OF LOVE TO/FROM GOD &, THEN, OTHER PEOPLE. IF THIS IS HOW GOD POSSIBLY MEASURES OUR SUCCESS, WHY DON'T WE?

Remember: GOD Loves YOU – even if you don't love Him!

4. Do the Old Testament Prophecies PROVE Jesus is the Messiah? Answer = YES!

For all those like "Doubting Thomas" who want to "see" it – to believe it, believers should simply ask them to look at the scientific, archeological, & mathematical evidence that Jesus is the Messiah beyond any reasonable doubt. Those who are waiting for the Messiah - are waiting for the Messiah to fulfill the following Major Prophesies:

- 1. To be born in Bethlehem (Micah 5:1); 2. From a virgin from the tribe of Judah – more specifically, from the House of David (Isaiah 7:14 & 9:6-7); 3. To be a prophet like Moses (Deut 18:15-18) & a priest Like Melchizedek (Psalm 110:4); 4. To HEAL, preach, & save (Isaiah 61:1-2); 5. To enter Jerusalem on a donkey (Zech 9:9); 6. Usher in a NEW COVENANT for Israel (Jer 31:31-34); 7. To be betrayed for 30 pieces of silver (Zech 11:12); 8. To suffer & be crushed for our iniquities (Psalm 22 & Isaiah 52-53); 9. Having His hands & feet pierced for our transgressions (Psalm 22 & Isaiah 52-53); 10. Having stripes of blood on Him so that we may be healed (Isaiah 53); 11. Yet- not one of His bones will be broken (Psalm 22); 12, 13, & 14. To be mocked & taunted; Yet to be silent before His accusers; to be tortured surrounded by 2 evil doers (Psalm 22 & Isaiah 52-53); 15 & 16. To have His garments cast lots for them & be buried in a rich man's tomb (Psalm 22 & Isaiah 53); 17. To rise from the dead (Psalm 16:10); & 18. To have EVERYONE bow down & worship Him, even those who can't keep their soul alive (Psalm 22)! Very sophisticated mathematicians have concluded that if Jesus fulfilled 9 out of these 18 major prophecies, the odds that HE IS NOT the promised messiah are one thousand trillion to one! Actually, there is a lot of archeological & scientific evidence proving that He fulfills all 18! That makes the odds ten to the power of 24 (one trillion times one trillion times one trillion) to one!

HELLO!! I THINK WE FOUND HIM!

This explosion of knowledge/studies in the fields of archeology, mathematics, & scripture has helped many in the scientific community to become "believers." Many world famous scientists were believers. Isaac Newton would be known as one of the greatest theologians of his time, if it wasn't for his work in Calculus & Physics. **However, no amount of scientific evidence can convince anyone to believe.** *"We have been saved by grace - through faith. It is a gift from God."* (Eph 2:8-9) Jesus did NOT say that He was *ONE of the ways* to Heaven. Jesus said, "I am THE WAY, & the TRUTH, & the LIFE. NO ONE comes to the Father but through Me!" (John 14:6)

To elaborate further: Every story in the Old Testament (AKA "Old Covenant"), correlates to THE STORY in the New Testament. Don't forget, God's living word states (with an old covenant prophecy) that many will have a "*veil over their eyes*. *They will hear & see the truth - & still not believe*"(Isaiah 6:10) Many of these people with "*a veil over their eyes*" may be very intelligent –as well as wealthy &/or successful on this earth! However, if you don't believe in Jesus Christ as the Messiah - you are "***FULL OF IT***!" ☺ I pray you come to know & accept Jesus Christ as the messiah –as your personal Lord & savior – as there is no greater Love in the world!

5. **Should believers in Christ celebrate "Passover?" The answer = Yes.** My "Non-Messianic" Jewish relatives celebrate Passover to thank God for having the angel of death "pass over" our ancestors (as they put the blood of a sacrificial lamb on their doors) during the time of Moses. Believers in Christ should celebrate Passover to thank God for having the angel of death "**pass over**" us eternally thanks to God for sacrificing the blood of the "Holy Lamb of God (Jesus)."

6. **Was Paul a sexist? Answer = Probably Not!** Many females are non-believers because of this misconception. Hopefully my explanation helps bring them closer to God (& God's Love).

Two thousand years ago, most women did not read. Two thousand years ago, men & women usually sat on opposite sides of the church/temple. Therefore, *I believe* the correct interpretations of 1 Tim 2:12 & 1 Corinthians 14:35 are the following:

- Anyone (man or woman) who is illiterate in a language should not teach anyone in that language.
- No one (man or woman) should yell across the church while the pastor (or priest) is giving the sermon.

Two of the greatest disciples of Christ was Mary Magdalene (as I discussed in chapter 1) & of course His mother Mary. Where were "the 12 male disciples:" At the cross (one of them – John the apostle was there –where were the other 11? To 1st see the empty tomb? To 1st bear witness to His resurrection? It was Mary Magdalene who Jesus gave the honor of reporting

His resurrection to the apostles!   Was there a more devout disciple of Christ?

Where were all these "devout" MEN?   Jesus fed thousands with almost no food.   Jesus performed miracles & healed diseases of many people in many towns.   Jesus raised Lazarus & a little girl from the dead.   Where were thousands of "devout" men who witnessed these miracles?   When the going got tough: the men ran away & the women stayed!   These facts are documented many places in the new covenant – including Paul's writings.

7.   Does the Bible state that earth can <u>only</u> be 5,773 years old?   Answer = No!

The 1st event to occur on earth was not documented in Genesis. It was in John 1:1-3 & 9. *"In the beginning was the Word, & the Word was with God, & the Word was God. He was in the beginning with God. All things came into being through Him. The world was made through Him!"*

Jesus told us *"My ways are not your ways."* I believe 2 Peter 3:8 may explain how this earth is over 5,773 years old. *"With the Lord one day is like a thousand years, and a thousand years like one day."* Isn't it possible to translate this mathematically? Aren't there 365.25 days in a year? Thus, can we say 1 year to God is like 365,250 years to man?   Thus, isn't it possible that 2nd Peter may justify an earth over 2 billion years old?   In addition, there are many theologians who believe in the "***gap theory***" of time in the Bible. The "gap-theory" states there is a gap in time between Genesis 1:1 & 1:2 (& this gap in time is where dinosaurs & the ice age may *possibly* be explained).   Either way, only God knows.

This is a great example of where God can use Christians to bring "scientific atheists" closer to Him.   Many scientific atheists are turned away from Him because many Christians will argue with them that there is no other answer to this question. The truth is there is scriptural & scientific evidence that: What we biblically consider "man" has been on this earth about 5,773 years; & the earth MAY be over 2 billion years old.

For centuries people have tried to (ignorantly –in my humble opinion) separate science from the word of God.   However, the word of God usually confirms most scientific truths -& most scientific laws confirm the word of God to be true in every aspect.   In addition, the world's most famous scientists in history were devout believers of the word of God.

You can tell these scientific atheists that there is only one absolute 100% way to find the TRUTH to this (& every answer).   If they accept Jesus Christ as their personal Lord & savior –they will be saved.   Then they can go to Heaven & ask Jesus Himself all the questions that science could not 100% prove to be true or not!! ☺

8.   Do we understand the "culture" of Jesus?   Answer = probably not.

55

Two thousand years ago (as well as today), society looked at Jesus like He was the Jewish carpenter's son from Bethlehem or Nazareth. Jesus tried to tell people where he was from. People did not understand. Do they understand today? I learned a lot of this from a sermon I heard by Dr. Myles Monroe years ago & it touched my life (& I hope it touches yours).

People would tell Jesus about their diseases. Jesus would try to show His culture to them. He would heal all their diseases. I'm paraphrasing: "Where I'm from there are no diseases! When you go to Heaven, you will have no diseases. You will have no blindness, no deafness, & no lameness." In Heaven, you will not have any pain, obesity, diseases or be "**_FULL OF IT_**!"

Jesus would try to show people His culture of LOVE. People didn't get him! They would say, "I love my family –but hate my enemies." Jesus tried to show them ("I'm paraphrasing): "In Heaven (& in the thousand year reign with Jesus on this earth - & ever after), there is:

- No hatred or un-forgiveness of others. In Heaven, there is only Love of everyone.
- No disease (including Chronic Pain, Obesity, or being "**_FULL OF_**" body, mind, or soul toxins!).

When they asked Jesus how to pray, He told them (in Matt 6:9-13): *"Our Father who is **in HEAVEN**, hallowed by your name. Your kingdom come. Your will be done: **On earth** as it is **in HEAVEN**…"*

Pilate <u>somewhat</u> understood where Jesus was from (John 18:33 – 19:11). Pilate asked Him, *"Are you the King of the Jews?"* Jesus answered, "*MY **KINGDOM IS NOT OF THIS WORLD**! MY KINGDOM IS NOT OF THIS REALM.*" Pilate then said to Him, *"So you are a king?"* Jesus answered, "*You say correctly that I am a King. For this I have been born, & for this I have come into **the world**, to testify to **the truth**. Everyone who is of **the truth** hears my voice."* Pilate said to Him, *"What is truth?"* Jesus was trying to explain to Pilate that **He is the truth**.

Pilate did not understand who Jesus was or where He was from. Pilate said to Him, *"Do you not know that I have the authority to release you, & I have the authority to crucify you?"* Jesus answered, "*You would have NO authority over me, unless it had been given to you from **ABOVE**.*"

People were amazed how Jesus knew "The Living Word of God" so well. They looked at Him like a 12 year old Jewish son of a carpenter from Nazareth. He tried to explain & show them that **He is** THE LIVING WORD OF GOD! No wonder He <u>knew</u> the Living Word of God! In the beginning, was *"THE WORD = Jesus!"* Jesus is *the truth.* Jesus is *"THE WAY!"*

9. Who killed Jesus? My biblically based answer = No one!

Jesus laid His life down for <u>all</u> humans (to fulfill the will of God the Father – fulfilling the "old covenant" prophecies) as the <u>**sacrificial**</u> Holy Lamb of God to take away the SIN of the world! One may argue that even *Caiaphas* (*the* *high priest of the temple the year* of Jesus' sacrificial crucifixion) knew/prophesied that Jesus was to *"die for the people* [**sacrifice Himself**] *- so that the whole nation not perish, but in order that He might also gather together into one the children of God who are scattered abroad."* (John 11:49-53)   Remember: Jesus was never killed. True: He **sacrificed Himself** to allow a horrific death of His flesh to fulfill prophesies of the "old covenant."   However, He has risen & lives eternally. God [the son] can never die!   Anyone who blames the Jews or the Romans for "**killing Jesus" is ignorant** of the abovementioned truths.

10. Is there proof of the Holy Trinity in the Old Testament?   Answer = Yes!

As mentioned previously, there are so many Old Testament messianic prophecies (that Jesus = God the Son = The Messiah fulfilled).   Here are some less known examples of the proof of the Holy Trinity in the Old Testament.

Gen 1:1 = *"In the Beginning, Eloh**im** created -."* Eloh**im** in ancient Hebrew represented "Gods" (most theologians equate this use of the word "Elohim" as God the Father - & God the Son). This strongly correlates with John 1:1-3 & 9.

Gen 1:2 = *"The* **Spirit of God** *was moving over the surface of the waters."* Is not God's Spirit Holy?

Gen 1:26 = *"Then God said, 'Let **US** make man in **OUR** image, according to **OUR** likeness."*   To whom was God, the Father speaking to (when He said "Us" or "Our")?

Gen 3:22 = *"Behold, the man has become **like ONE of US**, knowing good & evil."*

Gen 11:7 = *"The Lord (God the Father) said: Let **US** go down & there confuse their language."*

Ezekiel 36:27 = *"And I will put My **Spirit** with you."*

11. Does God cause or give us diseases?   My Answer = No!

Many people (including many rabbis, priests, & other teachers of God's word) ignorantly believe & teach that God causes people to get diseases! This is (I believe) diametrically opposed to the truth.   God does *allow* people to get diseases. God does *allow* people to bombard themselves with (&, therefore, become "***FULL OF***") direct body (as well as spiritual & intellectual) toxins.   God does *allow* people to not cleanse themselves of body, mind, & soul toxins. God does *allow* people to break all of the "10 Dietary Commandments" (illustrated in Chapter 5) on a daily basis –often three times daily!   God does *allow* the mother of a newborn to be "***FULL OF***" direct body toxins exposing the fragile fetus & newborn to become "***FULL OF***" these direct body toxins (predisposing the fetus & newborn to diseases)!

This allowance is because God loves us & gave us free will.   Robots (like the ones I invented in 1990) have no free will.   Therefore, robots can NOT love.   When you truly love God it is because He chose you & you chose Him.   God gives us gifts & we must always be thankful to Him for these gifts. Some people never "open" these gifts!

More proof that God does not give us diseases - include the following biblical facts:

- There is no disease (including obesity) or pain (physical or psychological) in Heaven.
- & there is no disease in His "Thousand Year Reign" on this earth (in the future). We will have a *"glorified body"* of perfect health (of our bodies, minds, & souls).

Remember, God is our heavenly Father who loves us. Remember: *God is Love*. If God did not love you for even a fraction of a second, then God would not be God! This is because God = love!

Blame diseases on Satan & your flesh. **Blame diseases** on your own fleshly will to:

- Be bombarded with & become "*FULL OF*" intellectual & spiritual toxins (SINS) that can lead to diseases – as well as obesity &/or chronic pain (Chapters 1 & 2);
- Be bombarded with & become "*FULL OF*" direct body toxins from the food we eat, the air we breathe, the water we bathe & swim in, etc. (Chapter 3);
- Be bombarded with & become "*FULL OF*" dietary toxins (Chapter 5);
- Break all of the "10 Dietary Commandments" (Chapter 5);
- & avoid cleansing our bodies from (staying "*FULL OF*") toxins via dietary & non- dietary methods (Chapters 5 & 6).

12. Should we still follow any dietary rules/laws – like the "10 Dietary Commandments" shown in Chapter 5? Answer = Yes.

Many people (including believers in Christ) ignorantly believe that –since we are under the "new covenant" (prophesied in Jeremiah 31:31-34), God doesn't care if we eat foods "***FULL OF***" direct body toxins (such as pesticides, antibiotics, & man-made genetically modified organisms, etc. in our food) – like ungrateful lazy gluttons (see Chapter 1)! These may be the same people who ignorantly believe that God doesn't care if we bombard our bodies with (& become "***FULL OF***") non-dietary direct body toxins (such as the thousands of industrial chemicals & toxic heavy metals in our homes, work places, etc.) shown in Chapter 3!

Many people ignorantly believe that God doesn't care if we consume &/or optimally absorb the most healthful, super-cleansing foods & supplements (capable of cleansing our bodies from direct body toxins – mentioned in Chapters 5 & 6)! Many people ignorantly believe that God doesn't care if we treat our bodies (*the temple of the Holy Spirit*) like sewers!

Many people ignorantly believe that God doesn't care if our bodies (including our intestines, liver, cardiovascular system, skin, etc.) are "***FULL OF***" toxicity! Many people ignorantly believe that God doesn't care if our brains are "***FULL OF***" direct body toxins (like aluminum, lead, mercury, pesticides, pharmaceuticals, etc.) causing chemical imbalances between serotonin & dopamine (which may lead to Parkinson's, Autism, ADHD, OCD, etc.)!

Do not get offended by the word "ignorant." I believe the original use of the word was not meant to be a derogatory term (like it used today in our culture). Don't forget: if you "do not know" of the abovementioned _facts_, then you are "**_FULL OF_**" extremely important misconceptions. Remember: **God cares** about your physical health **& loves you** more than any person or thing could ever love you. As mentioned previously, God wants you to achieve optimal health of your body (as well as your mind & soul)! God does not want you to be "**_FULL OF IT_**!" I strongly believe, it is God's will for us to read & follow this book's guidelines to help us cleanse (& optimize the health of) our bodies, minds, & souls!

IV.   "_YOU'RE FULL OF_" Anti-Godly Tax & Government Policies

Our anti-Godly tax & governmental policies are severely under-recognized mind & soul toxins. They destroy the health of the minds & souls (& eventually the bodies) of the:
- Hard-working honest Americans who are punished by them
- & the lazy liars (as well as the gamblers) who actually benefit from them!

"_A Nation of sheep will beget a Government of Wolves_" – Edward R. Murrow
The U.S. government (the IRS & other government agencies) have been "**_FULL OF IT_**" (for over 40 years) regarding the following bogus terms:
- "Inflation" (which has excluded food & energy for the past 40 years!); "Federal Income Taxes;" "Percent Unemployment" (which excludes workers who claim for disability); etc. Participation rate percentage is a more valid indicator of true unemployment/employment.

Similar to food, diets, nutrition, the word of God, & health (of our bodies, minds, & souls) – The U.S.A. government has <u>failed to disclose the truth</u> regarding our anti-Godly tax & government policies!

Since Americans have become _like sheep that have strayed_ farther away from God in our nation's history, we have created anti-Godly "Representatives," Tax & Governmental policies! Said differently: Our Anti-Godly tax policies, government policies, & political "representatives" that support them = are like **dirty diapers**. They need to be changed for the same reason!

One may question: Why include our nation's tax & governmental policies in a diet book? By now, you (hopefully) realize this is not just some simple diet book. This is because we are not simple beings. We are complex beings that must be cognizant of how governmental influences (such as tax incentives/rewards) can influence/hypnotize our minds, souls, & bodies!

One may also question: What do our nation's Anti-Godly tax policies have to do with our health?   Our Anti-Godly tax policies are an under – recognized toxin to our minds, souls, & bodies (including those who "benefit" from them financially!).   As mentioned throughout this book, there is an extremely strong connection between the health of your body - & the health of your mind & soul.   Our anti-Godly tax & Government policies create a huge financial "pain" to the majority of Americans – which may lead to "spiritual pain" in our minds & souls – as well as body pains!

When a country creates Anti-Godly tax policies, its' people become farther away from God.   I do NOT believe it is 100% the fault of the government that we are so far from God – as well as more diseased, obese, & in chronic pain than ever before.   However, the power of our nations' anti-Godly tax & government policies to leach into the health of our minds, souls, & bodies is severely under-recognized.

Remember a famous quote: "when America gets a cold, the world gets pneumonia!"   Thus, our nations' Anti-Godly tax policies have hurt (& may continue to harm) the health of possibly everyone in the world!

Consider the following analogy.   The U.S. economy is like your loved one who is **bleeding to death**.   One group of physicians (Republican "Representatives") recommends stopping the bleeding –but refuse to give a blood transfusion.   Another group of physicians (Democratic "Representatives") recommends giving the patient a blood transfusion – but outright refuse to stop the bleeding.   Most Americans (who love America/this "patient") believe they should do both.   And they should! Refusing to do both has led to (& will lead to) a blood "deficit" (i.e. "financial deficit") that continues to worsen.   It is not a coincidence that our economic growth has been "anemic."   Don't forget these so-called "representatives" (in the House of "Representatives" & the Senate) **work for us**!   Remember: United we stand!

Consider what "*shape*" our economy is in - due to our anti-Godly tax & government policies since 1997.   Our Democratic "Representatives" may want to "spread the wealth" from top down (creating a *pyramid* wealth distribution).   Our Republican "Representatives" may want to create a *spinning top (or upside-down pyramid)* economy.   Since 1997 (due to our anti-Godly tax & government policies), we have created an *HOUR GLASS economy* – squeezing the working middle class to help the wealthy investors (above) & lazy, lying dead-beats (below – as well as above the middle)!

There are thousands of versus in the Bible that pertain to money. God wants us to give generously & gladly.   God wants us to be good stewards of our money & spend wisely.   Some may foolishly repeat the question, "What does this have to do with the health of my body, mind, or soul!?"   Our anti-Godly tax & governmental policies have created a financial burden on most of our society.   This **financial burden** becomes a **mind & soul (&, eventually a body) TOXIN/burden.**   As this financial burden "**weighs us down**" (as we get more "stressed" over it) it predisposes us to **chronic pain, diseases &/or becoming "over-weight!"**

This is because **chronic stressors** (like the **chronic financial burden of our anti-Godly tax policies**) can cause our body's cortisol (a steroidal hormone released by our adrenal cortex in response to *stress*) levels to be elevated for a **prolonged period of time.**[6]   When elevated for a **prolonged period** of time, **cortisol** can predispose you to becoming "***FULL OF***":[6]

- Diabetes; **Weight gain & Obesity**; Immune system suppression; **Poor Digestion & ABSORPTION of food**; Atherosclerosis (due to constriction of blood vessels); Insomnia, chronic fatigue syndrome, thyroid disorders, dementia, & depression; Fertility dysfunctions; & even impotence!   The erectile dysfunction caused by this chronic stressor may be due to the fact that the sympathetic ("fight or flight") part of the nervous system is overly stimulated.   For a man to achieve a full erection, he must allow the parasympathetic (relaxation) part of the nervous system to "take over."   If he is too nervous/ "stressed out," he may not be able to achieve the full erection.   This "physiological stress reaction" is analyzed in greater detail in chapter 3.

The following relationship is severely under-recognized in our society:

- AS our nation has become more deficient in God (more "***FULL OF***" SIN) than ever before, we have become more deficient in the health of our bodies, minds, & souls – as well as our finances.   Said differently, as our "God deficit" has increased: so has our health, moral, intellectual, & financial deficit!   It is NO coincidence that our current nation's largest God deficit has led to our country's largest health, moral, intellectual, & financial deficit!

Has money become our nation's *MASTER!*?

One can argue that what infuriated the temple leaders most about Jesus Christ was **His interference with**:

- The unethical (anti-Godly) ways the temple [& the **temples leaders**] **made money** (Matt 21:12-13)
- & the political/**economic power of the temple leaders**. (John 11:47-53)

One can argue that this "love of money over God" was the #1 reason why the temple leaders insisted the Romans crucify Jesus!   Are our current leaders any better than the temple leaders – or the Romans – 2,000 years ago?   Are many Americans any better?

To confirm any of the below mentioned specific tax information, contact your certified accountant &/or simply go to the IRS website (www.irs.gov).   If you care about the financial health (strongly connected to the health of the body, mind, & soul) of America &/or yourself, you should know the following truths/facts (*for the truth shall set you free*):

- 1: Our tax & other government policies are anti-Godly.
- 2: Our tax & Government policies are more satanic (Anti-Godly) than ever before in our nation's history.

- 3: The above is true **because** Americans (& their so-called "Representatives") are "_FULL OF_ Intellectual & Spiritual Constipation!
- 4: These Anti-Godly tax & Government policies have contributed to the destruction of our:
  - ○ Economy (both our nation's & our personal finances);
  - ○ Personal relationships with our friends/family;
  - ○ & Health of our bodies, minds, & souls!
- & 5: my answer to correct them (based on scriptural & economical science).

1. **Our tax & other government policies are anti-Godly.**

Our anti-Godly tax & governmental policies "punish working" by "rewarding" the following anti-Godly sins: Laziness; Lying***; & Gambling

Many able-bodied Americans receiving state government assistance (via welfare: food stamps, free housing, Medicaid, etc.) & federal government assistance (via early tax-free SS disability, early Medicare benefits, reimbursements for health insurance premiums under the new "ACA," etc.) _may_ be considered "lazy malingers/liars" as these rewards are often greater than working!   ***This "lying" applies to able-bodied lazy malingerers who lie to receive disability &/or welfare benefits – as well the lies the IRS tries to deceive workers with by hiding the truth (that our tax & governmental policies truly "punish workers").   Remember: _the truth shall set you free._   By rewarding the abovementioned sins, our anti-Godly tax & government policies have helped make Americans:

- ○ More immoral & deficient in God
- ○ More diseased, disabled, obese, in chronic pain
- ○ & _Wicked slaves to our national debt_ (Proverbs 22:7)

Have we been hypnotized by our government to believe that these anti-Godly tax policies are acceptable?

Our tax & governmental policies **punish workers** –especially workers earning less than $114K/year (approximately in 2014 –each year this amount goes up slightly) by rewarding two types of economic vampires:

- **The lazy able-bodied malingerer** under age 65 (often in their 20s, 30s, 40s, & 50s) who _chooses_ not to work & receive:
  - ○ 2 years (or the remainder of their life if they _claim_ they were injured during a government job) of 60-80% of their tax free income; SS disability; Medicare benefits; Welfare benefits, etc.;
  - ○ &/or reimbursement for health insurance premiums under the new "Affordable Care Act" ("ACA" – which ironically is anything but "affordable");
- & **the wealthy investor for "gaining" 100%** of their money "received" that year via their long-term capital gains on their investments.   Our tax policies reward (over earning money) Americans for investing (some may refer to this as a form of "**gambling**") in the stock market – or other investment vehicles.   Our tax policies reward investors (over earners since 1997) for gains or losses in the stock market!   Said

differently, our tax policies reward investors (over earners since 1997) so that:

- o When you win = you win; & when you lose = you still win!

I realize we should not blame the investor who takes advantage of this anti-Godly tax policy. However, if you do not believe this is anti-Godly, then *"YOU'RE FULL OF IT"* (see below).

These economic "vampires" are rewarded in our anti-Godly tax & governmental policies leading to our nation becoming *enslaved to its' debt.* (Proverbs 22:7) These economic "vampires" have led to (**since 1997**), **America becoming "FULL OF:"**

- **Lazy liars & gamblers**
- **Welfare - since we reward welfare & punish work-fare**, we have become "*FULL OF*" more Americans on "poverty" - receiving more food stamps & other state government-funded welfare programs than ever before.
- **Disability – since we reward disability & punish work-fare,** we have become "*FULL OF*" more Americans receiving Disability benefits than ever before! This number has skyrocketed (not ironically) in 1997 when the government stepped in to start punishing workers more than ever before (see later on).
- **National Debt** – has grown to record highs (in 2014). This is because our tax & governmental policies punish workers - & rewarding the abovementioned "economic vampires." 1997 was the beginning of our down-fall as a country (see below).

What are the most damaging/anti-Godly (& anti-economical & anti-American) tax/governmental policy changes/events to ever occur in the past 50 years?

My answer = The "**ACA**" implemented in **2014** & **long-term capital gains** (on investments such as stocks, non-owner occupied real estate, etc.) **being cut from 28% to 20% in 1997 & 20% to 15% in 2002**![7] Investors have been rewarded tremendously from 1997 to current (2014) &, therefore, "workers" have been punished for all these years! If you look back from 1997 (the inception of the abovementioned anti-Godly tax policy) to current, our country has (with no coincidence) become more anti-Godly (more lazy, more immoral, more selfish, more diseased/"disabled," more obese, etc.)! Is this simply a *coincidence*?

The Jewish law states we should ALL tithe 10%. (Lev 27:30, Num 18:26, Deut 12:17) It does NOT say that people who gain millions of dollars/year with their investments (without working = "unearned income") should be exempt –or pay a much lower percentage! There was the story of the poor widow ("the widow's mite") who put two small copper coins (a cent) into the treasury. (Luke 21:1-4) Jesus said, *"This poor widow put in **MORE** than all of them (the rich). The rich put into the offering out of their surplus; but she out of poverty put in ALL that she had* *to live on."* God understands **percentages!** Is our country's situation much different than what happened at "that treasury" approximately 2000 years ago?

The **ACA** is, unfortunately, more socialistic & **anti-Godly** than any European or Canadian models of health care. It **punishes honest Americans (under the age of 65) who work** & **rewards lazy able-bodied Americans who choose not to work &/or lie** (do not report to the IRS) about the income they actually receive! The ACA also **punishes Americans for being responsible with their health** versus those who are irresponsible with their health & choose to abuse &/or neglect their health!

- The healthy & fit 55 year old man may pay twice the dollar amount in health insurance premiums as they did 1 year ago. However, he will pay the same amount (in the same county) as the 55 year old drug addicted, alcoholic, glutton (weighing over 300 pounds) man! If the 300+ pound man chooses not to work (or lie to the IRS re: his income): the federal government will actually reward him financially by reimbursing him most of his insurance premiums (via a "subsidy")!

Therefore, the ACA (unfortunately) sends clear messages to Americans under 65 (as implemented in 2014):

- You are being **punished** for working hard & taking responsibility for your health (following all "10 Dietary Commandments" & "10 non-Dietary Cleansing Methods");
- & you are being rewarded for being lazy, lying, & irresponsible (with your health & employment).

Our tax policies (since 1997) punish Americans who work (earned income) & **reward those who** "gain" their money via investments ("Unearned income"). We tax the **money we "EARN" at a higher rate** than the **money we don't "EARN" (gain via investments)**! President Reagan - & our "reps" in approximately 1986 worked together to "fix this" (by lowering long-term capital gains tax rates from 50% to 28% so that earned & unearned income would be taxed at somewhat "similar rates").[7] However, future Administrations (Clinton -1997 & Bush Jr. in 2002)[7] have created a huge "reward" (tax break) for "un-earned income" &, therefore, a punishment for earned income! This is true when you compare those who "earn" $1 million/year to those who "gain" ("un-earned income") $1 million/year. This is also true when you compare those who "earn" $75K/year versus those who "gain" ("un-earned income") $75K/year. This is why the media is "***FULL OF IT***!" It's not a war between the rich & the poor/middle class. It is a war between those who "earn" money versus those who "gain" money ("unearned income") – as well as "lazy malingerers" who receive benefits/money for faking disability.

Our tax policies (as mentioned above) **reward gambling** (risk taking) &, therefore, **punish working**. If you gain money via investments in real estate, stocks, etc.: you pay a much lower tax rate to the Federal government than if you earn money (since 1997). *"Lowering the tax on capital gains was **MEANT** to **encourage people to take the RISK** of investing money in companies, new* *ventures, & stocks, so as to promote economic growth & job creation."*[7] True, this **artificially** helped inflate the stock market – on both occasions (for a few years at least). However, at what cost?   In fact if you lose money in the stock market, you get a tax benefit/reward (most years, you can claim a net capital loss on investments up to approximately $3K/year)!

Long-term Capital gains taxes were reduced in 1997 from 28% to 20% & in 2002 from 20% to 15%.[7] This 15% long term capital gains tax stayed until 2013 (where it was still 15% for the 1st $450K gain - &, then, still *only* 20% after that).   This reduction in capital gains tax from 1996 to current (2014) can be seen as an annual 8%-13% "reward" for investors' overall long-term capital gains tax <u>rates</u> &/or a 29%-46% savings ("reward") in the investor's long-term capital gains taxes owed!   If you had the same $1 Million long term gain from 1997 to 2012, you would have paid 29% less (from 1997 to 2002) & then 46% less (from 2003 to 2012) in long term capital gains tax!   When you compound these tax savings (rewards) to investors from 1997 to current (2014), you have created **the largest income inequality in the U.S.** (currently worse than China's)![7]   Our country's anti-Godly tax policies have become the laughing stock of the world!   There was a time when the U.S. was responsible for the majority of the world's wealth!

Our policies also **reward disease, chronic pain, disability, & the lazy, able-bodied malingerers receiving federal government benefits (like early SS disability, early MCR benefits, subsidies, etc.) & state government benefits (like food stamps, welfare checks, etc.)**!   If you believe America does NOT reward welfare & disability/disease (like obesity), then *"YOU ARE FULL OF IT*!"   If you believe everyone receiving welfare &/or disability benefits (higher amount of SS at an earlier age; Medicare eligibility currently after 2 years on "disability;" tax-free income; & other tax benefits/deductions, etc.) are truly disabled &/or can't "find work," then *"YOU ARE FULL OF IT*!"

Our policies punish work-fare & **reward welfare.**   As per FOX news (on 8/24/13), many states **"reward"/give welfare benefits** greater than $25K/year (in 2013).   **Welfare benefits** (usually determined via means testing) may include the following state government benefits:
- "TANF" (Temporary Assistance for Needy Families).
- Food stamps (often $3K/year in many states).   There are adults living in their parents mansions (in Palm Beach County) receiving food stamps!
- "AFDC" (Aid to Families with Dependent Children).
- Free housing!   There are welfare recipients in Palm Beach County living in "free" (state government) housing with inter-coastal & ocean views. I can't afford to live in a home with ocean views – but our welfare recipients can – for free!?
- Medicaid. State Medicaid can act as a secondary insurance to Medicare. This can save the Medicaid recipients over $10K easily in health insurance premiums, deductibles, out of pocket health care costs, etc.   For example, many state Medicaid programs will pay a nursing home approximately $4,500/month (over $50,000/year) to take care of all the

needs of the long-term resident (they are referred to as "residents" – not patients – as the nursing home is where they live/reside)!   Some homeless people in the 40s & 50s choose to live in these nursing homes & the state Medicaid pays the nursing home for them to live there (they have to *claim* some medical disability).

When you add up the abovementioned Welfare benefits, it is easy to determine how FOX news came up with this number (close to $30K in certain states).   Again: I do not write this to push any political agenda as I believe both parties are at fault for our anti-Godly tax policies (see later).   I am not blue or red –I am red, white, & blue! ☺

When you consider the "***cost***" **of working (taxes, driving to/from work, stress, etc.**), these welfare benefits may be equivalent to a worker earning $45K/year!

Our policies punish work-fare & **reward disability**.   **If these welfare recipients also get disability benefits, the combined rewards may be greater than a worker earning** <u>**over $70K/year**</u>!   Since we are "punishing" workers, many able-bodied Americans have **chosen not to work** to receive welfare &/or disability benefits!   I do not believe everyone receiving welfare &/or disability benefits is a lazy malingerer.   However: if you believe these welfare & disability "rewards" do not influence one's decision to seek employment, then "***YOU'RE FULL OF IT***!"   If you believe these welfare & disability rewards are not directly toxic to our minds & souls (& eventually/indirectly to our bodies), then: "***YOU'RE FULL OF IT***!"

- From 1980 to 1990, the number of "former workers on disability" remained relatively unchanged (approximately 3 million).[8]
- <u>Since 1997 (no coincidence</u>) the number of former workers on disability has skyrocketed to a record high of 8.9 million in April 2013.[8]   This number is growing by over 75,000/month (in mid-2013) of new Americans receiving disability benefits (almost as much as new Americans gaining employment in the private sector)![8]
- <u>The percentage of these disability claims for "*chronic musculoskeletal pains*" (more subjective & difficult to disprove) has skyrocketed (& become the #1 reason/claim for disability) in the past 50 years (when claims were mostly due to more objective/confirmed diseases – like heart disease, stroke, etc.)!</u>[8]
- In 1961, "Back Pain & other musculoskeletal problems" made up only 8.3% of all disability claims.[8]
- By 2011, "Back Pain & other musculoskeletal problems" made up 33.8% of all disability claims![8]   As mentioned above, chronic musculoskeletal pain has a subjective component to it - & may be exaggerated so that the claimant receives all the financial rewards of disability!   Even if these former workers truly had some pain, they may get hooked on the pain medications.   Then they often become even more disabled due to their drug addictions!   <u>This is simply more proof to one this book's major concepts: as we have become more deficient in God – we have become more immoral, sinful, lazier, diseased, obese, & in more chronic pain!</u>
- Applications for disability rise & fall with unemployment rates (100% correlation since the 1980s)![8]   If you believe that is simply a 30+ year "*coincidence*," then "***YOU'RE FULL OF***

IT!" The disability "financial rewards" are tremendously greater than the unemployment benefits. In fact, one may argue, they are far better than the employee's benefits! This again proves my point: **America is punishing workers & rewarding disease/disability & lazy malingerers**! The media tries to con you into believing former workers faking their injuries to receive disability benefits - which "lowers the unemployment percentage number is a good thing!" However, the media is "*FULL OF IT*" as workers leaving the workforce (legitimately or illegitimately) to receive disability benefits are NOT a good thing! If you get hypnotized by the media to believe the above is "good for our nation" in any way, then "*YOU'RE FULL OF IT*!" ☺

- The ratio of "working-aged" Americans receiving disability benefits (6.5 for every 100 who have a job) in 2013 has doubled in the past 20 years (no coincidence **after 1997**)![19] This has made the U.S.A. an "entitlement country" in which we are "taking away" more than we are "putting in!"
- One-Sixth of **Medicare**'s budget in 2013 goes to paying for "working-age" **disabled**![8]
- Every month, 14 million Americans get a disability check from the U.S. government![8]

Workers injured "on the job" often receive 60-80% of their salary TAX-FREE for 2 years (then they become eligible to receive Medicare benefits – well before turning 65). If these employees work for the government, they may receive this "**TAX-FREE" money for life** – as well as other benefits (for life)! Sounds like a "life sentence" for the taxpayers! As younger people are signing up for disability benefits, the "Social Security Disability Fund" is going broke by 2016.[8] Remember: who pays for all this?! The SS Administration is being forced to increase the percentage of SS funds towards the "SS Disability Funds" & away from the "SS Retirement Funds!" Peter robs from Paul! In other words: our left pocket borrows from our right pocket! If you believe this is good for our overall economy, then "*YOU'RE FULL OF IT*!"

Due to the "rewards" of receiving worker's compensation, these insurance companies have created "Functional Capacity Evaluations" (FCEs – often performed by Physical Therapists trained in this –like myself) to test if the employee/claimant is a malingerer (& to what extent)! In other words, the worker's compensation insurance companies want to find out how "*FULL OF IT*" the employees/claimants are!

I'm not saying that all Americans on disability or welfare are a bunch of lazy malingerers. Unfortunately, the true malingerers hurt the system for the truly disabled/injured severely on the job –as well as those on welfare truly seeking employment in the private sector. However, we can't deny the fact that these "**rewards**" may have a subconscious (& toxic) effect **to lure &/or keep someone on welfare &/or "disability**!"

Our tax policies **punish workers (since 1997) for earning** an annual income ("net profit" for self-employed) of **UNDER approximately $114K**! Our policies **reward workers for earning OVER $114K (in 2013)**.

Can ALL of our economic "bubbles" (overall stock market 1997 to 2000 & again from 2002 to 2007; Real estate market 1997 to 2006 January;

etc.) **be caused, at least in part, by our tax & governmental policies?**
Answer = Yes!   In 1997, the government rewarded Americans with a $250K tax-free gain (if single) or $500K tax-free gain (if married) for gains they made with real estate they lived in 24 out of the last 60 months of the date of sale. The long-term capital gains tax breaks stock investors received have also been shared by real estate investors since 1997.   All of the abovementioned tax policy "rewards" led to "bubbles" in those sectors – as well as "bubbles" in more people receiving: disability, early SS, early Medicare, welfare; tax breaks for investors gaining "un-earned" riskier investment gains)!   Therefore, our anti-Godly tax & Governmental policies have contributed to **the following anti-Godly "bubbles" that exist currently (in 2014):**

- National debt <u>bubble</u>
- Americans under age 65 receiving disability benefits (Medicare at a "working age;" SS Disability; etc.)
- Americans receiving welfare/Medicaid benefits (food stamps, etc.)
- Discrepancy in wealth between American upper-class investors versus the rest of us!

If you do not believe the **above four bubbles** exist or are toxic to our minds, souls, & bodies: then "***YOU'RE FULL OF IT***!"   Alan Greenspan once coined the phrase: "Irrational Exuberance" regarding stock investors (due, in part at least to the Anti-Godly tax rewards for investors &, therefore, "punishment" of workers)!   Many Americans actually quit jobs in the late 1990s to become "day-traders."   Many people actually quit jobs from 1996 to 2006 to become real estate investors.   Americans currently have "**IRRATIONAL APATHY/Acceptance**" to these bubbles.   Americans, & their so-called "representatives," really don't seem to care much about these anti-Godly tax bubbles!   It is irrational for Americans to be so apathetic of the over $50,000/American of national debt (in 2014) we all "owe."   Consider the following analogy of an American who:

- Earns $35K/year but spends $50K/year
- Owns a house worth $300K but owes $500K on it
- & does not have any money in savings or retirement & no family members with money who can help that American financially!

It would be **extremely irrational to be apathetic** to those facts!

American's irrational apathy regarding our "*flood*" of national (&/or personal debt) – as well as all other body, mind, & soul toxins we are "*FULL OF*" – is analogous to those who drowned in the flood during the days of Noah!   God warned those people for 40 years.   How many more years do we need?   Indirectly, these "bubbles" **punish hard-working, anti-gambling, honest workers**!   To better explain how our tax & governmental policies punish workers, consider the following analogy:

68

If an uncle (call him "Uncle Sam") has 10 nieces & 10 nephews (no sons or daughters) decides to give ("reward") 50% of his $1 Million inheritance to 1 nephew & the other 50% (divided equally) to 5 nieces – this punishes the other 14! Doesn't it?

What makes this analogy horrific is that this "rewarded" nephew who doesn't work is already wealthy (gaining his money purely via investments)! In addition, the 5 rewarded nieces are lazy, obese (due to laziness & gluttony), drug-addicted, binge-drinking malingers - who "choose" not to work (receiving financial rewards such as: Medicaid, food stamps, health insurance subsidies, disability benefits such as: early SS, & early Medicare)! The other 14 nieces/nephews are responsible with their health & earn their money by working &, therefore, "Uncle Sam" punishes them!? What message is this from our Government?

And we wonder why our nation has turned away from God?!

Other ways our tax policies are Anti-Godly include the lies (which are sins as you know) the IRS (Internal Revenue Service) deceives us with. *The truth shall set you free.* Therefore, we should all know *the truth* – as well as these IRS lies/deceptions!

The 1st lie to us = the term "Effective Tax Rate"

Does the IRS believe the taxpayers are stupid or gullible? The IRS is "*FULL OF IT*" as they have successfully fooled most taxpayers with a term called **"Effective Tax Rate."** This is a bogus term meant to deceive the U.S. taxpayer (especially those earning under approximately $114K per year in 2014) into thinking they are paying less in total "Federal" taxes to the IRS! This is only the percentage of what the IRS calls "**federal income taxes**" (paid to the IRS) compared to your AGI (Adjusted Gross Income). "*Federal Income Taxes*" is also another bogus term meant to deceive the U.S. taxpayer (especially those earning under $114K per year in 2014) into thinking they are paying less in total "Federal" taxes to the IRS! Neither of these numbers (In my strong opinion) affects the spending (or saving) habits of over 90% of American workers! We have been lied to about this year after year. What does God say about nations that lie continuously?

The "Payroll Tax" (AKA Self-employment tax or "FICA" tax for) is a **TAX** based on your net profit (or "earned **INCOME**") that goes to **FEDERAL** government agencies (supposedly MCR & SS)! However, the IRS does **not** consider this "*Federal Income Tax*!!!?" Again: What does God say about nations that lie continuously?

What affects MOST Americans spending habits is their "**TAXABLE INCOME!**" Some may find this boring, but it needs to be explained as it is destroying the health of our minds, souls, & bodies. Gross income does not affect your personal spending habits as much as net income (or "net profit" for the self-employed). Net Profit does not affect your personal spending as much as your AGI (Net profit minus SEP IRAs - & other tax deferred retirement accounts). AGI does not affect your personal spending as much as TAXABLE INCOME! Taxable Income is approximately the money you have left AFTER all your personal & work-related tax deductions! If you believe AGI or net income affects your personal spending habits more than taxable income, then "*YOU'RE FULL OF IT*!"

However, **the following definitions need to be updated (& added, respectively) so that everyone gets a more TRUTHFUL understanding of their tax burden: "Total Income;" "TAXABLE INCOME;" "TOTAL Federal Income TAXES PAID to the IRS;" &, therefore, "True Effective Tax Rate."**

69

The below & abovementioned updates/changes may help the IRS to not be so **"FULL OF IT!"**

   "Total Income" should be defined as total "earned" + "unearned" income. This would include things like net profits & salaries – as well as dividends, & capital gains (long-term & short-term) on investments & assets, etc.

   "Taxable Income" should be defined as this abovementioned "Total Income" minus all personal & business tax deductions.

   "Total Federal Income Taxes Paid" should be defined as ALL the income taxes paid to the IRS that goes to the <u>Federal</u> Reserve &/or any other <u>Federal</u> government agency or department. Local & State income & sales taxes are not included here. This is because every state has a different "state income &/or sales tax." We want to compare apples to apples. This would, therefore, include "***federal income taxes***" (a truly bogus term as mentioned above) + "***self-employment taxes***" (or the employee's part of the FICA tax if employed) + "***AMT***" – if applicable + "***dividend taxes***" – if applicable + all "***capital gains taxes***" – if applicable.

   "True Federal Income Tax Rate" is a term that should be created or the term "Effective Tax Rate" <u>SHOULD</u> be (changed & to "True Effective Tax Rate") defined as the abovementioned "Total Federal Income Taxes Paid" as a percentage of the abovementioned "taxable Income." This gives every voter, producer, consumer, investor, & everyone else a **more truthful** understanding of what people are truly "receiving" (in the form of what we currently call "earned" – as well as "unearned income") have left over after personal & business deductions, & are truly paying in total federal income taxes on that "taxable income."

The Self-Employed Americans with a net profit under $114K per year (in 2013) were in the highest "True Federal Income Tax Rate!"   In fact, the less an American "earned" (under $114K per year), the higher their "True Federal Income Tax Rate" usually becomes! How do you believe God feels about that?! They pay (to the IRS) the highest percentage (the highest "TRUE Federal Income Tax Rate") of "TOTAL Federal Income TAXES" (Self-employment Taxes + "Federal Income Taxes," etc.) as a percentage of their true "TAXABLE INCOME!"

   For example #1: if a self-employed worker "received" $52K in gross income – but it cost that person $10K to earn that money: their "net profit" was $42K. If they had $17K in personal allowable deductions (real estate taxes + mortgage interest + charity donations, etc.): their "**taxable income" would be $25K. They would pay (in 2013 or most any of the past 10 years –**except slightly lower in 2011 & 2012)_**a "True Federal Income Tax Rate" of over 40%** (over $10K in "Total Federal Income taxes paid" out of a taxable income of $25K)! That leaves that worker $15K for items that are not tax deductible – like principal on the mortgage, groceries (for him & family), etc. Is it any wonder why dollar stores & <u>low cost fast food restaurants</u> (serving high calorie, nutrient-deficient food "***FULL OF***" artificial chemicals, pesticides, etc.) are doing well - & real estate prices aren't back to the high of January 2006!? Do you see the connection between our anti-Godly tax policies & the rise of obesity & diseases?

   For example #2: my **TAXABLE INCOME in 2010 was $47K**. I paid in "TOTAL Federal Income TAXES" $21,600 ($8K for "federal income taxes" + $13,600 for "self-employment tax").   These "Total Federal income Taxes" were 46% of my true taxable income!   Thus, **my "True Federal Income Tax Rate" or "True Effective Tax Rate" was 46%** (same as what it would be for all the past 10+ years except for 2011 & 2012)!   Subtracting the $21.6K in "total Federal Income taxes" from my "taxable income" of $47K leaves $25.4K to live on.   As God told us to be good stewards of our money, I put $5K into a ROTH IRA (one of the best retirement plans us "poor people" have at our disposal).   My mortgage takes an additional $7K away in principal payments.   That left $13K to live on that year for non-tax deductible items (like food, groceries, etc.)!   I think I'll keep my old broken down car!

The 2ⁿᵈ lie to us = the government stopped including food & energy in their "INFLATION" calculations decades ago!   Look at commodity prices. Look at food prices (more than doubled in prices in many instances in the past 10 years). Unless you live on a farm & have solar panels for your only source of electricity, the prices of food & energy have affected your wallet every day in the past 10+ years!   Groceries, car repairs, & other necessities leave me with approximately $3K per year left over. You wonder why we aren't fixing up our homes, buying cars sooner, etc.!   What the lower 90% (in income/wealth) ARE spending money on = the necessities (like those sold @ warehouse markets & "dollar stores").

When the spenders have less money to spend, we spend less!   Baseball is no longer America's favorite past-time.   It is spending!   But if 90% of Americans have less money to spend money on, we stop spending money!   This slows down the economy -& can even cause a recession/depression.   *A recession is when your neighbor loses their job. A depression is when you lose your job*!

It is inconceivable that the "self-employed" with an annual "TAXABLE INCOME" of $47K may pay (to the IRS) over 8-31% more (than millionaires & billionaires) in TOTAL Federal Income TAXES as a percentage of their true "taxable income"!   I always like to shock people by telling them: "I am in the highest 'True Federal Income Tax Rate' in this country!"   Most people are not aware of the abovementioned deceptions by the IRS.

Consider the following examples:

Consider **millionaire #1** who "receives" 100% of their $10 Million/year as "long-term capital gains" ("unearned income") in investments.   They may have had $100 Million in stocks that went up 10% to create that $10 Million gain.   That millionaire would only **pay approximately 15% ($1.5 Million)** in "long-term capital gains tax" (what I would call "Federal Income Taxes") **to the IRS** (15% from 2003 to 2012 – increased to 20% on the gains over $450K or so in 2013)!   What is worse, that millionaire avoids the anti-Godly "self-employment tax" (or "FICA" tax if they were employed).   They avoid paying/contributing towards this "self-employment tax" (which is composed of a "SS" = Social Security & "MCR" = Medicare tax) - yet they will be eligible for Medicare & SS when they reach the age of eligibility!   **This millionaire (percentage-wise) paid** (from 2003 to 2012) **a 31% lower** (approximately 28% lower in 2013) **"True Federal Income Tax Rate" or "True Effective Tax rate" than I - & most other *poor* "self-employed earners!"**

It is inconceivable (Anti-Godly & Anti-economical & Anti-American) that our tax policies punish Americans for *earning* an income - & rewards **wealthy Americans** for gaining "*un-earned*" income!

71

Consider **millionaire #2**. Even if **a millionaire** (in 2010) was self-employed & "earned" 100% of their $10 Million as a "net profit" – they would have paid a self-employment tax of approximately $0.3 Million (2.9% for Medicare tax+ approximately $13K for SS tax) in 2010. If that same millionaire had the same personal deductions ($53K) as I did (they don't –they probably have a lot more to lower their "taxable income" even more), the **total federal income taxes** (in "federal income taxes + self-employment tax") owed to the IRS would be approximately **$3.7 Million** in 2010 (or $4.2 Million in 2013) – which equals **37.1% of their taxable income in 2010** (or 42% of their taxable income in 2013). I had a "taxable income" of $47K & paid 46% of my taxable income to the IRS in TOTAL Federal TAXES (self-employment tax + federal income taxes) in 2010! **This self-employed earner with over 200 times my taxable income paid a 9% lower "True Federal Tax Rate" than I did in 2010**!

This is not "class warfare." **Why does millionaire #1 pay 100+% less in "true federal income taxes" than millionaire #2 since 1997**?! Is this an example of rewarding the wealthy & possibly the "lazy!?"

Don't be fooled by thinking that employed individuals get off easy. If I was "employed" in 2010 (& all other factors equal somehow –as this would have changed a lot of variables –which I will not bore the reader with), I would have probably saved approximately $5K in TOTAL TAXES owed to the IRS. This probably would have lowered what I paid to the IRS in total federal income taxes to approximately 35% (as a percentage of my taxable income). This 35% "True Federal Income Tax Rate" is similar to what millionaire #2's "True Federal Income Tax Rate" would be if they were employed. This "imaginary employed" individual would STIIL have paid a 15% higher "True Federal Income Tax Rate" than "millionaire #1!" Also, **the employed person adds under-recognized tax burdens/costs to the employer**. The employer pays:

- A worker's compensation "tax;"
- An unemployment "tax;"
- & **HALF** the self-employment tax (AKA "FICA") of that employee!

Don't get too mad at your boss for not giving you that raise you were looking for! Thus, are you really "saving" as an employee (versus self-employed)? Don't forget, your employer is a consumer also.

This is the truth! *The truth shall set you free.* No matter how you twist the numbers, it is anti-Godly – as well as anti-economical for us as a nation!

This tax savings (for the wealthy) have created greatest shifts of wealth in my lifetime!

Consider the following facts about the federal taxes paid (federal income plus payroll taxes) to the IRS (in 2011) by the richest Americans (the 238,000 American households with **taxable incomes** of $1 million or more in 2011):[7]

- 3% of them paid NO "INCOME" TAXES!
- 10% of them paid LESS THAN 15%! Warren Buffet says he pays federal taxes of only 17.4% in 2010, half the rate of his secretary!
- This is because "the truly rich" receive most of their money as capital gains on investments & assets, rather than as salaries or other forms of income.

In summary, the four governmental &/or tax policies I believe are the most "Anti-Godly" are (for the past 10 – if not 17 years – including 2014):

- **1, OUR Self-Employment TAX (our Medicare + Social Security Tax)**!
  Workers (especially the self-employed) are punished for earning less than

$114K (in 2013) per year! The "payroll tax" is 15.3% (reduced to 13.3% in 2011 & 2012) for self-employed earners making less than $114K (in 2013) per year. This "**self-employment tax**" equals the SS tax + the Medicare tax. It is roughly equivalent to the combined contributions of the employee & employer under the "**FICA tax**." Self-employment Tax (or "FICA") is 7.65% (reduced to 5.65% in 2011 & 2012) for the employee making less than $114K (in 2013) per year. The employer must pay the other 7.65% of this tax. **Earners making millions or billions of dollars per year pay/contribute the same DOLLAR amount to Social Security as earners making $114K per year (in 2013)!** We don't need to be math geniuses to figure out how wrong (SINFUL) this is on every level. Keep in mind: many millionaires avoid this tax completely by "*receiving*" their money as gains on investments & assets! Perhaps the IRS actually got one term accurate: "unearned income!" ☺

- **2, Millionaires & billionaires can pay a long-term capital gains tax of 15% to the IRS** (for the past 10 years – increased to 20% on amounts over $450K in 2013) **& avoid the Self-employment tax (or FICA tax)**! By paying a total of 15% (via capital gains tax) to the IRS, they may pay approximately a 31% lower "True Federal Income Tax Rate" than the self-employed worker (or approximately 15% less than an employed worker) with a taxable income of $47K per year! We don't need to be math geniuses to figure out how wrong (SINFUL) this is on every level. Not to get political, but Reagan's administration created tax policies so that "earned income" is taxed at similar rates as "unearned income." President Clinton's administration (& our "representatives") lowered the capital gains tax from 28% to 20% in 1997, & President George W. Bush's administration (& our "representatives") cut it down further to 15%.[7] The stock market & real estate market benefitted (for a while) from both of these cuts. But at what price? Remember: **when you reward investors over workers, you PUNISH workers**!

- **3, The tremendous governmental –induced financial rewards (illustrated previously) for receiving disability & welfare benefits has created a "bubble" which is exhausting the Medicare & Social Security (as well as state government's) funds making America a "*slave to its' debt & lenders*** (Proverbs 22:7)!" We have to ask ourselves: are we making it too beneficial & too easy to claim/receive welfare & disability benefits. Why do we have life-long **tax-free** income for disabled former U.S. government employees? Why is there no gap between worker's compensation & receiving SS disability & Medicare? Why are we giving away so many benefits for being disabled &/or diseased!? It seems like there are no penalties & tons of rewards!

- **4, The way the "Affordable Care Act" (ACA) has been implemented in 2014** is most definitely anti-Godly due to the following:
  - ○ It **rewards irresponsibility & punishes responsibility of one's personal health**
  - ○ & it **rewards laziness & punishes workers**. The message of the ACA is, unfortunately: If you abuse your body – avoid exercise, eat junk food, & avoid work: The government will reimburse most of your health insurance! If you exercise regularly, eat an extremely healthful diet (following the "10 Dietary Commandments"), & work

73

hard: You'll have to pay much more in 2014 (versus 2013) to insure your health!   Someone has to pay for the irresponsible!

If you believe these four abovementioned tax & governmental policies are NOT anti-Godly, then "*YOU'RE FULL OF IT*!"   Remember, God is NOT a Democrat or a Republican.   If you believe any American "millionaire" (earning or "un-earning" $1 Million+ annually) or "billionaire" should pay a 31%, 21%, 15%, 10%, or even 1% lower "True Federal Income Tax Rate" than a worker with a taxable income of $50K: then "*YOU'RE FULL OF IT*!"   Again, see earlier where I discussed "more truthful definitions of what 'taxable income' & 'total Federal Income taxes" should be.

Is the "average" millionaire TRULY paying a lower "True Federal Income tax rate" than the "average" working middle class?   YES!?   However, we don't really know the true answer to this question because we do not have the term "True Federal Income tax rate" available yet!   One may ask: "Why not!?"   Why shouldn't we be able to know the truth!?   Don't we deserve the truth!?   Won't *the truth set us free* (from the wilderness of tax ignorance)?

- The 238,000 American households with "**taxable incomes**" of $1 Million or more (in 2011) paid an average of 29.1% in federal income + payroll taxes.[7] Should we compare a millionaires' "taxable income" to a working "middle-class" household's "net income?"   That would be HORRIBLE MATH!   We can do better than that!

- What is meant by the word "MAKING?"   You will hear people (like the abovementioned person in example #1) use the words: "I *make* $52K per year (because 100% of their self-employed income comes in the form of a $1000 check weekly).   If it "costs" that person $10K to earn that annual $52K, their net profit may only be $42K.   If they had personal tax deductions of $17K (mortgage interest, real estate taxes, charities, etc.), their annual "taxable income" may only be $25K. Their "True Federal Income Tax Rate" would be over 40% (even in 2011 & 2012 with the 2% reduction in self-employment tax for the employee)!

- This is why we need to change the definitions the IRS tells us to get a more truthful picture of what "True Federal Income tax rates" Americans are truly paying.   See my "more truthful definitions" mentioned earlier.   We need to compare apples to apples.   **The facts are most workers earning less than $114K per year (in 2014) are paying a much higher "True Federal Income Tax Rate" than many millionaires & billionaires**!   These workers are also "paying" for able-bodied lazy malingerers receiving disability &/or welfare benefits!

Is our nation's debt enslaving us? Yes.

Proverbs 22:7 says *"the borrower becomes the Lender's SLAVE."*   America's debt is at record highs of over $17 trillion (in 2014)!   Individual American's have more financial debt.   Both of these are huge burdens to Americans.   These **financial burdens become toxins to our mind, soul, & body**!   We develop a slave mentality.   We basically have become slaves to other countries as they loan us more money than ever in America's history. The *lenders become our master*! Thus, America has become a slave to money & the lenders we owe money to!

Has America's debt caused us to become "wicked slaves?"   Yes.

Psalm 37 says *"a wicked person borrows money & does NOT return it!"*   Where I am from, this is called stealing!   See Psalm 37 does not say a wicked person borrowed once or twice & did not return it.   Psalm 37 implies that wickedness involves a "trend" of borrowing & not returning!   Our nation continues to borrow money from other nations & NOT return it!   There is a trend there!

> **2.   Our tax & government policies are MORE satanic (anti-Godly) than ever before in our nation's history!**

As mentioned above, the working "middle class" (especially the self-employed earning under $114/year in 2014) has become *"the widow's mite"* of our nation!   Consider the following historical tax-facts:[7]

- The top marginal income tax rate was 91% during the 1950s, 70% during the 1970s, 35% in the 2000s, & **39.9% in 2013**.   Long-term capital gains tax was lowered from 28% to 20% in 1997, & cut down further to 15% in 2002 (in the first term of George W. Bush's presidency).   When you consider that many wealthy individuals gain their money ("unearned money") via investments (versus "earning")**, the rich currently have historically low tax rates**.
- These historically low tax rates (on the rich) are the major reason why the rich are SO MUCH RICHER than they used to be (read on).
- **The rich are so much richer than ever before**.   Don't be misled by the fact that the wealthiest 1% of taxpayers alone pays 21% of total taxes (including payroll, state, & local taxes),   This is because the rich are so much richer than they used to be!   **The top (wealthiest) 1% of Americans also earns 21%** of the total income in the U.S. - & **hold 33%** of the country's cumulative wealth!
- Due mostly to these anti-Godly tax policies, **INCOME INEQUALITY** in the U.S. has SOARED since the 1970s & is now more marked than China, according to the data compiled by the CIA!   The top (wealthiest) 10% of Americans own 73% of the total wealth in our country!   The "tax savings" (lower "True Federal Income Tax Rates") for the rich (compared to the working middle class) has created a compounding wealth effect!   It has also created a compounding *poverty effect* on the workers with annual "taxable incomes" under $75K.   **Our three income classes have become: the rich, the poor, & the broke!**
- More than half of the U.S. senators & members of the House (of "un-representatives") are part of the top 1% (in wealth)!!!!!

> **3.   Are America's Anti-Godly tax & government policies due to:**

- **Our so-called representatives' Toxic Minds & Souls (being *"FULL OF"* Intellectual & Spiritual Constipation)?**
- **Or Our Citizen's Toxic Minds (being *"FULL OF"* Intellectual Constipation)?**

We currently have the best example in my lifetime of: *"Taxation without representation."*   We must Love & even pray for our so-called government "representatives."   However, we should not love their SINS.   These "reps" may be considered (from 1997 to current 2014) the most over-paid (top 1%), under-worked, inefficient, & unproductive *workers* in America.   And they are supposed to represent us!?   I do not think so.   There is no coincidence that their approval rating in the past 10 years has been under 25%.   They get pensions & health insurance after they get fired (voted out).   We would never get these pensions or health insurance if we got fired for doing a lousy job!   They were (& may be) allowed to break laws that we would serve jail time for.   They refuse to take a pay cut −despite the people they claim to represent taking a huge pay cut.   They receive millions of dollars in "contributions" & never let the public know about it (they don't let us know who gave what amount. Nor do they let us know exactly what they did with all that money)!   Are Lying & Stealing Acceptable SINS for our Nation's "Representatives?"

Who exactly do these "representatives" represent?!

Most Americans do NOT feel it is Good or Godly that:

- Americans are being punished (especially in 2014 due to the ACA) for working & being responsible with their health.
- Americans are being rewarded (especially in 2014 due to the ACA) for choosing NOT to work & being irresponsible with their health!
- America has become a bunch of **wicked SLAVES** to our lenders as our debt hits record highs!
- The rich <u>are able</u> to pay a 15-31% <u>lower "True Federal Income Tax Rate"</u> than the working "middle class." See my more "truthful definitions" of "True Federal Income Tax Rate" mentioned earlier in section 1 of this topic. Even the wealthiest Americans (like Warren Buffet) know this is bad for the economy & adds to our nation's debt.
- The number of Americans receiving disability benefits has skyrocketed (since 1997 – no coincidence)!   We are **rewarding disability**. This is bad for our economy (once again **punishing workers**) & adds to our nation's debt.
- **Welfare benefits/"rewards**" may be greater than $25K/year (in 2013 in many states). This is similar to **punishing a worker** for earning approximately $45K/year or less (considering the "cost" –taxes, stress, driving, etc. of working)!
- **Many Americans receive the combined "rewards" of welfare & disability**!   This may be similar to punishing a worker for earning $75/year or less. If you believe these welfare & disability "rewards" aren't toxic to our debt, economy, minds, & souls (& eventually/indirectly to our bodies), then: "*YOU'RE FULL OF IT!*"

Are our minds so polluted ("*FULL OF*" spiritual & direct body toxins) that we are less intelligent?[5]   **Most Americans have "Intellectual Constipation!"**   I would estimate 99% of American adults are not even aware of the "abovementioned Anti-Godly tax & governmental policies." I would estimate that 99% of American adults are not aware that "Affirmative action" is the most anti-Semitic law ever created. Think about it.

In addition, I would estimate 99% of American adults do not know the answers to the following questions:

- What is the correct spelling of "FUCHSIA" or "RHYTHM?"
- What is the answer to the multiplication of 48 times 52? It is 2496. When you multiply any even number below 52 by 52: you divide that number by 2 for the 1st 2 digits & double that number for the last two. I realize most adults need a calculator for this. Now you don't!
- What is the answer to the multiplication of 63 times 57? It is 3591. This is called "The difference of two squares" [A brilliant college professor of mathematics (Bernard Atlow) introduced this formula to me].   60 x 60 = 3600. 63 – 60 = 3. 60 – 57 = 3. 3 squared = 9. Thus, 3600 – 9 = 3591. Most people need a calculator for this. Now you don't.   Has technology made us lazy physically & mentally?
- What is a "PEG Ratio?" This is the foundation to "fundamental analysis" when choosing stocks to purchase. This is why most individual investors & mutual funds DON'T beat the S&P 500 Index!   The PEG Ratio = (Price divided by earnings) divided by "growth rate" of net earnings. If a stock has a "P/E" of 20 & its' earnings are

expected to grow at 20% annually, it is fundamentally considered "fairly valued" (A "PEG" ratio of 1.0).   If you did not know this most simple basic "stock fact," you really should have a financial advisor help you with your investments!

- 6 + 4 x 2 = 14 (It's not 20).   6 – 4/2 = 4 (It's not 1)!   This is called the "Orders of Operation."   This is basic mathematics.   IT often reads as "PE MD AS" (or "Please Excuse My Dear Aunt Sally").   Parenthesis or Exponential is calculated before Multiplication or Division – which is calculated before Addition or Subtraction.   If you understand chess, this makes more sense.   Your pawns have "less value" than your rooks & bishops – which have less value than your Queen.   If you understand our government, this makes more sense.   Our President & vice President have "more value" than the senators & our "representatives" - which have more "value" than we the "peons!"   At least it seems that way!   Our lack of understanding in the basics of mathematics may be one reason why we get stuck with these "anti-Godly" (& "anti-economical") tax & government policies!

- A payment of $800 per month on a $400K mortgage with a 6% mortgage interest rate does NOT include Taxes or Insurance.   It also doesn't include Principle (& probably doesn't include Interest either).   Think about it.   If you had a fixed rate 6% mortgage: the interest alone would be $2K per month!   The $800 per month payment was usually called a "minimum payment" (similar to your credit card options).   By paying this minimum payment, you would create "negative amortization."   In other words, the next month you would owe $402K.   After 2 years, you could owe over $448K.   If the value of your home grew to $600K (like in 2000 to 2005), you would make a profit.   If the value shrunk to $250K (like in 2006 to 2009), you would be "under water!"   Most people did not understand (nor were even told) what kind of mortgage they were getting!   Greed was on everyone's part!   Many bankers, buyers, mortgage & stock brokers were **greedy.**   If you have a net income of $25K per year, what are you doing buying a $1 Million mansion anyway!?   Did that greed turn our nation closer or further away from God!?   Most (if not all) of us who own homes have suffered since 2006.   The mortgage industry in early 2000s turned the safest investment into the riskiest!   There is no coincidence that these loans (debt) are called "**TOXIC**!"

To expand on this concept, because 99% of Americans do not understand the abovementioned basics in mathematics, they don't even realize how "anti-Godly" & "anti-economical" these tax & government policies are!   They don't realize that they have been conned by paying a higher "True Federal Income Tax Rate" than the rich.   Recent studies have concluded that U.S. education (Kindergarten through grade 12) ranked similarly internationally to some third world countries![10]   This proves again a central theme/concept of this book: **as our God deficit has hit record highs so has our intellectual (as well as our financial, moral, & health) deficit**! I'm hoping the above helps bring all the readers of this book into the top 1% (at least intellectually) of our nation & world.   I'm hoping the above can help us all get closer to God & God's Love.

4. **These Anti-Godly tax & government policies have contributed to the destruction in our:**
   o **Economy (both nationally & our individual finances);**
   o **Relationships with friends, family, etc.;**
   o **& Health of our bodies, minds, & souls!**

As mentioned previously, our nation's three income classes have become: the rich, the poor, & the broke!   These tax & government policies have turned our country from having streets

77

paved with Gold, to streets of homeless beggars.   When our nation was "under God," we were blessed to be the most prosperous nation in the world.   As America has forgotten about the giver of our blessings, we have fallen into financial & economic diseases that have hurt us all!   Our nation's debt becomes our personal debt.   Our debt has made our nation "wicked slaves" (as per psalm 37 & proverbs 22:7).   I pray our nation gets closer to God & God's Love (by implementing my tax & governmental policies mentioned later).

Workers are being punished for earning less than $114K (in 2013) per year!   Money is only relative (like Albert Einstein may have said).   The government decided (decades ago) not to include energy or food when calculating what they call "inflation numbers."   However, food & energy inflation hurts the poor & broke dramatically more than the wealthy!   We all know energy & food prices have skyrocketed in the past 40 years.   We all know the bottom 90% financially are struggling & the top 1% never had it so good!   *Should our tax policies continue to punish those who "earn" money & reward those who receive money from "unearned income (dividends & capital gains)? Should our tax policies continue to reward the rich (& the lazy able-bodied welfare & disability recipient) & punish the worker earning less than $114K (in 2013) per year?!!   Should our government reward lazy malingerers (liars) & punish honest workers!?*

America & Americans have the largest debt they have ever had.[11] Since approximately **1997 (no coincidence)**, American's household debt as a percentage of GDP & disposable personal income has increased by over 30%![11] Our tax policies have turned us from God & made our nation *wicked & enslaved to its' lenders*!   Psalm 37:21 says: *"The WICKED borrows AND does NOT PAY BACK!"*   We are basically STEALING from our country's current & future bank/reserve!   America (& Americans) has become a *SLAVE to our lenders* (Proverbs 22:7)!   Do we Love the able-bodied welfare-recipients of our society that get rewarded by the government for not working?   Do we love the able-bodied malingerers who receive tremendous disability benefits in their early 60s (or 50s, 40s, 30s, & even 20s)!   Do we Love the rich who take advantage of these anti-Godly tax policies?   Remember, it IS NOT THE FAULT OF most MILLIONAIRES that pay a lower "True Federal Income Tax Rate" than ever before - & even pay less than the "poor middle class!"   The rules are set up by our so-called government "representatives!"

Our financial bankruptcy is related to our moral bankruptcy.   Enabling buyers to put nothing down on a house (& "walk" away without ever paying any principal) punishes those who put 20% (or more) down & pay off their debt.   Our moral bankruptcy has led to **most Americans (except for the top 1%) becoming either "TAX BROKE OR HOUSE BROKE!"**

Consider the truthful attitude many "middle class" households on their tax burden with the following analogy:
-   The 1st 2 weeks of the month that they work = go towards **taxes** to the IRS & State Income Taxes (if applicable).
-   The 3rd week of the month that they work = go towards the rent of their home or the mortgage of their home (part of which includes real estate **taxes** –which go to the local government).
-   The 4th week of the month that they work = go towards the rising prices of necessities (part of which they pay a state sales **tax**, a "road **tax** on gasoline," etc.)
-   The last 2 days of the month that they work = credit card debt &/or taking the family out to a restaurant.   Enjoy your bucket of fried chicken, French fries, & 72 ounces of soda!

Do you now realize the strong connection between money & your health?!
Are you sure you are NOT a government employee (without the benefits)?
The Amish lifestyle is sounding better & better each year!
Tax Fact: 47% of the U.S. population pays no *"federal income tax"* at all![7]
How is that possible?

-    Many of these are ultra-poor/"**broke**" (often elderly or truly disabled or workers earning less than $50K/year). Remember, our nation's 3 income classes have become: rich, poor, & **broke**! In addition, the IRS' definition of "federal income tax" is a bogus term. Consider a married couple or single parent with 2 kids working 5 days a week with a net profit of $30K per year. These people are "**tax-broke & house-broke**." They pay over $4K (approximately 15.3% of this net profit - lowered to 13.3% in 2011 & 2012 - & back up to 15.3% in 2013 & 2014) "self-employment tax" (or half of this approximately $4K if they are employed as the "FICA tax"). Don't forget this **over $4K in "TRUE Federal Income Taxes"** goes to some "*Federal* Government Agency" (supposedly, MCR & SS "funds")! They may have over $30K of personal deductions (child tax credits, real estate taxes, mortgage interest, SEP IRA or other "tax deductible retirement programs," & health-care expenses - over 7.5% of their Adjusted Gross Income) to lower their "taxable income" to zero! Therefore, they would pay "*no Federal Income Taxes.*" However, their "**True Federal Income Tax Rate" would be infinity** ($4K in "Total True Federal Income Taxes Paid" to the IRS as a percentage of $0 "taxable income" = infinity)!

     These people are not lazy dead-beats! These are low income families working their tail off just to pay the bills! 100% of these American's earnings go towards supporting their children, themselves, local & state governments (via real estate taxes & sales taxes), the federal government agencies (like SS & MCR via the "self-employment" or "FICA tax"), &/or the bank that owns their mortgage! These Americans are house &/or tax-broke! American's tremendous household debt is a financial burden that hurts the health of the economy & our bodies!

-    A very small percent of the Americans that pay no "federal income taxes" (as defined by the IRS) are actually **millionaires** (approximately 7,000 in 2011)![7] They make their million(s) purely on capital gains on assets & investments. They do pay a capital gains tax to the IRS of 15% (increased to 20% on the gains over $450K or so in 2013). Despite the fact that these millionaires did NOT (& may never) contribute (pay in taxes) towards Social Security or Medicare, they will still receive these "entitlements" when they are of that age (if they aren't already)! Really? Do they really "deserve" it for free? Are our tax policy makers actually telling us that these millionaires (who did not contribute towards Social Security or Medicare) can't afford to contribute towards Medicare &/or Social Security?!

-    However, some of Americans are able-bodied & *choose* not to work. They are **lazy &/or too proud** to earn low-paying jobs. Remember: **laziness & pride are 2 under-recognized sins**. Many able-bodied people will claim: "the only jobs out there are low-paying jobs (where you must work 40 hours per week to earn $15K per year). Why should I bust my tail to earn $15K per year – when the government GIVES me more than that (for NOT working!) in: food stamps, Medicaid benefits, & other welfare benefits!? With the **financial rewards** so great for receiving **welfare benefits**, many of these able-bodied Americans are **lazy malingerers that *choose* not to seek employment**.

Perhaps the elephant in the room are the 8.9 million (as of April 2013) former American workers who receive disability benefits.[8] Many of these people are honestly disabled. However, we can't ignore the strong (30 year) direct correlation between unemployment rates & disability applications![8] With the financial **rewards so great for disability**, many of these people are lazy malingerers (**liars & deceivers**) discouraged from working! Remember: **laziness & lying/deceiving those of the truth are sins**.

   Working "middle class" households (which are now considered "poor") should be upset/disappointed (as I believe God is upset/disappointed that this nation which has been "under Him" for so long –that He has, therefore, blessed & prospered for so long) that their relatively high "True Federal Income Tax Rates" go towards:

- **Enabling tax breaks for investors** – including, but not limited to, the top 1% richest Americans! These "rich" are often ignorantly referred to as "greedy-thieves." That is dividing & inaccurate. It is a war between those who "earn" money versus those who gain money via investments ("unearned income"). Investors –including, but not limited to the wealthy, simply have smart accountants & are applying a Godly sense of being good stewards of their wealth. Remember, the rich (for the *most* part) did NOT create these anti-Godly tax policies! As already mentioned, this is anti-Godly, anti-economical, anti-American, immoral, & has contributed to destroying the health of our bodies, minds, & souls!
- & **enabling the lazy/proud/deceptive able-bodied** (I don't like the word "dead-beats" or "government financial leeches" –but they are often described as such) **malingerers** to receive state & federal government rewards for being lazy, proud, & often deceptive/dishonest! Remember, these people did NOT create the anti-Godly tax policies. They are simply taking advantage of them!

So which of the above bothers you (the working "middle-class" household members) more? Perhaps this the question more voters need to take into consideration when they vote? Remember: we are supposed to LOVE everyone (the rich, the lazy/proud/dishonest able bodied, the tax policy makers, etc.). Remember: "**United** we stand!" Remember: "**One country, under GOD!**"

Most people are cognizant of the fact that chronic pain, obesity, & other *preventable* causes of disease/death (such as smoking & binge-drinking alcoholic beverages) are causing a financial burden to society (see chapters 3 & 4). However, we should also be aware that the financial burden on over 90% of Americans (due mostly to our anti-Godly tax & government policies – in my strong opinion) has become a causative factor in disease(s) (including obesity & chronic pain).[6] Consider the following **examples of how our tremendous financial deficit (personal &/or national) may lead to our health deficit**:

- The "poor" (& even those not so poor due to our "fast-paced" society) **eat more fast foods**. Fast foods usually cost less & don't require time (which in our society is equated with money - "time = money"). However, fast foods are usually very high in calories & low in nutrients. Your brain tells your body to continue to eat – as your body does not absorb the nutrients it needs. This leads to over-eating & predisposes you to obesity – as well as a whole host of other diseases.
- **Being anxious, "stressed-out,"** &/or depressed (all sins) over your own personal (or the nation's) financial deficiency can **lead to diseases, obesity, &/or chronic pain** (see chapters 3 & 4).[6] As already discussed in chapter 1 (as well in the beginning of this section), stress increases cortisol production –which causes you to store more fat.[6] Stress also stimulates the sympathetic ("flight or fight" response) nervous system (the

exact opposite nervous system response optimal for digestion). Stress, therefore, leads to poor digestion & absorption of the foods you consume. Stress, therefore, leads to intestinal putrefaction (which becomes a breeding ground for harmful microorganisms & other toxins). Stress, therefore, leads to a slower metabolism –which predisposes you to obesity (& many other diseases).[6]

As mentioned at the beginning of this chapter, **the strong relationships/connections between God, your health, finances, & morality are severely under-recognized in society**. By now, I have (hopefully) effectively demonstrated these connections.

- Our nation's largest **God deficit** has led to our largest:
  o Health, Intellectual, Moral & Financial deficits! Because we (as a nation) are more deficient in God: we are more obese, in chronic pain, &/or diseased – as well as less intelligent, more immoral, & more broke (more in debt[11])! Because we have strayed farther away from God in our nation's history, we are less blessed. If you believe this is simply a coincidence, then "***YOU'RE FULL OF IT***!" However, if one was to play "devil's advocate" & remove our "God deficit" from the equation - they would have extreme difficulty reputing the following relationships:
- Our nation's largest **health deficit** has led to our largest:
  o Intellectual, Moral, & Financial deficits. Because we are more obese, in chronic pain, &/or diseased: we are less intelligent, more immoral, & more broke!
- Our nation's largest **intellectual deficit** has led to our largest:
  o Health, Moral, & Financial deficits. Because we are less intelligent: we are more obese, in chronic pain, diseased, more immoral, & more broke!
- Our nation's largest **moral deficit** has led to our largest:
  o Health, Intellectual, & Financial deficits. Because we are more immoral (sinful): we are more obese, in chronic pain, diseased, less intelligent, & more broke!
- Our nation's largest **financial deficit** has led to our largest:
  o Health, Intellectual, & Moral deficits. Because we are more financially burdened (more in debt[11] & more stressed): we are more obese, in chronic pain, diseased,[6] less intelligent, & more immoral!

Hopefully we all see the connections! If you believe these body-mind-soul connections are simply "coincidences" (versus "**God-incidences**"): then "***YOU'RE FULL OF IT***!"

When you have **personal financial debt it increases stress - which can lead to obesity, chronic pain, disease,[6] & quarrels amongst spouses/family members**. You try to work more/extra hours ("over-time") to get slightly "ahead" of your expenses. However (due to our taxes being relatively high compared to "the rich"), it has become harder than ever to "catch up" with our finances. In addition, it leads to "personal relationship debt" (see below). The burden of this personal financial & relationship debt weighs you down like carrying around a 200 pound sack of debt on your back! This "stress" is a toxin to your mind, soul, & body!

America has become extremely money-oriented to replace the Love of God with the Love of money! Our self-worth has become dependent on our net financial worth! Americans will actually commit suicide when they lose their money (their "master"). Many Americans who lose their money (via investments or con-men/women) will often tell people, "I lost everything!" As money has become "the master" of most Americans, many Americans have lowered their morals to do whatever it takes to gain money! Lovers of money (versus God) will be willing to do SINFUL acts (steal, lie, deceive, be selfish & greedy) to gain money. Have we noticed how many "con-men" (& "con-women") have popped up since 1997? When our government rewards Anti-Godly behavior, should we really be shocked that so many Americans behave anti-Godly!? These are not coincidences!

This can lead to us "owing" time, love, & energy to our friends & family. Thus, we get "**personal relationship debt**." Our personal financial debt can also lead to our health deficit. We exercise less, eat more "fast foods" &/or processed toxic foods! When you are on your death bed, you probably are not going to wish you spent more time at the office. You are probably going to wish you spent more time:

- With friends & family; Giving more love to others; Bringing more people closer to God & God's Love; Reading & listening more to God's word; & treating your body more like *the temple of the Holy Spirit* it is.

Don't go to your physical death bed with any of these regrets. Don't let Satan, "the world," or our so-called "representatives" get in the way of what God has called you to do! But we should fight the fight so the government can represent us & God better by changing these anti-Godly tax & government policies! Remember: Salvation comes from Bethlehem – not Washington D.C.!

Jesus Christ led one of the busiest schedules. He healed ALL diseases, casted out demons, performed miracles (like raising people from the dead, walking on water to show the power of faith to His disciples, feeding thousands with food for only a dozen or so). He always had time to listen to His disciples –as well as to anyone else. While suffering an excruciating physical death, He still worked (helping someone enter the kingdom of Heaven; forgiving those who mocked & crucified Him, & comforting His mother & John)! He always has time to listen to you. He wants to hear from you! He wants ALL (including our nation's "representatives") to come to Him!

If America's so-called "Representatives" can create Satanic/Anti-Godly tax & government policies, what's to stop Americans from acting like Satan! If America's so called "Representatives" are irresponsible & "wicked" (as per psalm 37) with our country's debt, why should individual citizens be responsible with our personal financial debt?[11] If our "Representatives" are unethical & irresponsible, what's to stop "our neighbors" from selling or buying irresponsible mortgages & investments?! *"Love your neighbor"* is currently considered abnormal in America. "Screw (Con) your neighbor" is the new norm!

If you believe it is Good (or Godly) to be over-worked, over-whelmed, &/or continuously over "stressed," then "***YOU'RE FULL OF IT***!" One of God's 10 Commandments is to rest on the Sabbath.   Many Americans are forced to work 7 days/week just to "make ends meet."
If you believe buying an excess of material possessions will make you happy: "***YOU'RE FULL OF IT***!"
If you believe "over-buying" where you have credit card debt you can't pay off at 18-30% interest is a good thing: "***YOU'RE FULL OF IT***."
If you believe God wants you to be poor, you may be ***FULL OF IT***!   Money is NOT the root of all evils.   *The **love** of money is*!   The more financially blessed you become, the more of a blessing you can be to others!   Money is mentioned in the Bible more than the word prayer.   When you tithe, you are sowing a seed & will be blessed exponentially!   God blessed you to be a blessing to others.

If you own insurance on your home, automobile, life, & health – but have NOT "insured" your soul = "***YOU'RE FULL OF IT***!"   This may be the easiest time in our world's history to accept Jesus Christ as Lord (as your personal savior).   There is more technology/information available to us to become "in Christ."   By accepting Jesus Christ as your Lord & personal savior, you "insure" your soul for eternity!   It **doesn't cost you anything**!   He already PAID the price!   *It is FREE – for Him to set you free!*

5.   **So what's MY answer to "correct" our Anti-Godly tax & government policies?**

Based on our earlier discussion (& MY OWN Interpretation of the Bible & economics):

-   **ONE: Lower the SS tax by 5.3% to 10%** (2.65% lower for the employee & 2.65% lower for the employer) & **make it a flat tax (PERCENTAGE-wise) WITH NO EARNINGS CAPS**!!!   If self-employed workers earning a net annual income of UNDER $114K pay a SS tax of 12.4% (of their "net profit"), then self-employed workers earning a net profit of OVER $114K should pay the same SS tax of 12.4% (of their net profit).   What is $13,640 to a millionaire (it is 1.36%)!?   What is $13,640 to a self-employed worker earning an annual net profit of $10 Million (it is 0.136%)!?   MY proposal lowers the SS tax rate, eliminates the "cap" (approximately $114K/year in 2013) & makes the self-employment tax (AKA: "FICA") a flat 10%: all self-employed earners pay the 10% (& all employed workers would pay 5% - & all employers would pay 5%). This puts more money in the hands of more than 90% of all American employees & employers.   Don't forget BOTH - the employer & the employee - are consumers!   Thus, **the "Self-employment TAX" (AKA "FICA") becomes a "Godly" 10%**.   What percent is a **"tithe"** again!?

-   **Two: Change taxes on "unearned" income (such as dividends & all "capital gains" on investments & assets) to rates similar to our "earned income" (resembling the "marginal tax rates" system)!!**   This way – the tax rate on "un-earned" money will be *somewhat similar* to "earned money" (similar to what Reagan did in the last 2 years of his presidency).   This makes it a fairer tax (in my opinion) in which we are **no longer punishing workers**!   Thus, annual gains under $40K or so on "un-earned income" on investments & assets would still be taxed at historically low levels (overall, under 20% when you understand how the "marginal tax rate" is applied. The more you gain, the higher a percentage of "capital gains tax rate" you pay. Reagan did this in the 1980s & it worked until 1997 when we lowered capital gains to 20%[7] (which, as mentioned previously, rewarded investors & punished workers)!

- o Long-term capital gains should be taxed similar to how short-term capital gains are taxed (as "ordinary income" utilizing the "marginal tax rate" system). If the government wants to reward long-term investing (versus short-term volatility), the IRS can offer a 10% (versus a current possible 100%) reduction in taxes owed for long-term capital gains. For example: if you had a short-term gain of $10 Million (sold in 2013), you would owe approximately $3.92 Million in short-term capital gains taxes. If you had the same long-term gain (sold in 2013), you should owe approximately $3.528 Million (versus the current $1.975 Million) in long-term capital gains taxes.

Some may foolishly be fearful that either of these may cause a "sell-off" in the stock market. I believe strongly that it would not. In fact, doing all 5 of these corrections would most likely result in great stock market growth. Have our historically low capital gains tax rates resulted in great (sustained) stock market gains in the past 12 years? They haven't! They may have created an artificial tax incentive "bubble" (which eventually burst)! In March of 2000, the "Nasdaq Index" was at approximately 5,000 (& the "Dow" was at 15,000)! In addition, the stock market is a future indicator of the economy. These 5 changes would result in great economic growth, reduction of our debt, & confidence (in my strong educated opinion). Thus, it should (read on) result in great stock market growth!

- **Three: Increase the eligibility age for Americans (currently under the age of 60) to receive Medicare & SS by 5 years to get us closer to PSALM 90's age 70**! The fact that the government has identified certain ages when we receive Medicare & Social Security benefits (full or partial benefits) negatively affects (as a direct mind & soul toxin – as well as an indirect body toxin) how we view our health as we age. If we *BELIEVE* age 62 or 65 is *OLD*, then we start acting old! We stop exercising as much. We stop taking care of our health as we have been told: "Once you are on Medicare, your health is the government's problem!" Isn't 70 the new 50? Are not people living longer? Haven't most 90 year olds received more money from Medicare plus Social Security benefits than they ever put in in their lifetime?

- **Four: No more welfare without workfare & increase the years needed to be eligible for "Disability Benefits" (like Medicare eligibility; a disability SS at an early age; & tax breaks, etc.) by 2 more years**. If you are able-bodied & choose not to work: you should not be financially rewarded. Remember: laziness, pride, & dishonesty are SINS! They are also not good for our economy! This may hurt some people who are truly disabled. *** But too many people have "scammed" these federal systems too long (as the financial rewards are huge) & the system is broke. As mentioned previously, the massive influx of Americans (younger than ever before – often in their 40s) onto disability benefits will cause (& is already causing) long-term economic harm![8,9] Don't be fooled by low unemployment numbers as over 75,000

84

(& growing) former American workers <u>leave the workforce each month to receive disability benefits</u>![8]

*** Some may foolishly argue that this is not fair to people who truly become disabled.   Private insurance companies can offer some form of "disability insurance gap plan" (which the worker &/or employer can pay for) to help workers pay for these 2 extra years they are truly disabled.   This way, people will have **2 additional years –without any federal government "rewards" for claiming disability**.   This will dramatically reduce the number of Americans who eventually receive these Federal government financial rewards & encourage people to **return to the work force**!

- **Five: Change the IRS' Definitions of "Taxable Income" & "Effective Tax Rate" or Create a New Term For your "TRUE Federal Income Tax Rate!"**

Remember, the TRUTH shall set you free. We should demand honesty (**disclosure of the truth**) from our tax policies (as well as our tax policy makers)!

The **most truthful definition of "Taxable income" should be**:

- ALL "earned + unearned income" minus all personal & business allowable deductions.   As I discussed earlier, "effective tax rate" (just like how the government calculates "unemployment percentages" or "inflation" or in recent decades) is a bogus term meant to deceive taxpayers that they are paying less in taxes than they actually are.   The "**True Federal Income Tax Rate" should be used (already mentioned in section 1 of this topic)**:
  - "Total Federal Income Taxes Paid" to the IRS divided by the abovementioned definition of "taxable income" multiplied by 100%. "**The total federal income taxes paid**" to the IRS" would include: "self-employment tax" or "FICA tax" + "federal income tax" + "AMT" - if applicable + "Capital Gains tax" – if applicable + "Dividend tax", etc.   This "True Federal Income Tax Rate" is the number that all **producers, consumers, voters, & investors (& EVERYONE else) SHOULD be made aware of**!   This is the number that effects demand & supply curves!   This would give everyone a more truthful understanding of how much money an individual "made" or "received" ("earned" via "work" or "unearned" via dividends &/or gains on investments), had left over (after all personal & business & tax deductions), & paid in federal taxes as percentage of this money left over!   By being more truthful, we may bring our nation closer to the truth!
  - **Six: Give people lower health insurance premiums for being responsible with your health**. Car insurance companies give out "safe driver discounts."   Home owner's insurance companies give out discounts for "safer" homes (away from flood zones or the ocean, hurricane shutters, etc.).   Health insurance companies should offer lower premiums for people who are & have been responsible with their health. We should reward (not punish) responsibility for our health.

What do I know? God simply raised me up (from a "slow child") to be one of the top 20 college students in this country (who tutored fellow classmates in micro-economics –one of the most fascinating courses I ever took in college explaining how to be the best consumer by purchasing only what you need & the best producer by selling in bulk)! ☺   However, only God knows everything!   Remember, **our tax code has more words in it than both the Old Testament & New Testament combined!**   Where are our minds?

Just by doing these 6 SIMPLE changes, I believe we can:

- ○ Get our nation's fiscal "house" in order. We can **eliminate the deficit** & even have a tremendous surplus in 14 years or much less (probably 10 years). Similar to our physical health, there needs to be a BALANCE in our economic health.
- ○ Lower true unemployment dramatically. When you put more money in the hands of the employees – as well as the employers – you are putting **more money in the hands of the consumers**! Since our economy is 70% consumer-based,[11] the consumer will spend more. When the consumer spends more –this increases demand for the producer.   The producer usually has to hire more people to produce more. Then those hired people have jobs & more money - & they will spend more also! This creates a perfect economical circle of expansion.
- ○ Lower the number of people receiving welfare & disability benefits. When we stop "rewarding" welfare & disability so much (& start "rewarding workers" more), millions of Americans will seek employment. The best solution to welfare = work-fare. Therefore, this will also lower "true" unemployment.
- ○ Grow the U.S. stock market. Since the stock market will see the economy growing, the stock market will grow also. If all 5 of these changes were implemented, the "S & P 500 Index" & "DOW Index" should grow (assuming no Global disaster or "The Rapture" occurs before then) over 400% in 14 years!
- ○ Help the housing market recover. When we increase the spending (& number) of the abovementioned consumers, we increase the demand from all producers (including those in the real estate market)! If all 5 of these changes we implemented, the average residential real estate should at least double (unless "The Rapture" of the church occurs before then) in 14 years.
- ○ Bring our nation closer to God & God's Love.
- ○ Optimize the health of our economy/finances – as well as the health of our bodies, minds, & souls.

Another option (which would be more dramatic & hurt the livelihoods of many in the accounting profession – as well as others) would be:

- - A 10% (tithe) federal sales tax & tax rate on all earned & unearned income without any personal deductions allowed. This might work.

However, it would require an overhaul of the entire tax code.   The question would be: "who do we hurt?"   In other words, what deductions would we eliminate?   If we eliminated real estate taxes & mortgage interest as a tax deduction, wouldn't that hurt the real estate market?   If we eliminated charity as a tax deduction, wouldn't that hurt charities that are already suffering?   The answer is not always that simple.   However, my above 5 suggestions are very simple to do – I believe - & will help our entire country the most.   I believe EVERYONE directly &/or indirectly benefits –even if they can't see or perceive it right away.

The above suggestions are just some of the things our "representatives" can work together to help our nation.   This unfortunate division in our country is destroying us.

If you believe it is good that our country gets divided politically: "*YOU'RE FULL OF IT*."   The Devil wants to divide & conquer.   Remember: "<u>United</u> we stand. America is one country - <u>under GOD</u>!"   America should learn from the Old Covenant relationship my Jewish ancestors had with God.   When America – like the Israelites in the "old covenant" - was a "*United country under God*" (following God & God's living word), God helped America become the greatest country in the world.   *If we are divided as a nation: What power are we under*?!

Are you ("You" includes the media, our "representatives," you, & everyone else we know) helping our country get more united "under God" (or more divided – under Satan)?!

Why can't our so-called "representatives" work together to fix this SINFUL mess & bring our nation closer to a "country under God!"   As I have mentioned previously, it is no coincidence that our nation's largest God deficit has led to our largest financial/economical, intellectual, moral & health (of our *bodies, minds, & souls*) deficits!

CHAPTER 3: *"YOU'RE FULL OF"* more Direct Body Toxins than ever before

I. **You're Bombarded with (&, therefore, *"FULL OF"*) More Direct Body Toxins than ever before = an under-recognized & *Modifiable* Cause of Diseases, Obesity, & Chronic Pain**

By the end of reading this chapter, you should understand the following:
- Every human on God's planet is "***FULL OF***" more direct body toxins ("***IT***" - AKA: "environmental, material, physiological, &/or biological toxins") - as well as the mind & soul toxins ("***IT***") illustrated in Chapters 1 & 2 - than ever before.
- How to best avoid non-Dietary direct body toxins ("***IT***").
- "***YOU'RE FULL OF***" Diseases, Obesity, &/or Chronic Pain because: "***YOU'RE FULL OF IT***!"
- &, lastly, "***YOU'RE NOT FAT: YOU'RE FULL OF IT!***" I chose this as the title of my book because being "***FULL OF IT***" is currently (in my opinion) the greatest health care crisis of the 21st century! The question is at what level/extent does the accumulation of these direct body toxins (combined with the mind & soul toxins) **exacerbate or cause diseases** [including chronic body pain &/or Obesity] in YOU!? Too many people believe in the lie that if they are thin: then they are healthy & have no toxins in them. Said differently, "***YOU'RE FULL OF IT***" – whether you are obese or thin!

"***YOU'RE FULL OF***" **more direct body toxins than ever before in the history of the world**

In the last 100 years, earth (created by God) has become increasingly more "***FULL OF***" pollution via direct body toxins. Therefore: No matter how careful we are or where we live on God's earth, we are all "***FULL OF***" some level of direct body toxins (a form of "***IT***"). As we have become bombarded with (& "***FULL OF***") more direct body toxins, we have become less healthy, more diseased, in more pain & more obese. As stated throughout this book I do not believe the following relationship is a coincidence:
- As our **God deficit** is larger than ever before in our nation's history (referenced in chapter 2), so is our **health (as well as our financial, intellectual, & moral) deficit**! When you compound/accumulate & combine the mind & soul toxins (discussed in chapters 1 & 2) with the direct body toxins we are "***FULL OF***", the result is: we are **less healthy, less fit, more diseased, more obese, & in more chronic pain** than ever before in our nation's history.

Our "Representatives" receive **money** from companies to allow them to pollute our air, water, food, appliances, toys, buildings, & homes with many of the tens of thousands of new toxic chemicals introduced into our environment in the past 100 years!   As mentioned in Chapter 2, we have replaced God with money (**Money has become America's master**).   Is it any wonder we are more diseased & obese (as well as in more pain, less intelligent, more immoral, & more broke) than ever before in our nation's history?

As we continually **break God's 10 Commandments**, we also pollute our bodies by:

- **Breaking the "10 Dietary Commandments"** mentioned in chapter 5
- Bombarding our bodies with Anti-Godly direct body toxins (this chapter)
- Avoiding all of the "10 Non-Dietary Cleansing Methods" (chapter 5)
- & avoiding all of the "Super-Cleansing Foods & Supplements" (Chapter 6).

To reinforce my title: as we have become more "***FULL OF***" ***mind & soul*** toxins, we have also become more "***FULL OF***" direct body toxins!

*"In the Beginning **God** created the heavens and **EARTH**"* (Genesis 1:1).

As the people of this earth (especially in our nation - in the past 100 years) have strayed farther away from God, we have polluted the earth (one of God's creations).   This is NOT a coincidence.

Anti-Godly direct body toxins are polluting/contaminating the water, air, food, beverages, buildings, & homes all across this planet (that God created).   These anti-Godly direct body toxins include, but are not limited to:

- Industrial chemicals (We either import or produce ourselves). American industrial manufacturers make & import around **75,000 different chemicals**, 3000 of which are produced at over a million pounds per year![1]   If you believe these manufacturers test all these chemicals for health safety, then "***YOU'RE FULL OF IT!***"
- Toxic Heavy metals (like arsenic, lead, mercury, & cadmium)
- Pesticides (found in the air we breathe, food we eat, & even our water supplies)
- Herbicides
- Cigarette smoke (including passive smoking – AKA "2nd hand smoking")
- Radiation (from X-rays, CT scans, treatment of cancers, etc.)
- Pharmaceuticals (illegal, legally prescribed & over-the counter). Remember: western medicine often treats diseases (caused by being "***FULL OF***" **toxins**) with more **toxins**!
- Alcohol (especially binge drinking) – as well as Stimulants
- EMF (Electro-Magnetic Field) pollution –from cell phones, computers, televisions, "smart meters," electric blankets, & almost every appliance found in the home[2,3]
- Food additives (such as preservatives, artificial colors/flavors, pesticides, etc.)
- & possibly "**natural**" non-organic **foods & dietary supplements**. "Natural" is NOT synonymous with Organic! Many "natural" foods, beverages, & dietary supplements contain toxic herbicides, pesticides, artificial sweeteners (including mercury-filled aspartame), genetically modified ingredients, artificial preservatives, high fructose corn syrup, artificial coloring, & other anti-Godly ingredients![4]   It has been estimated that the average American eats 24 pounds of artificial sweeteners (such as mercury-filled aspartame) per year![5]   It has also been estimated that 29 million pounds of antibiotics (which equates to 80% of the nation's antibiotic use) are added to our animal feed every year![4] One can easily argue, breaking all of the "**10 Dietary Commandments**" (see Chapter 5) are the most detrimental direct body toxins we become "***FULL OF!***"

Has technology made us healthier & smarter or lazy gluttons?

Technology has allowed many mentally & physically challenged to rise-up to become more independent.   Information technology has also allowed easy access to information.   This may make many of us mentally lazy as we don't learn math & other subjects or "challenge" our brains.

If you believe that physical laziness & gluttony are the only 2 causes of diseases, then "***YOU'RE FULL OF IT***!"   Their avoidance is very important (both part of "Dietary Commandment #1").   However, as technology has dramatically increased in the past 100 years, the vast variety & amount of direct body toxins we are bombarded with (& "***FULL OF***") has increased exponentially!   Thus, we need to need to try multiple ways to avoid & cleanse our bodies from these direct body toxins.

The bombardment & "storing" (being "***FULL OF***") direct body toxins in our intestines (& the rest of our body) has a damaging accumulative effect on our health.   As we are drowning in a ***flood*** of direct body (as well as mind & soul) toxins, we must build "an arc" of salvation from these **direct body toxins** by:

- Trying our best to recognize & avoid the direct body toxins we are being bombarded with (this chapter);
- Following the "10 Non-Dietary Cleansing Methods" (chapter 5);
- Following the "10 Dietary Commandments" (Chapter 5);
- & Consuming "Super-Cleansing Foods/Supplements" (Chapter 6).

Consider the following example: If you don't empty your bowels of the intestinal putrefaction (waste matter stored in the intestines), it becomes a breeding ground for harmful drugs, microorganisms, & other toxins.   This intestinal putrefaction, therefore, predisposes one to diseases (including obesity &/or chronic pain) - & possibly even remaining addicted to the drugs "***YOU'RE FULL OF***!"

A common misconception is that only overweight people store direct body toxins.   It is true that the more body fat a human has, the *more likely* they are to have more toxic heavy metals in them.[1]   However, thin people may be even more "***FULL OF***" direct body toxins than overweight individuals.   Where, why, & how we store (become "***FULL OF***") the direct body toxins we are exposed to MAY have something to do with our genes.   However (in my strong opinion), it has more to do with:

- The types & amounts of direct body toxins we have exposed ourselves to – as well as the ones we are currently exposing ourselves to (this chapter);
- The intellectual & spiritual toxins we have been exposed to (&, therefore "***FULL OF***") – as well as the ones we are currently exposing ourselves to (chapters 1 & 2;
- Not following any of the "10 Non-Dietary Cleansing Methods" (Chapter 5);
- The breaking of the "10 Dietary Commandments" (Chapter 5) on a daily (if not multiple times per day) basis;
- & the avoidance of ALL the "Super-Cleansing Foods/Supplements" (Chapter 6).

The Bodies of Every Human on this planet (God's creation) are bombarded with (& "*FULL OF*") more direct body toxins than ever before – predisposing us to more diseases, obesity, & chronic pain.

Dr. Sherry Rogers (in her book *Detoxify or Die*)[6] & Dr. Linda Greenfield (in her online self-instructional program for Healthcare Professionals entitled: *Over the Edge: Biological Stress & Chronic Conditions*)[1] illustrate how all **food, water, air, animals, & humans** in this world are currently "***FULL OF***" direct body toxins!

When you store (become "***FULL OF***") these direct body toxins for a prolonged period of time, you may worsen (& even cause) chronic diseases such as:[1]

- o Cancers; Neurological diseases (such as ALS, Alzheimer's, Multiple Sclerosis, & Parkinson's Disease); **Chronic pain;** Lack of healing; & psychological conditions such as depression, panic attacks or inability to sleep.

This is because prolonged physiological toxicity can have a **compounding (& even multiplying) deterioration** to our health. For example, the presence of lead (found everywhere in our environment) makes mercury 100 times more toxic![1]

The following **14** examples prove we are "***FULL OF***" more direct body toxins than ever before:

1. Analysis of the **exhaled breath of humans** showed:[6]
   - o **89% had benzene** (a carcinogen found in **polluted air, cigarette smoke, crude oil, gasoline, perfumes, hair spray, after shave lotions, & most shampoos**) & **93% had perchlorethylene** (a carcinogen found in dry cleaning products & industrial solvents).
   - o An estimated **92% of Americans** over the age of 6 carry detectable levels of **BPA (bisphenol-a)** the hormone-mimicking chemical.[7] We are exposed to BPA & the equally (if not more) dangerous sister chemical **BPS** from a number of things, including:[7]
     - ▪ **Plastic water bottles**
     - ▪ **The inner lining of canned foods**
     - ▪ **Paper money**
     - ▪ **& even BPA-free receipts** (may contain BPS).

BPA & BPS have been linked to diabetes, breast cancer, **obesity, & other diseases**.[7] Canada has already banned BPA as toxic, & the FDA finally banned BPA in baby bottles nationwide.[7]

2. U.S. EPA studies of humans (tested) showed that **100% had**:[6]
- **Stored in the fat of their bodies:**
   - o **Dioxins** (a compound in "Agent Orange" – the herbicide used in Vietnam that led to 400,000 deaths & diseases), **PCBs** (Polychlorinated Biphenyls in **old fluorescent lights & appliances** – linked to cancer & nervous system problems),[1] **dichlorobenzene** (found in **polluted air, cigarette smoke, & crude oil** – linked to anemia, blood cell & bone marrow damage),[1] & **xylene** (found in **gasoline & airplane fuels**)!
- **Stored in the tissues of their bodies:**
   - o **Styrene** (a carcinogen found in **Styrofoam cups**). This is believed to be one of the many reasons why childhood cancers have increased so dramatically.[1,2,6]
- **Stored in their blood:**

- Heavy toxic metals like mercury (found in our air, seafood, & dental amalgams), lead (found in our air via dust of eroding paint & water via plumbing), aluminum, & cadmium (found in our air via exhaust pipes, seafood, & dental alloys).[1]

These toxic heavy metals were found in 100% of people all over the world! The most common cause of toxic heavy metal poisoning is from **arsenic** – which is found in **water supplies worldwide** (accumulating in **seafood**) & from the workplace.[1]

The symptoms of **heavy metal toxicity (similar to industrial chemical toxicity)** progress slowly & can cause, exacerbate, &/or mimic:[1]

- *Degeneration of most organs & systems*
- *Alzheimer's disease, Parkinson's, Multiple Sclerosis, & most autoimmune diseases*
- *Muscular Dystrophy*
- *Mental disturbances – like Depression, panic attacks, & insomnia*
- *Allergies;*
- *ADD, ADHD, & autism in children*
- *Cancer (100 years ago, cancer caused approximately 3% of all deaths in Europe & less in America. Now cancer kills approximately 23% of all Americans.)*
- ***Chronic Pain;*** *Lack of healing; Impaired cognitive, motor & language skills; Learning difficulties, nervousness, depressed moods & emotional instability; Insomnia, nausea, lethargy, &/or feeling ill.*

3. **America's Food is "*FULL OF*" toxins** banned by other countries (& considered a crime if ever found in the foods of some countries). Here is an example of 6 food ingredients allowed in the U.S. – while banned in other countries:[8]

- **Azodicarbonamide** can be found in our frozen dinners, boxed pastas, bread, & packaged baked goods. It is also used to bleach flour & yoga mats - & is known to induce asthma.
- **Brominated vegetable oil (BVO)** can be found in sports drinks, sodas, & makes carpets flame retardant. BVO can build up/accumulate in human tissue & has been linked to hearing loss, schizophrenia, growth problems, birth defects, & major organ damage. Over 100 countries ban BVO –but not the United Shame of America!
- **Potassium Bromate** can be found in baked goods & may increase the risk of cancer, & damage to the kidneys or nervous system.
- **Olestra (Olean)** can reduce fat absorption – as well as vitamin depletion, cramping, & anal leakage (that doesn't sound good at all)!
- **Arsenic (a poison)** can be found in our non-Organic chicken (except in Maryland) to make it look pinker & prettier?!
- **Artificial Colors** can be found in everything from cereals to candy -& even cheese. Food coloring has been linked to brain cancer, ADHD, & nervous system damage.

The United Shame on you America does not even warn the consumers of the potential harm of these toxic ingredients allowed in their foods! These are just 6 examples of why "Dietary Commandment #2" is so important - & how so many Americans break this Commandment on a daily basis (see chapter 5).

4. **America is "*FULL OF*" Pesticides & herbicides.** Remember: **Insects don't cause cancer!!** 2.6 billion pounds of pesticides are spread on America annually (that's 10 pounds per American)![1] Pesticide exposure has been shown to increase the risk of Parkinson's disease by over 300%[9] – as well as many other neurological diseases.[10] Being "*FULL OF*" pesticides or

92

herbicides have been shown to increase the risk of cancers[10,11] & even atherosclerosis.[12]

5. Even our **water** is "***FULL OF***" direct body toxins.

More than 60,000 different chemicals contaminate our water supplies.[1]   In a study of 954 cities, approximately 33% of the drinking water was found to be contaminated.[13] One pesticide, atrazine, was found in 96% of all surface water system tests by the pesticide industry itself.[13]

6. Our "**Western Medicine**" is "***FULL OF***" toxins (drugs, radiation, etc.) to treat & diagnose chronic diseases (caused by being "***FULL OF***" toxins – see chapter 4)!?   I have great respect for allopathic & osteopathic physicians, but we can't deny the fact that our society accepts & even demands our health care system evaluates & treats chronic diseases with toxins.   Below are just a couple of examples.

-   We all know that almost **every pharmaceutical** has short-term & long-term side effects.   These pharmaceuticals end up in our water supplies (somewhat due to patients ignorantly flushing them down the toilet), food (via the animals drinking this water & the vegan-food supplies are usually watered with unfiltered water), & the air we breathe!

-   Hospital body scans (x-rays, CT scans & MRIs) expose us to especially high **EMF (Electromagnetic field)** pollution.[2,3]   One MRI may deliver EMF pollution equal to 100 conventional x-rays![2]   Studies imply the possible association of EMFs with birth defects & cancer.[2,14]

-   We treat chronic pain with pharmaceutical painkillers versus getting to the root cause of the pain.   Americans have become "***FULL OF***" **Prescription Painkillers** & it is killing us literally & financially:[15,16]

    o   Drug overdose death rates in the U.S. have more than tripled since 1990 - & most of these deaths were caused by prescription painkillers.   Before you blame the prescribing physician or even the patient, consider the following fact: more than 75% of people who misuse prescription painkillers use them *prescribed to someone else!*   **This is a societal problem –as well as a health care problem. Our society "irrationally accepts" & are apathetic to this health care crisis.**

    o   Deaths in the U.S. (from 1999 to 2010) from *prescription painkiller overdoses among women have increased more than 400%, compared to 265% among men*.   This correlates perfectly to the **300% increase (from 1999 to 2010) in the sale of these painkillers**! Rates are also higher amongst people of low income, mental illness (like **depression**), & those with a history of substance abuse.   Women may be more likely to dangerously combine mental health drugs (like antidepressants & sleep drugs) with painkillers.

    o   These painkiller drugs were involved in more deaths in 2008 than cocaine & heroine combined.

    o   The misuse & abuse of prescription painkillers was responsible for more than 475,000 emergency department visits in 2009, a number that nearly doubled in just five years.

    o   As mentioned in chapter 2: "Back Pain & other musculoskeletal problems" has become the #1 reason (33.8% of all disability claims in

93

2011) for the skyrocketing increase of former employees receiving disability.[17]   As mentioned in chapter 2, this has become a tremendous financial burden to our nation.   Many of these people on disability are prescribed painkillers – leading to an addiction (for the patient – as well as the patients "friends").   This may be a major reason why we are "***FULL OF***" more painkillers than ever before!

7.   Americans have become "***FULL OF***" **the spectrum of cardiovascular diseases**: from blood clots causing heart attacks, strokes, & pulmonary emboli – to bleeding causing bruising, anemia, hemorrhagic strokes, & gastrointestinal bleeding.   Because Americans have become "***FULL OF***" more blood clots, diseases caused by blood clots, &/or diseases that increase the risk of blood clots: America has become **Blood Clot Paranoid &, therefore, "*FULL OF*" more ANTICOAGULANTS (both natural & pharmaceutical) that may increase your risk of bleeding &/or anemia!**   This is analyzed further in "Dietary Commandment #6" in chapter 5!

Americans have become "***FULL OF***" more:

Blood clots causing: Deep vein thrombosis, pulmonary emboli, strokes or transient ischemic attacks from a blood clot in or going to the brain, heart attacks ("myocardial infarction" or "re-infarction" – if repeated) caused by a clot in a coronary artery, obstruction of any blood vessel from a blood clot, etc.

&/or **diseases that increase your risk of a blood clot** such as: Atrial fibrillation, peripheral artery disease, coronary artery disease, etc.

This has something to do with the facts that (shown in "Dietary Commandment #6") we have become (especially **in the past 40 years**) "***FULL OF***" more:

- Emotional stress (due to the excessive mind & soul toxins we are "***FULL OF***" – shown in chapters 1 & 2)
- Direct Body Toxins (mentioned in this chapter – including cigarette smoke, etc.)
- Diabetes; Obesity; Physical Laziness (a sin) –as well as avoiding all the other "non-dietary cleansing methods" shown in chapter 5; & breaking all the "10 Dietary Commandments" (especially consuming refined carbohydrates, trans-fats &/or hydrogenated oils) shown in Chapter 5.

As we have become "***FULL OF***" more venous & arterial blood clots (as well as more diseases caused by blood clots &/or diseases that increase our risk of these clots), **we have strayed to one side of the cardiovascular disease spectrum to become blood clot paranoid**.   Our blood clot paranoia has caused us to become "***FULL OF***" more anticoagulants than ever before!   Anticoagulants (both natural & pharmaceutical) may benefit you by **preventing** the **occurrence or growth of blood clots**. Anticoagulants possessing "**thrombolytic**" characteristics: may actually help **dissolve blood clots**.   However, **anticoagulants may also potentially harm/kill you by increasing the risk of bleeding &/or anemia.**

Natural anticoagulants causing an increased risk of bleeding (&/or anemia) has become an extremely under-recognized public health problem!   Natural anticoagulants can have great health benefits - including, but not limited to, **the prevention of blood clots** (some natural anticoagulants like "nattukinase" may actually help to prevent & even **dissolve** current blood clots –mentioned in "Dietary

Commandment #6" in chapter 5).   However, **natural anticoagulants may increase the risk of bleeding &/or anemia when taken**:

- In excess; with each other; with prescribed &/or Over-The-Counter pharmaceutical anticoagulants; near the time of surgery or trauma; &/or by someone who already has a bleeding/hemorrhagic disorder.

In the 1970s: Americans had available to them only a few pharmaceutical anticoagulants (such as aspirin) & a few "natural" anticoagulants (such as garlic, ginger, & vitamin E).   **The number of different "natural" & pharmaceutical anticoagulants (as well as** other substances that can increase the risk of bleeding &/or anemia) has **skyrocketed in the past 40 years**!!   In addition, the percentage of people who regularly consume them has also increased dramatically!   As the world has become more integrated in the past 40 years, Americans are regularly consuming natural anticoagulants (often ignorant of their bleeding &/or anemia risks) from sources across the globe.   Many of these "natural" anticoagulants were not part of the American's diet (or even available) in the 1970s.   In the 1970s, were Americans even aware of chia or flaxseed oil (or other foods/oils high in omega 3 fatty acids), devil's claw, dong quai, gingko biloba, nattukinase, turmeric, &/or white willow bark (just to list a few)!?

The **list of natural anticoagulants** – as well as our need to **create an optimal healthy BALANCE between preventing blood clots and preventing bleeding (& anemia)** is analyzed in tremendous detail in "Dietary Commandment #6" (Chapter 5).

8.   Even our **homes & office buildings** are "***FULL OF***" direct body toxins.

- **Flame retardant chemicals** (over our **furniture, computers**, etc.) pollute our air, end up in our food chain, & are toxic to the thyroid, developing brain, & developing endocrine systems.[1,6]
- An average **carpet** outgases volatile organic compounds (VOCs) like **formaldehyde, dioxins, PCBs, etc.**[6]
- It has been estimated that **indoor pollution** (from **asbestos, formaldehyde, benzene, trichloroethylene & other VOCs**) may be causing **50% of illnesses** worldwide).[18]   **Trichloroethylene** (found in **adhesives, paint removers, correction fluids, & spot removers**) pollutes our air, water, & can harm our: liver, kidneys, immune system, & fetal development.[1]   *If you experience headaches on a regular basis & the reason can't be pinpointed, consider the pollution in your home or office as a possible cause.*[18]
- Toxic **EMF** (Electromagnetic Field) pollution also comes from **electric blankets, microwave ovens, hair dryers, cell phones, smart meters, television sets, - & to a lesser extent radios, lamps, & alarm clocks.**[2,3]   When we become "***FULL OF***" EMF pollution:[3] *Our body's voltage is raised & this can cause a great many symptoms most likely due to the result of a "**stress response**" - & that stress trigger being the EMF pollution*!
- **Radon** may be found in our homes & buildings.   If the levels of this toxic radioactive gas (an indirect decay of uranium or thorium) are high enough, it can lead to lung cancer.   Radon is considered the 2nd leading cause of lung cancer (blamed for about 21,000 lung cancer deaths/year in America) - & the **leading cause of lung cancer in non-smokers** (blamed for about 2,900 lung cancer deaths/year in American non-smokers)![19]   Radon levels are typically higher on the first floor of houses & buildings – as it is a gas that rises often from house/buildings built on soil or concrete which possessed a high concentration of uranium or thorium.   Radon levels are also highest when

95

there are no windows that can be opened to "let the gases out." The U.S. EPA has estimated that 1 out of 15 homes have dangerously high levels of radon.[19]

9. **Our babies are _"FULL OF"_ more direct body toxins &, therefore, more diseases than ever before**! The _sins_ (being exposed to & "_FULL OF_" direct body toxins) mostly _of the mother_ are paid (suffered) by **their babies**.

The biological father's toxic load can definitely damage the DNA of his sperm &, therefore, harm the baby from the moment of conception. In the "Old Covenant," the sins of the biological <u>fathers</u> were often paid (suffered) by their sons. (Ex 20:5; Ex 34:6-7; Numbers 14:18, 33; Deut 5:9,10; 1Kings 21:29; & Jeremiah 32:18) Jesus ended these generational curses. (Jeremiah 31:29-31; & John 19:28-30) However, the sins mostly of the biological _mother_ (being "**_FULL OF_**" direct body toxins) are **currently** paid/suffered by her babies (after conception)! One of the most significant ways a fertile woman can **_cleanse_** herself of direct body (AKA "physiological, material, &/or environmental") toxins she is "**_FULL OF_**" = is to have a baby! However, the baby _pays_ the price. This is written to inspire all of us & not to offend.

- Newborns are currently "**_FULL OF_**" more disease-causing direct body toxins than ever before. Thanks to the fall of Adam, all humans are born into sin. (Psalm 51:5 & Romans 5:12) Thanks to our largest God-deficit, we are born "**_FULL OF_**" more direct body toxins than ever before:[20]

In 2004, 2 major laboratories found an average of 200 (out of a total 287 tested) industrial toxic chemicals in umbilical cords after the cord was cut. Most of these industrial chemicals have shown to be: Carcinogenic (to humans & animals); Toxic to the brain & nervous system; & causing birth defects or abnormal development in animal tests.

Exposure of a fetus to environmental toxins is a greater concern because:[20]

- _Body systems are developing._
- _It takes <u>less pollution</u> [direct body toxins] to create <u>greater problems</u> for the child (compared to the mother). The EPA concluded, after a review of 23 studies of early life exposures to cancer-causing chemicals, that carcinogens average <u>10x the potency for babies</u> than adults, & that some chemicals are up to 65 times more powerful![1]_
- _& these problems escalate throughout the rest of the child's life predisposing the child to more diseases._

Here are some sad statistics from the World Health Organization (in 2005) proving the above:[20]

- **Asthma, autism,** _attention deficit & hyperactivity disorders_ **(ADD & ADHD), childhood brain cancer & acute lymphocytic leukemia** _have all increased over the past 30 years._
- _Five to 10 percent of American couples are **infertile.**_
- _Approximately **50% of ALL PREGNANCIES end up in MISCARRIAGE**!_
- _As per the Centers for Disease Control (CDC), approximately 4% of babies are born with **birth defects**._

- *The incidence of **childhood cancer increased by 27%** between 1975 & 2002, with the sharpest estimate for brain & nervous system cancers (a 56.5% increase) & acute lymphocytic leukemia 68.7% increase.*

Don't give the mothers "Jewish Mother's Guilt" as it is **the toxic environment** that deserves a lot of the blame for the damage to the children.   This may be seen as the environment poisoning the bodies of the mothers – which, unfortunately, they pass on to their babies.   However, it should also be seen as the environment poisoning the children after they come out of the womb & are no longer breast-fed.

10. Proof that the damage to our children's bodies are from **the toxic environment** include the following examples:

- Our water, air, & food are "***FULL OF***" direct body toxins - & (as stated previously) these toxins are more potent in children than adults.
- One study of 100 children found 99% of them had detectable levels of pesticides in their systems.[9]   The only child who didn't ate organic food![9]
- The average 6 to 11 year old is "***FULL OF***" the pesticide chlorphyrifos (a nerve damaging hormone disrupter) twice the level of adults & 4x the level the EPA has deemed "acceptable."[21]
- A 2003 study of pesticides in Iowa & North Carolina found that parental exposure to pesticides increased the risk of cancer in their children.[21]

Feel better mothers?   See: it *IS* the responsibility of the mothers, fathers, & our entire society to do our best to avoid all direct body toxins (as well as mind & soul toxins) for the health of everyone!   It has been said: *it takes a village to raise a child*. I would say: it takes everyone in the world to make a conscience effort to raise a healthy baby, child, & adult (& even pet). ☺

11. **Americans are "*FULL OF*" more "Chronic Diseases" than ever before**.

According to the CDC, "Chronic Diseases" (like heart disease, cancer, stroke, diabetes, arthritis, & neurological diseases such as Parkinson's, Alzheimer's, & Multiple Sclerosis) are non-communicable illnesses that are prolonged in duration, do not resolve spontaneously, & are rarely cured completely.[22]

Chronic diseases are caused by the body being in a state of "*chronic inflammation*" from the **accumulation** & **compounding** of the **combination** of the ***body, mind, & soul*** toxins reaching at or above the "***FULL OF IT*** Level of Disease, Obesity, &/or Chronic Pain."   This "***FULL OF IT*** Level ..." is analyzed further in Chapter 4.

The CDC's report on Chronic Disease in 2009 stated the following alarming statistics:[22]

- Chronic diseases are believed to be triggered by **DIET, LIFESTYLE HABITS, & ENVIRONMENTAL TOXINS**.   CHRONIC DISEASES account for **more than 75% of U.S. health care spending**!
- 70% of Americans die each year from chronic diseases.
- Heart disease & stroke are the 1st & 3rd leading causes of death, accounting for more than 30% of all U.S. deaths each year.
- Cancer, the 2nd leading cause of death, claims more than 500,000 American lives each year.
- **Baby boomers have 3 times the cancer rate of their grandparent's generation**![1]   This rate increases to 6 times for smokers.[1]   The WHO as far

back as 1965 estimated that at least half of all cancers are due to environmental causes (food additives, pesticides, industrial chemicals, toxic heavy metals, etc.)![1]

- In 2005, **50% of every American adult had at least one chronic illness**, while about 25% of people living with a chronic illness experience significant limitations in daily activities.
- The percentage of U.S. children & adolescents with a chronic health condition has increased from1.8% in the 1960s to over 7% in 2004.
- Diabetes is the leading cause of kidney failure, non-traumatic extremity amputations, & new cases of blindness each year among U.S. adults aged 20-74 years.
- **Arthritis** is a major cause of **chronic pain** & the most common cause of disability – limiting activity for 19 million U.S. adults.
- Obesity has become a major health concern for people of all ages. Nearly 20% of Americans aged 6-19 & over 33% of adults are obese. See chapter 4 for more on the topic of obesity.

12. **Americans are "FULL OF" 4 Health damaging (but modifiable) BEHAVIORS** that the CDC considers are responsible for much of the illness, disability, & premature death related to **chronic diseases** (such as **heart disease, stroke, cancer, diabetes, & arthritis**).[22,23] These **4 health damaging BEHAVIORS are**:[22,23]

- 20% of American adults & high school students **smoke cigarettes**.
- More than 33% of U.S. adults **fail** to meet minimum recommendations for **aerobic physical activity** based on the *2008 Physical Activity Guidelines for Americans*. As illustrated in chapter 1, this "laziness" puts us at great risk of heart disease, diabetes, & cancer.[24,25] This "laziness" (an under-recognized sin –less than 150 minutes/week of moderate exercise) is killing more Americans (& humans world-wide) than cigarette smoking![24,25]
- More than 75% of U.S. adults & 80% of high school students **fail to eat five or more servings of fruits & vegetables per day**.
- Over 15% of U.S. adults aged 18 or over engage in "**binge-drinking**" (5 or more alcoholic drinks for men & 4 or more for women during a single occasion) in the past 30 days. Remember, drunken-ness is an under-recognized sin (already mentioned in chapter 1). In fact all of the above 4 behaviors are under-recognized sins (already mentioned in chapter 1).

13. **Americans** (as well as most people in the rest of the world) are "***FULL OF***" **MALABSORPTION**: an under-recognized direct body toxin & physiological **STRESSOR**.

As America (& the rest of the world) strays farther away from God's 10 Commandments, we have also strayed (not ironically - in my opinion) farther away the "10 Dietary Commandments" illustrated in Chapter 5)! Breaking all (or even just one) of the "10 Dietary Commandments" can lead to poor absorption & digestion of the food you consume. This mal-absorption & poor digestion can create the following health problems:

- **Intestinal Putrefaction** – which can create a breeding ground for harmful microorganisms & storage site for drugs, toxic heavy metals, & the other direct body toxins mentioned previously in this chapter.

- **A slower metabolism**. This can also be due to the abovementioned intestinal putrefaction. This slower metabolism & intestinal putrefaction can lead to more mal-absorption, poor digestion, & (therefore) even more intestinal putrefaction & even slower metabolism. This harmful cycle can lead to **diseases, obesity, &/or chronic pain**.
- Added toxic load &, therefore, elevates your "**_FULL OF IT_** **Level of Diseases, Obesity, &/or Chronic Pain**" (analyzed further in chapter 4).
- &, therefore, **tremendous physiological stress** to the body. This can stimulate a "physiological stress reaction" (mentioned below) – which can exacerbate &/or cause diseases, obesity, &/or chronic pain (if you reach the "**_FULL OF IT_** **Level**" –analyzed further in chapter 4). Many scientists believe that mal-absorption & poor digestion of the foods we consume are the most significant direct body toxins we face. Mal-absorption & poor digestion may **cause us to age** (looking, feeling, moving, & thinking older) & deteriorate our health more than any other direct body toxin.

Optimal absorption & digestion (as well as cleansing intestinal putrefaction) are just some of the major benefits one may receive by following the "10 Dietary Commandments" in chapter 5.

14. **Our bodies are bombarded with (& "_FULL OF_") _STRESS_ from these psychological & physical toxins/_STRESSORS_.**

The psychological toxins/stressors (described as mind & soul toxins in chapters 1 & 2) & **direct body toxins/stressors** put our bodies under constant prolonged "stress." When our bodies are "**_FULL OF_**" these stressors for a **prolonged** period of time, our body has physiological responses including, but not limited to:[1] Our sympathetic nervous system ("Flight or fight") dominates. This can cause:

- An increased heart rate & blood pressure which predisposes us to an increased risk of heart attacks and ischemic strokes.
- Decreased life of red blood cells leading to anemia & lowered oxygenation
- Increased sugar & fat levels and a **tendency to gain weight**
- Poor digestion & absorption of food –as well as reduced intestinal motility (so we become more "**_FULL OF_**" intestinal putrefaction –as well as ulcers & nutrient deficiencies)
- Increased anxiety, sleeping difficulties, & accelerated neural degeneration.

When elevated for a **prolonged** period of time, cortisol (a steroid hormone released by the adrenal cortex in response to stress) can predispose a person to:[1,26]

- **Weight gain & obesity;** Diabetes; Immune system suppression (predisposing us to cancers & impaired disease resistance); Poor digestion & absorption of food (so we become more "**_FULL OF_**" intestinal putrefaction). As mentioned above, this creates **more physiological stress** to the body. Thus, the harmful **cycle continues**.
- Atherosclerosis – with increased blood pressure
- Insomnia, chronic fatigue syndrome, thyroid disorders, dementia, depression
- & even fertility dysfunctions.

A prolonged increase in cortisol increases dopamine (a neurotransmitter similar to adrenalin) levels in the brain which are <u>associated with</u> neuroses & psychoses (including schizophrenia).

A loss of DHEA (DHEA is a precursor to many hormones) which can result in <u>more fatigue</u>, bone loss, <u>loss of muscle mass</u>, depression, **chronic pain**, decreased sex drive & impaired immune functioning.

As one can comprehend from reading the abovementioned short & long-term damage caused by these **stressors**:

- Any of these symptoms or diseases can cause other symptoms & possibly lead to other diseases (as well as obesity &/or chronic pain).
- "Stress" is a psychological & physical phenomenon.
- No <u>physical </u>disease or symptom lives on an island without at least one <u>psychological </u>component to it.
- Every <u>psychological</u> disease/disorder carries at least one <u>physical </u>component to it.
- To reinforce our strong body, mind, & soul connection – consider the fact that many people "***FULL OF***" direct body toxins are also "***FULL OF***" mind & soul toxins (such as a "toxic personality")!   The question is: which came first!?
- It is not simply being "***FULL OF***" only one toxin in our body, mind, or soul that causes disease(s) –including obesity, chronic pain - & death.   It is the <u>accumulation</u> & <u>compounding</u> of the <u>combination </u>of all the different types & amounts of ***body, mind, & soul*** toxins that you become so "***FULL OF***" – that you reach the "***FULL OF IT* Level of Disease, Obesity, &/or Chronic Pain.**"   This is analyzed further in Chapter 4.

<u>Are we looking at Diseases all wrong</u>?

Are direct body TOXINS (from radiological tests & pharmaceuticals) the best way to evaluate & treat diseases caused by TOXINS!?   Is this how we treat our body (*the temple of the Holy Spirit*)?

- **Consider some neurological diseases.** Why does the brain stop producing enough dopamine in the person with Parkinson's?   Why do the myelin sheaths of nerves disintegrate in the person with Multiple Sclerosis?   Why does plaque form in the brain of the person with Alzheimer's?   I believe the "storing" (Being "***FULL OF***") of direct body toxins (harmful microorganisms, industrial chemicals, heavy metal poisons, food additives, drugs, pesticides, pollutants, etc.) - in our brains, central nervous systems, or anywhere else in our bodies – (as well as the spiritual & intellectual toxins we are "***FULL OF***") brings us to this "***FULL OF IT* Level**" of these neurological disease(s)!
- **Consider Atherosclerosis** (also known as Arteriosclerotic Vascular Disease) = a hardening of the arteries specifically due to multiple plaques within the arteries.   It can lead to: PAD (Peripheral Artery Disease); CAD (Coronary Artery Disease); Renal Artery Disease; Angina Pectoris; Heart Attacks; & Ischemic Strokes, etc..   What caused the hardening of the arteries?   What caused the plaque within the arteries?   It has been hypothesized that atherosclerosis is an **inflammatory** process initiated in the arterial vessel wall in response to retained low-density lipoprotein molecules, which then become susceptible to oxidation by **"free radicals"** - &, then, become **TOXIC **to the cells![27,28]   The damage caused by the oxidized LDL molecules trigger many **immune responses** which over time can produce **plaque**![27,28]
- **Consider Hypertension** (High Blood Pressure). Are medications that may increase the risk of atrial fibrillation & heart failure the best way to treat high blood pressure?

- **Consider High Cholesterol**. Are medications that may increase the risk of liver, brain, & muscle damage the best ways to treat high cholesterol?
- **Consider most Cancers**. How & why did the tumor(s) get there in the first place?   Are treatments that may kill healthy living tissue the best way to treat cancer?   Are we truly comparing quality of life (as well as longevity) when we consider effectiveness of these treatments –compared to a completely natural approach?
- **Consider Diabetes**.   Why are the person's blood sugar levels so consistently high?   Are Diabetic medications that may increase the risk of weight gain (which may increase your risk of Diabetes) the best solution?
- **Consider Hypothyroidism**. Why is the thyroid under-active in the first place? Are thyroid hormones that reduce your body's iodine levels - the best way to treat an iodine deficiency (or an excess of – being "***FULL OF***" - fluoride, chlorine, or bromine)? [29]
- **Consider Obesity**. Why or how did you get this way? This is discussed further in the next chapter (chapter 4).
- **Consider Chronic Pain**. Why or how did you get this way? This is discussed further later in this chapter.   How we get diseases, obesity, & chronic pain is also analyzed in chapter 4 (where the "***FULL OF IT* Level of Disease, Obesity, &/or Chronic Pain**" is analyzed).
- **Consider Non-Traumatic Orthopedic Diseases/Dysfunctions**. This is discussed in the next section.

I can go on & on listing different disease processes –showing how we often treat diseases with direct body toxins.   I have a lot of respect for my friends who are allopathic & osteopathic physicians.   Many of them have been "called by God" to do what they do.   God wants us to use the natural & the super-natural.   However, our nation has looked at health/disease in the wrong way for years.   It has become a cultural problem.   We **demand** our health care providers evaluate & treat our diseases with these toxins!   We live in such a polluted man-destroyed environment, that we often need man-made drugs to treat the man-made diseases!   Remember: **Optimal health is NOT the absence of disease**.   It is the optimal functioning of every living cell in your body.

Health & fitness are not the same.   Consider the marathon runner who dies at age 45 of a heart attack.   He was extremely fit –but not healthy. Like everything, we need a BALANCE.

As our knowledge in health care, science, & technology have dramatically increased (in the past 100 years), the amount of direct body toxins (as well as intellectual & spiritual toxins) we are bombarded with (& become "***FULL OF***") has also dramatically increased.

TESTING Methods to determine the "LEVEL" of Direct Body Toxins "*YOU'RE FULL OF*" include:
- **Hair analysis**. Dr. Lawrence Wilson, M.D. of "The Center for Development" considers hair a "soft tissue" in which most **toxic heavy metals** we are "***FULL OF***" are found.[30]   Therefore, Dr. Wilson considers **hair analysis the most accurate** (as well as a non-invasive, safe, & inexpensive) method of measuring

toxic heavy metals our bodies are "***FULL OF***!"[30]   **Everyone** tested by his laboratory in the past 30 years has been found to be "***FULL OF***" toxic heavy metals![30]   The following people were found to be "***FULL OF***" more toxic heavy metals than others:[30]

- o **Miners, electricians, plumbers, mechanics, smokers, & seafood eaters**!

His view is shared by the **U.S. EPA** – which reviewed 400 studies of hair analysis for toxic heavy metal detection & concluded the following: "*Hair analysis is an accurate test for arsenic, cadmium, lead (useful for low level lead exposure in children), & mercury – as well as for chromium, copper, nickel, selenium, tin & vanadium .*"

Dr. Wilson's view on hair analysis is shared by Phyllis Balch, C.N.C. (from her book entitled ***Prescription for Nutritional Healing, 5th Edition***):[31]   Hair analysis "*offers an **accurate early** assessment of the concentration of toxic (as well as beneficial) substances – making it possible to identify & treat toxicity before overt symptoms appear. The correlation between toxic substances in the **internal organs (& cells)** of the body & concentrations in **hair** has been found to be much more reliable than blood or urine sampling. This is because <u>urine & blood analysis</u> shows the level of <u>circulating minerals</u>.*"

- **Blood, Urine, & Sweat analysis** of toxic heavy metals & other physiological toxic elements.   However, these tests present with the following problems:[30]
  - o **Blood analysis** (including red blood cell testing) is considered "inaccurate & invasive."
  - o **C-reactive protein (CRP)** is a popular & highly sensitive test of the body's "**inflammatory load**."   The limitations to this test include:[1]
    - ▪ It is relatively non-specific. It will <u>not</u> identify which direct body toxins "***YOU'RE FULL OF***."   It will reflect low-level inflammation & increases with any type of infection.
    - ▪ & "silent inflammation" occurs long before it can be detected by CRP.
  - o **Urine analysis** (including a "urine challenge test"- in which a synthetic chelation agent like EDTA, DMPS, etc. is injected & then urine is collected for 24 hours afterwards to test for toxic heavy metals) is considered "*inconvenient, costly, & inaccurate.*"
  - o **Sweat analysis** for bio-toxins may be considered the superior of these 3 as toxic heavy metals (such as arsenic, cadmium, lead, & mercury) have been found to be more concentrated in sweat (& sometimes undetectable in urine & blood analysis).[32,33]   Bio-monitoring for toxic elements through the blood &/or urine testing alone may underestimate the total body burden of such toxic metals.[32,33]   However, sweat analysis only provides a short-term view.   The test would need to be repeated daily or at least weekly to gain a long-term picture (like only hair analysis does).

Other testing methods considered inaccurate by Dr. L. Wilson include:[30]

- **Stool Testing**: *inconvenient & inaccurate.*
- **Liver biopsies**: *invasive, painful, costly, time-consuming, & may not be accurate!*
- **Electronic & Energetic methods (include electro-acupuncture, radionics, kinesiology methods, & electronic scans such as the thalus, vega, etc.):** *unreliable.*

As illustrated throughout this chapter - & repeated by Dr. L. Wilson, M.D. - :[30]
"_**Thousands of toxic chemicals**_ _(or chemicals of questionable – often untested – safety) are spewed or dumped or even intentionally added to our **air, water, & food each & every day**. Therefore, detecting the levels of these chemicals is even more difficult to detect than toxic heavy metals because almost all are difficult to analyze by chemical means. Since these toxic chemicals are, unfortunately, **ubiquitous** (& **increasing daily in quantity & variety**) – assessing normal or baseline levels is almost impossible!"_

Hypothetically: If we _could_ accurately test for the tens of thousands of toxic industrial chemicals – as well as the toxic heavy metals – in humans currently versus any time in the past, the results would indubitably show that we are "_**FULL OF**_" more of these direct body toxins than ever before. In fact (as previously mentioned), the tens of thousands of toxic industrial chemicals we are currently "_**FULL OF**_" were not even introduced to our environment 100 years ago. Unfortunately, this trend is continuing so that future generations will be even more "_**FULL OF**_" these direct body toxins than currently! This may lead to this book's sequel in the year 2030 entitled: "_**YOU'RE even MORE FULL OF IT now than you were in the 2010s**_!"

II.   "_YOU'RE FULL OF_" Poor POSTURAL Habits – an under-recognized Toxin

God can use me to write an entire book on this topic. Health Care Professionals & the rest of society have **under-recognized the powerful impact POSTURE has on our health!** The health (of your body, mind, & soul) can also dramatically affect your posture. Posture can be reflective of our attitudes (our minds & souls). If you are under a great amount of psychological "stress," you are predisposed to a "forward head posture" (& all the health detriments that are associated with this posture – see later). If you are depressed, lonely, or feel unsupported: you may round your shoulders & predispose yourself to the abovementioned forward head posture. If you have a large abdomen, you may develop a "sway back" posture (see later).

       Poor postural habits are under-recognized toxins to our bodies (as well as our minds & souls)! Posture is like the weather. Weather (& **posture) can be extremely healthful** – like a sunny & 75 degrees Fahrenheit day in January on the beaches in Florida. Weather (& **posture**) **can also be very harmful** - like a 150mph hurricane that destroys your home **& kills you**!

       Realize **posture is dynamic**. Therefore, radiological pictures of your spine are only showing a "static picture" of you. Radiological pictures of you tell you what you look like at that ONE MOMENT (& one position –standing, or lying down or sitting) in time. Many people have "good posture" lying down & harmful postural habits when standing or sitting!

       Is it possible to be "big-boned?" To an extent = somewhat. The **3 major body types** include:[34]

- Ectomorph: usually long limbs & thin frame. Joints tend to be less stable & more mobile than the other 3 frames.
- Mesomorph: medium frame.
- Endomorph: largest frame. Joints tend to be more stable & less mobile.

As you can see, these body types are more important for the physical therapist analyzing one's arthrokinematic joint mobility (than it is for your appearance).   With over 35% of American adults obese, it can become challenging to figure out what body type/frame they truly have. You can achieve optimal health & fitness (& appearance) with any "body-type" (frame) you may currently have (or had years ago).

We go from the height of Goliath to that of Matthew! At approximately age 55, the intervertebral discs (the spongy discs between the bony vertebrae along our spine BEGIN to shrink).[34]   In addition, we develop poor postural habits & more osteoporotic compression fractures in our bony vertebrae (often in the thoracic vertebrae) as we age.   These are the 3 major reasons why we lose height after approximately 55 years of age.[34] We don't go from 6' to 5' from age 54 to 56. The shrinking process happens gradually.

Is our "shrinking" good news or bad news?   **The good news** is that those in the late 50s suffering from herniated discs (that are TRULY causing a problem such as nerve compression –most herniated discs do NOT cause nerve compression in most people)[34-37] may see these herniated discs (&, therefore, their dysfunction) shrink as they age.   Physical therapy & home recommendations can help tremendously to eliminate nerve compression. However, IF nerve compression worsens - often due to the patient's severe difficulty to change their postural habits – surgery may have to be considered (to save the nerve!).

The **bad news** is that the discs shrink (known as "DDD" = "Degenerative Disc Disease") after approximately the age of 55 for most adults![34,37]   This can leave less space for the:
- Nerves to travel through/between the bony vertebrae (the inter-vertebral foramen).   Thus, this increases the risk of spinal nerve compression – especially in the neck & low back regions of the spine (due to the natural lordotic curvature). Spinal nerve compression can lead to any amount of weakness, pain, &/or abnormal sensations along the entire pathway of the compressed nerve(s).
- Spinal cord - especially in the neck & low back regions (due to the natural lordotic curvature). Thus, this increases the risk of cervical & lumbar spinal stenosis. Since the spinal cord is the "trunk" from which the nerves "branch" off from, spinal stenosis can cause any amount of weakness, pain, &/or abnormal sensations.

- Intervertebral joints. Thus, this "DDD" increases the risk of cervical & lumbar "DJD" ("Degenerative Joint Disease"). This can lead to pain (especially with spinal movement) of these degenerated joints.
- Arteries in the back of the neck that "supply" the brain. God gave most of us 2 arteries in the front of the neck (called internal carotid arteries) & 2 arteries in the back of the neck (called vertebral arteries) that "feed/supply" the brain. This compression of the arteries to our brain can lead to forgetfulness, decreased cognitive skills, & even ischemic strokes (or "TIAs" = transient ischemic attacks).

The bottom line about our posture is that **we can't away with poor postural habits after age 55**! Don't be fooled if you are under 55 & believe you should take posture seriously only when you turn 55! As previously mentioned, poor postural habits don't happen overnight! The danger of wearing high heels is NOT that it will cause nerve, spinal cord, or joint compression dysfunctions **under age 55**. The danger of wearing high heels is that you usually develop a "poor sway back" postural habit (of excessive lumbar lordosis) that will be extremely difficult to change when you hit age 55 (& can no longer "get away" with it). As mentioned below, this poor sway back postural habit can lead to lumbar spinal stenosis.

The BAD NEWS about the DDD that occurs as we age (over approximately 55 years old for most people) **becomes HORRIFIC/DEADLY news when we have either or both of the 2 below mentioned POSTURAL dysfunctions**. These are the 2 most common postural dysfunctions (in my opinion) that are destroying the health of our bodies (the temples of the Holy Spirit) – especially as we get older.

Posture Problem #1 = A "sway back" low back postural dysfunction habit.

This is medically known as an increased lumbar lordosis or a backward bent low back posture. I start with the low back (versus the neck) as the low back/pelvis can be seen as the _foundation_ of the spine. I have had many patients with one-sided sciatica (or other forms of lumbar-sacral radiculopathy) due to a pelvis height (or leg-length) discrepancy or a side-bending of their lumbar-sacral spine. By the way, clinicians should always measure for pelvic height (or leg length) discrepancies standing - if the patient is able to stand (things change dramatically when the "_FEET HIT THE GROUND_!")!

As mentioned above, we can't get away with a sway back (increased lumbar lordotic posture). This turns the "bad news" about lumbar DDD to become "horrific" –possibly life threatening news! As mentioned previously, the excessive compression to only the sensory part of the nerve(s) can lead to "excruciating" pain, numbness &/or other abnormal sensations.

Consider what can happen due to the excessive pressure on only the motor part of the low back nerves. This weakness sounds so innocent.

However, it can be deadly!   As a specialist in orthopedic - manual therapy physical therapy – as well as lymphedema management, I have seen thousands of patients having both lumbar spinal stenosis & bilateral (both sides) leg edema (swelling). This weakness in your legs' muscles predisposes you to edema as your muscles are not pumping the venous & lymphatic fluid back up to the right atrium of your heart.

Over time, this inability of leg muscles (especially feet & ankle muscles) to "pump up" the venous & lymphatic fluid leads to some weakness of the vein valves (along with some varicosities) diminishing the negative pressure action a person's vein valves have on encouraging the venous return.   This leads to **edema - &, therefore, predisposes one for**:[38]

- A **discoloration (often brownish or reddish)** on the lower legs (as the "junk"/waste products of the body are not being pumped "up" from the calves to the heart)
- "Venous-stasis ulcers" – due to the abovementioned reasoning.   Skin & the deeper tissues of the legs need arterial supply (of healthy nutrients, oxygen, etc.) as well as removal of the waste matter of the circulatory system carried "up" from toes to the heart (right atrium) via the veins & lymphatic vessels.   If the "waste matter" stagnates (doesn't get carried back up), these "venous-stasis ulcers" may develop &/or interfere with their healing process.   One may say the circulatory system is similar to the gastrointestinal system: **it's all plumbing**!
- **Pain** – simply from the edema as pain & edema are "married to each other."   This is different from "true lymphedema" – which is due to removal or damage to lymph nodes.[39-40]   True Lymphedema (unlike edema) doesn't hurt when pressure is applied to the limb. [40]   In addition, true lymphedema (unlike edema) usually does NOT respond well to diuretics.[40]
- **Blisters; Weeping; & Cellulitis** – infections may be considered more of an immediate danger than most cancers!
- **Varicose veins; Thrombophlebitis; &/or a DVT (Deep Vein Thrombosis)**![38]   DVTs are the primary cause of **pulmonary emboli – which can be FATAL**![38]   Thus, a sedentary, obese (as obesity also leads to weakness of the vein valves) 70 year old person with a sway back posture (causing lumbar spinal stenosis) increases the risk of edema – as well as all the above mentioned health concerns that go along with edema (which includes death)!

This sway back posture makes your belly & buttocks "stick out" & APPEAR larger than they actually are. This sway back posture may have been a habit from years (often decades) before age 55. Consider a young 30 year old who is pregnant, has a large belly, or wears high heels. A robot would fall forwards! But our human brain tells us to compensate by arching our low back into a backward bent (sway back) posture!   This poor postural habit may exist for years AFTER pregnancy, your belly has slimmed away, or you stopped wearing high heels!

Based on the above, **this POOR sway back (low back - backward bent) POSTURE can make you "_FULL OF_"**:
- Joint compression **PAIN** in the low back!
- Nerve compression **PAIN** in the low back &/or leg(s)!
- **Numbness &/or abnormal sensations** in the leg(s)!
- **Weakness – even paralysis** in the leg(s) &/or low back muscles! This weakness predisposes you, therefore to becoming "_**FULL OF**_" **muscle strains** (partial tears of the muscles) & even **complete tears of the muscles** of your leg(s) &/or low back! This legs' muscle weakness also predisposes you to becoming "_**FULL OF**_":
  - **Edema** –with the toxins/"junk" of our circulatory system "pooling" in our leg(s)! This edema can (as mentioned above) lead to: **Edema pain, skin discolorations, blisters, weeping, Cellulitis, Varicose Veins, Thrombophlebitis, &/or a Deep Vein Thrombosis (DVT). This DVT (as mentioned above) can lead to a Pulmonary Emboli – which can be FATAL!**

Are you finally convinced that a poor low-back postural habit is TOXIC to the body?

If you have weakness in both legs – due to lumbar spinal stenosis – causing edema in the legs, your physician may recommend physical therapy. The physical therapist should evaluate – amongst other things – your posture, edema, sensation, pain questionnaire, muscle strength, & the arthrokinematic mobility of your low back vertebrae to forward bend to decrease the pressure off the lumbosacral nerves.

If the lumbosacral joints are hypo-mobile in forward bending, the physical therapist may use ultrasound as a deep heat modality – followed by joint mobilization to increase the mobility.[34] The physical therapist can train you how to **change your posture to decrease the sway back (low back "backward bent") posture***** – decreasing the pressure on the lumbosacral nerves & joints – in standing, sitting, and lying down.[34] The therapist may use motor nerve electrical stimulation –as well as therapeutic exercises (often ankle pumps with feet above/superior to heart 30 minutes per day –in the middle of the day) – to increase the strength of the weak leg muscles to improve the muscle pumping return of the venous & lymphatic fluid –thus decreasing edema. When approved by the patient's cardiologist (or PCP = primary care physician), the physical therapist may use edema reducing massage techniques, compression wraps - &/or stockings to reduce the edema.[40] Pneumatic compression pumps (when approved by the patient's PCP or cardiologist) can also be used to help "pump" the venous & lymphatic fluid to reduce the edema.[40]

***One of the most difficult home exercises I ask my patients to do is to change their sway back (increased lumbar lordotic) posture. As mentioned previously, they may have had this poor postural habit for decades (from pregnancy, wearing high heels, obesity, not "using" their abdominal muscles to "flatten" their low backs & "hanging" on their powerful iliofemoral ligaments)! These patients benefit from receiving postural re-education to "retrain" their abdominal muscles to "flatten" their low backs to help reduce the pressure off the low back nerves & joints.

One of my favorite postural retraining exercises is to have my patients thrust their pelvis forward or lift their belly buttons or belt buckles upwards (usually practiced standing as this is usually when the nerve compression via gravity is greatest). It's all about control of your muscles. What I've said for years: *"It's NOT so much the SIZE of the belly or tushy (buttocks) - that predisposes one to lumbar spinal stenosis or makes it difficult to reverse lumbar spinal stenosis. It is how you severe you are 'sticking them out' - that predisposes you to lumbar spinal stenosis. Thus, it is how you are able to 'stick them' back in –that can help reverse lumbar spinal stenosis!"* Postural retraining is not something you do once a day. Retraining your posture must be done throughout the day until you feel "comfortable in your new postural home."

Posture Problem #2 = A "forward head" postural dysfunction habit. This is medically known as a "backward bent" neck posture – or an "increased cervical lordosis."

As mentioned previously, we can't get away with this "forward head posture" as we age over 55. In fact (I strongly believe), we should never be in forward head posture at ANY AGE!

The abovementioned poor sway back posture can lead to an increased thoracic kyphosis ("hunched over") posture. Your brain is smarter than you think it is. Your thoracic spine (above or "superior" in anatomical terms) compensates for this backward bent (sway back) low back posture by adapting a forward bent/"hunched over" (increased thoracic kyphosis) posture!

The abovementioned "hunched over" (increased thoracic kyphosis) posture would cause a robot's eyes to face the ground. You compensate (once again) to look straight ahead by going into a "forward head" (an excessive cervical lordosis) posture – lifting your chin more than a fist distance from your chest. This poor neck posture may lead to **TMJ (Temporo-Mandibular Joint) dysfunctions** as it creates a greater effort on these muscles to open & close the mouth to chew food. This poor neck posture can (especially after the age of 55) cause excessive pressure on the neck nerves. This can, therefore cause **weakness, pain, &/or abnormal sensations anywhere the neck nerves travel to/from (from the head to the fingertips)**.

This poor neck posture (especially after the age of 55 – as mentioned previously) can also create excessive pressure on the two vertebral arteries in the back of the neck that supply the brain. If one's internal carotid arteries (the other 2 arteries in the neck that "supply" the brain) are clogged, this poor neck posture may cause **light-headedness, dizziness, impaired cognition, &/or possibly even predispose one to an ischemic stroke (or TIA)!**

Based on the above, this POOR forward head (neck backward bent or increased cervical lordotic) POSTURE, can make you "_FULL OF_":

- Joint compression **pain** in the neck!
- Nerve compression **pain** in the neck, head, &/or arm(s)!
- Nerve compression **numbness &/or abnormal sensations** in the head, neck, &/or arm(s)!
- **Weakness** – even paralysis in the arm(s) &/or neck muscles! This can predispose you to partial (& even complete) tears of the muscles of your arm(s) &/or neck. These partial tears, therefore, predispose you to becoming "_**FULL OF**_" muscle strains in your arm(s) &/or neck! This muscle weakness in your arms may also predispose you to:
    - **Edema** – with the TOXINS/"junk" of our circulatory system being pooled in our arm(s)! This is much less common than the edema seen in the legs - as the arms are usually close to the same height as the heart & the legs are farther below (as explained via the brilliant "Bernoulli's Equation"). However, upper extremity edema can possibly lead to the same previously mentioned health concerns (**cellulitis, DVTs,** etc.) as leg edema.
- **Light headedness, dizziness, impaired cognition**, &/or possibly even an **ischemic stroke (or Transient Ischemic Attack = "TIA")** from compression to the vertebral arteries!

Are you finally convinced that a poor neck postural habit is toxic to the body?

If you have cervical spinal stenosis (or any cervical radiculopathy – pinched neck nerves causing symptoms that radiate) a physical therapist can evaluate & treat you (similar in manner to the above-mentioned lumbar spinal stenosis).

For decades I have taught good neck posture to be "approximately a fist distance or less between chin & chest (top of chest = suprasternal notch)." When sitting, we should have the back of our head supported on the back of the chair. Avoid bifocals when on a computer as this tends to encourage you to be in bad neck posture.

When sitting or lying down, a fist distance or less between chin & chest is what I consider good neck posture. Look up with your eyes – not your chin. Listen with your ears –not your chin. If your spouse is taller than you are, have them sit or squat to kiss you!

When standing, a fist distance between chin & chest is what I consider good neck posture.

When should I have more than a fist distance or less? My answer is NEVER! Realize if the patient's joints don't allow them to move into good posture, the patient would benefit from having the physical therapist evaluate & treat their neck (same as mentioned above with their low back).

Optimal posture includes the **ears, shoulders, & hips in line with each other** when viewed from the side (or "lateral") view. This is just another great reason why God created Adam & Eve. You can ask your "Adam" or your "Eve" to view you from the side to see how optimal your posture is! Keep in mind, optimal posture is necessary for optimal health –as well as attitude & appearance.

Besides poor posture being a toxin – **toxins can also predispose one to poor posture**! Having a large abdomen - "***FULL OF***" intestinal putrefaction & other toxins - will predispose you to a sway back posture (increased lumbar lordosis – as mentioned above). Being "***FULL OF***" mind & soul toxins (such as guilt, low self-esteem, anxiety, depression, etc.) – may predispose you to having rounded shoulders - & a forward head posture!

Poor posture can also predispose you to mind & soul toxins! As mentioned above, having a sway back low back posture may actually predispose you to laziness (as you may have muscle weakness), depression (as you are in chronic pain &/or can't do as much as you did in the past), lower self-esteem, & even apathy (to exercise, health, or possibly even our morals)! Having a rounded shoulders & forward head posture may actually make you feel less confident, anxious, low self-esteem, etc.! Therefore: **the cycle of toxicity continues** as body toxins cause mind & soul toxins (as mind & soul toxins cause more physiological toxicity)!

These sound extreme – but they are possible. Just see how you feel when you bring your shoulders back & stick your chest out. Do you feel better emotionally & physically when you are hunched over with rounded shoulders or when your shoulders are back (not all the way) & chest is out & up?! Whom would you prefer to be seen with (as well as dance with or marry): the partner with poor posture or good posture? I am not preaching materialism or praising appearance. However, consider the following analogy:

-    One "**temple**" is decrepit with broken furniture, leaky roof, & wet flooded carpets.
-    & the other "**temple**" (despite being the same age) looks beautiful with apparently new paint, roof, furniture, carpets.

Which temple are you more attracted to (to praise & worship God in)? Remember: *your body is the **temple** of the Holy Spirit*!

Christians should be more aware of how others view us. This has to do with our posture also. ***Straighten up & rise up & be proud*** (with good posture & faith) that you are a child of God.   The Holy Spirit dwells in your body.   Therefore, be proud of your body.   You are a child – a representative – of the most Loving & Powerful Shepherd in the world!   He loves you more than anything will ever Love you!

III.   *"YOU'RE FULL OF"* More Chronic Pain than ever before

Here are some reasons why:
- *"**YOU'RE FULL OF**"* spiritual "pain" (sins – mentioned in the 1st 2 chapters) in your mind & soul that is a "psychological stressor" that exacerbates &/or causes chronic body pains (as well as diseases & obesity).   Remember: treating your body (*the temple of the Holy Spirit*) like a sewer *"**FULL OF**"* direct body toxins is also a sin.   These Sins are under-recognized stressors that can <u>compound & accumulate</u> to make you reach the *"**FULL OF IT** Level of Chronic Pain"* (as well as Disease &/or Obesity).
- America is *"**FULL OF**"* financial rewards (analyzed in Chapter 2) for having chronic body pain!   As mentioned in Chapter 2, "**Chronic Back Pain** & other chronic musculoskeletal problems" **has become the #1 reason (33.8% of all claims in 2011) for receiving disability benefits** in America.[17]   **In 1961,** 25.7% of all disability claims were for heart disease, stroke, etc. - & **only 8%** were for "back pain & other musculoskeletal problems."[17]
- *"**YOU'RE FULL OF**"* direct body toxins (from industrial chemicals, heavy metals, drugs, harmful microorganisms, etc. –mentioned previously in this chapter) –found in the air we breathe, food we consume, water we drink, bathe, & swim in, etc.   These direct body toxins can <u>compound & accumulate</u> (to <u>combine with</u> mind & soul toxins) to make you reach the *"**FULL OF IT** Level of Chronic Pain"* (as well as Disease &/or Obesity).   *"**Pain** is the body's response to a more silent & un-noticeable underlying (**toxic) inflammatory load**."*[1]
- *"**YOU'RE FULL OF**"* prescription pain killers.   As mentioned earlier in this chapter, there has been a **300% increase** (from 1999 to 2008) in the sale of these strong **prescription pain killers**.[15]   These prescription pain killers may possess addictive, withdrawal, & a "**drug tolerance**" quality in which the drug becomes less effective at reducing the person's pain.   The patient (or the person taking these prescription pain killers – prescribed to someone else) may truly be in severe chronic pain – despite taking more of these toxic painkillers!   Remember: most of these prescription painkillers just "mask the pain" & are temporary in nature.   Because our society *believes* this is the *answer* to their chronic pain, their chronic pain persists!

- "**_YOU'RE FULL OF_**" poor posture (an under-recognized direct body toxin) - that can predispose, exacerbate, & even cause chronic body pain (as well as diseases & obesity)! This was analyzed previously.
- "**_YOU'RE FULL OF_**" more obesity than ever before. There is a strong relationship between the increase in our obesity rates & the increase in our body pains (as well as other musculoskeletal problems).   The increased physiological "load" of obesity can increase the compression of our joints, nerves, spinal cord, intervertebral discs, & menisci. Obesity can also interfere with your ability to perform exercises (such as postural, stretching, & aerobic exercises) that can help reduce or eliminate your chronic pain &/or other musculoskeletal problems. Thus, obesity can predispose, exacerbate, or even cause chronic body pain (as well as other musculoskeletal problems).
- "**_YOU'RE FULL OF_**" more **diseases – including depression** - than ever before.   Many diseases may also interfere with your ability to perform exercises that can help your chronic pain &/or other musculoskeletal problems.   Depression (considered a psychological **disease** –but may also be considered a spiritual disease) may be another risk factor for **chronic pain**.   "*Most patients with **chronic pain** are **depressed**, & most of the depressed patients had **depression** before the onset of **chronic pain**.*"[41]

Throughout this book: the body, mind, & soul connection has been shown & will be analyzed further in Chapter 4.   The strong (under-recognized) connection/relationship between our increased chronic pain, obesity, & diseases (especially depression) is also analyzed further in Chapter 4.

IV.   How to Best *Avoid* becoming *"FULL OF"* Non-Dietary Direct Body Toxins

The best ways to avoid direct body toxins & "detox" (cleanse your entire body) are to:
- Follow the "10 Non-Dietary Cleansing Methods" (Chapter 5)
- Follow the "10 Dietary Commandments" (Chapter 5)
- Consume "Super-Cleansing Foods/Supplements" (Chapter 6)
- & follow some easy & practical ways to attempt **to avoid non-dietary direct body toxins - we can all do:**

1.   Try to Avoid Pesticides & Herbicides.

Pesticides & herbicides are not only sprayed on our foods & beverages. Realize the government pays to have planes &/or helicopters spray the air we breathe with pesticides in an attempt to kill mosquitos carrying certain disease-causing viruses (such as the West Nile Virus).   If our air "carries" (in the form of gas & liquid via rain) pesticides (& other toxins), it makes you wonder if anything is truly "100% Organic!?" Avoiding the spraying of pesticides & herbicides in or around your homes are important to reducing the risk of cancers,[2,10,11] neurological diseases,[2,10] & atherosclerosis.[12]

      Realize your earthly work bosses may not be receptive to avoiding pesticides &/or herbicides being sprayed in your work environment.   In fact (when I was a "Director of Rehabilitation" for a clinic in SE Florida), Medicare (Yes, the Federal Government) required that we HAD to have a contract with a pesticide company in order to treat patients under Medicare!   We are of this world, but must try not to be "of this world."   Their spraying (as previously mentioned) exposes us to neurotoxins, oncological-, & arteriosclerotic-causing TOXINS![2,10-12]

      As will be discussed in chapter 5, all food you consume should be "100% Organic!"   This will hopefully make it as close to God's creation as possible. This will be discussed further in chapter 5.

2. **Open the windows of your home & office (if allowed) every day** for a certain period of time.

In my opinion, windows should only be closed for security reasons (especially when sleeping or not present), temperature, & humidity reasons.   As previously mentioned in this chapter, our homes & buildings are "***FULL OF***" direct body TOXINS from:

- Flame retardant chemicals (over furniture, computers, carpet, etc.); radon (& other harmful gases); EMF pollution (from appliances, "smart meters," etc.); adhesives; mold; mildew; paint; paint thinners; & even certain paraffin candles; etc.   Opening the windows may allow many of the gaseous toxins (like Radon, etc.) to "leave" – at least temporarily our homes & workplaces. Testing your house for Radon (possibly buying a Radon test kit @ the hardware store for $10-15) may end up protecting you & your family from the 2nd leading cause of lung cancer![19]

Keep in mind, leaving the windows open too long in hot & humid climates may increase the risk of mildew &/or mold (which can be extremely harmful to your health).   There is that concept of "balance" again.   **Drying the shower walls (with a towel) immediately after showering may help prevent mildew & mold in the shower.**

      You may be able to CLEANSE the air within your home with God-given air purifying plants.   In the late 1980's, NASA found the following ***5 plants*** to be some of the most effective at cleaning the air of the benzene (often found in paint on the walls), formaldehyde (commonly found in drapes), & trichloroethylene (found in spot removers & other household products):[18]

- One: **Chrysanthemum** (*Chrysantheium morifolium*) – removes/cleanses air of benzene & formaldehyde.
- Two: **Gerbera daisy** (*Gerbera jamesonii*) – removes/cleanses air of benzene & trichloroethylene.
- Three: **Bamboo palm** (*Chamaedorea sefritzii*) – removes/cleanses air of formaldehyde.
- Four: **Red-Edge dracaena** (*Dracaena marginata*) – removes/cleanses air of benzene & trichloroethylene.
- Five: **Spider plant** (*Chlorophytum comosum*) – removes/cleanses air of formaldehyde.

Five other plants NASA found most effective at purifying the air (removing high concentrations of indoor air pollutants such as cigarette smoke, organic solvents, & possibly radon) include:[42] **Peace lilies; Mother-in-law's tongue; Ficus; Snake plants; & Devil's ivy.**

It has been suggested that 1 of the abovementioned 10 plants per 100 square feet may provide the best air purification for your home.[42]

You can further reduce your exposure to indoor air pollution by doing the following:[42]

- *Remove/leave shoes outside* the entrance door to your home.
- Replace toxic chemical cleaners with *God-given varieties (such as 9 parts water & 1 part white vinegar; as well as grain alcohol; &/or a lemon/baking soda combination*).
- Clean your air conditioning filter & check chimney (if applicable) for buildup.
- Replace toxic commercial fragrances & air fresheners with God-given varieties.

3. **Avoid Chlorine, Fluoride, & Bromine by: Filtering your drinking & bathing water; Using a fluoride-free toothpaste (after age 20); & Avoiding bakery products.**

As per Dr. David Brownstein, M.D. (in his book *Iodine: Why you need it, Why you can't live without it*, 2nd Ed.), one may benefit from:[29]

- Taking a supplement or consuming food sources of iodide & iodine (**if deficient** – as too much iodine may be harmful);
- Avoiding/reducing the chlorine & fluoride (found in drinking, bathing, & swimming water);
- & avoiding bromine (found in bakery products & medications – such as inhaler medications).   Dr. Brownstein suggests that there is very little evidence of Fluoride preventing cavities after the age of 20.

Dr. Brownstein states that the correct balance (of reducing or eliminating our fluoride, chlorine, & bromine; & increasing the iodine/iodide to the right levels) may:[29] Improve the immune system; & possibly decrease the risk of hypothyroidism, thyroid & breast cancer, & fatigue!

Fluoride (found in our tap water, toothpastes, & pesticides) consumption is believed to **directly stimulate hardening of the arteries[29] (AKA "atherosclerosis"** –the #1 cause of death in the Western world)![43]   Fluoride intake is also associated with a decreased IQ in children & cancer (contributing to over 10,000 cancer deaths since 1977)![44]

Due to the above, the U.S government is calling for decreasing the levels of fluoride added to our water supplies.[44]   However (due to "Cryolite" – a sodium aluminum fluoride sticky fluoride-based pesticide sprayed on non-organic foods), common non-organic foods (like iceberg lettuce) may contain 180 times more fluoride than tap water![45]

Make sure your **kitchen faucet is "LEAD-FREE"** as many kitchen faucets (even new ones) are still made of (Yes, even in the year 2014) *"leaded brass alloy!"*   These kitchen faucet manufacturers admit in their brochures/instructions that *"lead will be in the water* coming out of the leaded brass alloy faucet. We can reduce the lead exposure by trying to avoid using the warm/hot temperature water!"*   One manufacturer only uses leaded brass alloy for ALL their kitchen faucets! Isn't it bad enough that our city has lead pipes to allow the water to enter our house?   Now we have to watch out for the kitchen faucet manufacturers! Should this even be allowed? Isn't lead-based paint illegal? There are lead-free kitchen faucets (like "*Pfister*") available & I would recommend them for my friends & family! ☺

4. **Drink & eat out of clear, colorless glass - & avoid canned goods, drinking out of plastic (especially if reused or exposed to sunlight) & Styrofoam.**

You can't live in a plastic bubble! Even if you did, the inhalation & contact of the plastic *inside* the bubble would probably be more harmful than what is *outside!* We already live in a plastic & toxic bubble! Even our 100% organic fruits, seeds, nuts, & vegetables are sold in plastic containers! **Before eating these foods, they should be washed (even if the plastic container states "Pre-washed") with filtered water from the sink** (to hopefully remove most of the plastic residue as well as any mold, bacteria, yeast, etc.). Some **plastic bottles** contain bisphenol A – an artificial hormone that acts like estrogen (& can **increase body fat** in men &, therefore, **increase the risk of obesity** -& all obesity-related diseases –like **atherosclerosis, diabetes, disability,** etc.)![7]

Don't be fooled by plastic bottles that read "BPA-Free" (Bisphenol-A free). Many of these plastic bottles have substituted BPA for "BPS" (Bisphenol-S). BPS may actually have worse effects to environmental & human health (because of its' relative inability to biodegrade)![7] Opt for fresh or choose glass jarred goods over canned goods (as canned goods are a major source of BPA & BPS).[7]

Cooking food in the microwave with plastic dishes/containers may increase toxic exposure to you & the food! Repeated washing & re-use of plastic water bottles may accelerate the breakdown of the plastic, increasing your exposure to potentially harmful chemicals.[2] Wrapping food with plastic wraps (or aluminum foil) may increase toxic exposure.[2] Opt for storing food in the refrigerator in clear colorless glass bowls (with clear colorless glass on top of the bowl).

5. **Washing hands with antibiotic-free & chemical free "natural" soaps.**

You can keep these "natural" bar & liquid soaps in clear, colorless glass dishes & bottles. Antibacterial soaps often contain the carcinogen triclosan (that can be absorbed through the skin & pose a risk to the liver) – which reacts with chlorinated water to become chloroform (similar in makeup to dioxin)![2,6] Using regular (chemical free) soap, sufficiently heated running water, & thorough scrubbing will probably do the job just as well with no side effects.[2]

Some additional considerations for **hand washing** (that most people do not follow) include:

- Scrubbing fingernails (keeping them short & clean to make them inhospitable for bacteria & fungus) & the finger's web spaces.
- When finished hand washing, rinse hands with water running from forearms to fingernails.
- Wash hands before & after touching food (including dirty dishes).
- Wash hands before & after using the toilet.
- Wash hands before touching commonly used areas like a doorknob, elevator button, handrail, etc.
- Wash hands after removing gloves, handling chemicals, etc.

- Wash hands before & after shaking hands. Perhaps we should be more like the "1960s" & HUG versus shake hands! ☺
- Wash hands before touching near mucous membranes – such as nose, eyes, etc. This includes blowing nose & putting on & taking off eye contact lenses. **When you sneeze, wash your hands & face!** A fool would state that they don't need to wash their hands because they *don't have a cold*! It is still body fluid. You may not have a urinary tract infection –but you should still swash your hands after urinating!

6. **Avoid artificial (with un-natural perfumes & other toxic chemicals) skin care products, cosmetics, hair & nail care products, shampoos, soaps, perfumes, shaving cream, & suntan lotion!**

Most so-called "moisturizers" contain alcohol (which dries your skin)! The fragrance industry routinely uses over 500 toxic substances![2] According to the Environmental Working Group (EWG), approximately 75% of commercial sunscreens contain toxic chemicals that are linked to cancer & disrupt hormones.[46] Toxic chemicals rubbed on your skin are readily absorbed into your bloodstream. There are natural, chemical-free alternatives for all of these products.[2,46] Extra-virgin coconut oil (possibly with an SPF of 10) may be a healthful alternative for sunscreen.[46]

7. **Avoid mercury/amalgam dental fillings - & replace them with safer alternative materials**.[2]

The true composition of dental amalgam is about: 30% silver; 20% copper, tin, & zinc; & 50% mercury – a heavy metal toxin.[31] Insisting on a dental dam, continual suctioning, goggles, & air mask over the nose may reduce the exposure to the toxic mercury liquid & vapor when having them removed. This is between you & your dentist(s). Ultimately, the decision is yours.

8. **Avoid &/or limit the exposure to EMFs (Electromagnetic Fields) from electric blankets, microwave ovens, hair dryers, cell phones, "smart meters," television sets, & computers.**

As discussed earlier, hospital body scans (x-rays, CAT scans & MRIs) expose us to especially high levels of EMFs.[2,6] In addition, every plugged-in household appliance emits EMF pollution.[6] One does not have to live like the Amish or the Mennonites (though they may have the healthiest lifestyles)! Most cell phones have speaker phones that can be held from a distance. One can stay away from the other household devices when in use. When sleeping:[6] - Unplug all unnecessary appliances & keep all plugged-in appliances (& cell phones) away from your head. You may have to sleep with your head on the "foot" of your bed if you have appliances plugged-in on the opposite side of the wall where the "head" of your bed is to help avoid the EMF pollution! If you can sleep on the sand of the beach (you're your skin touching the sand) that may help "ground" your body to reduce the damage from the EMF pollution (see below).

As per Dr. Linette Beck, AP, DOM (www.becknaturalmedicine.com/):[6]

- *When our bodies are "**FULL OF**" EMF pollution, our body's voltage is raised (**positively charged**) & this can trigger the harmful "**physiological stress response**."*

- *The **earth is highly negatively charged**, so having your **bare feet touch the ground** (recommended at least 6 hours/day) neutralizes our bodies. Therefore, literal "grounding" ourselves helps us avoid &/or reduce the damage caused by the EMF pollution – which reduces the stress response.* (this is mentioned again in chapter 5)

Are the promoters of wireless products (like the "smart meters" from your electric companies; cell phones, etc.) "***FULL OF IT***?"   The Bio-Initiative Report (www.bioinitiative.org) indicates there is negative biological impact at EMF emissions 1,000-10,000 times lower than what the wireless promoters say is safe. Dr. Beck recommends & has a "Smart Meter Electromagnetic Radiation Blocker" to dramatically block the EMF radiation from your smart phones.

9. **Try your best to avoid the "Poor Postural Habits"** mentioned earlier in this chapter.

Remember, I have hopefully shown how these poor postural habits may predispose, exacerbate, or even cause: **Chronic body pains (nerve, joint, muscle, etc.); Obesity; & diseases** (like strokes, depression, lumbar & cervical spinal stenosis, radiculopathy/neurogenic neuropathy, pulmonary emboli, etc.)!

10. **Avoid the 4 most health damaging health BEHAVIORS (as per the CDC) that Americans are "*FULL OF*"** – mentioned earlier in this chapter.

These modifiable health behaviors (to greatly reduce the risk of chronic diseases such as heart disease, stroke, cancer, diabetes, & arthritis) include:[22,23]

- Avoid cigarette smoke by yourself –as well as second-hand smoke.
- Avoid binge drinking.
- Avoid physical laziness by exercising moderately at least 150 minutes per week.
- & eat at least 5 servings of fruit & vegetables per day (following the "10 Dietary Commandments" illustrated in Chapter 5 - of course")!   I realize this last behavior is a "dietary" method of cleansing/avoiding direct body toxins/diseases.   However, it is listed by the CDC as one of the 4 most modifiable behaviors to help avoid chronic disease.   Therefore, it is mentioned here.

CHAPTER 4: Why "_You're FULL OF_" more Diseases, Obesity, & Chronic Pain than ever before

After reading the 1ˢᵗ 3 chapters, you should understand that EVERY HUMAN (especially Americans) on God's earth is currently, unfortunately, "_**FULL OF**_" direct body toxins ("_**IT**_") – as well as mind & soul toxins ("_**IT**_").   The question is at what _level_ does the accumulation & compounding effect of the combination of these toxins ("_**IT**_"): cause or exacerbate diseases, obesity, &/or chronic pain - in YOU!?   By the end of this chapter (if you haven't come to these conclusions already), there should be enough evidence to support the following concepts:

- That the cause of obesity is the accumulation & compounding of the combination of the direct body (as well as the mind & soul) toxins reaching the "_**FULL OF IT** Level of Obesity_" for that person.
- There is also a "_**FULL OF IT** Level_" for **diseases –as well as chronic pain** – for each person.
- "**YOU ARE FAT (- as well as diseased &/or in chronic body pain)**: because "_**YOU'RE FULL OF IT**_!"
- Although we are _living_ longer, we are _not thriving_ longer.   We are living longer – but with a lower level of health & fitness.   We are "_**FULL OF**_" **more obesity, diseases, & chronic pain than ever before** in the history of our country (& the rest of God's earth) because we are more "_**FULL OF IT**_" (body, mind, & soul toxins) than ever before!
- "_**YOU'RE NOT FAT, YOU'RE FULL OF IT**_!"   I chose this as the title because being "_**FULL OF IT**_" is the largest health crisis (in my opinion) that is destroying the health of our bodies, minds, & souls!   Said differently, "_**YOU'RE FULL OF IT**_" whether you're fat or thin!

I.   "_**YOU'RE FULL OF**_" Myths about Obesity & Nutrition

As mentioned in the "Preface" of this book, we are currently at a time when _"people will turn their ears **away from the truth** & will turn aside **to myths** in accordance to their OWN desires – in order to have their ears tickled!"_ (2Tim 4:3-4)

Many of the following **nutritional myths** (as mentioned in chapter 2) are analyzed in greater detail in Chapters 5 & 6.   Chapter 6 describes the good ("super-cleansing") versus the ugly regarding fats, proteins, carbs, etc. However, it needs to be outlined here, so people get a preview of the truth & understand that they have been conned &/or believed the following _"myths (in accordance to their OWN desires) – to have their own ears tickled!"_   Some of the **Nutritional MYTHS** (which have led to a dramatic **increase in OBESITY – as**

118

well as Diseases &/or chronic pain) we have become "***FULL OF***" include the following:

- *The majority of your diet should be **grains**!*   Even the current (2013) USDA FDA recommendation ("My Plate" –which replaced "My Pyramid" in June 2011) recommends 25% of your "plate" be grains![1]   *Grains contain very little (if any) fat & cholesterol &, therefore, consuming 25% (or greater if we go by the "**USDA Food Pyramid" of the 1970s**) of "your plate" as grains will make you thin, lose weight, & healthy!*
- *We should replace healthful **saturated fats** (like extra-virgin coconut oil & probiotic goat's milk yogurt) with harmful **Hydrogenated oil & trans-fats** from vegetable sources!*
- *All **fats** are equal in healthfulness/harmfulness.*
- ***Fats** – even healthful fats like raw nuts & edible seeds should be avoided as they will make you fat & unhealthy!*
- *All **fiber** sources are equal in healthfulness/harmfulness!*
- *All **carbs** are equal – non-organic orange juice is equal to a raw organic orange.*
- ***Food combining** doesn't matter – as long as the food tastes delicious to satisfy your OWN desires!*
- *All **soy**-based foods are healthful!*
- *All **foods & supplements** are equal in healthfulness/harmfulness whether they are: raw or fried with hydrogenated oils & trans-fats; organic or sprayed heavily in pesticides, genetically modified (&/or injected with hormones &/or antibiotics); salted or unsalted; sugar-added or no sugar-added; combined appropriately with other foods; eaten in a peaceful or stressed-out state of being; eaten in a God-thankful or God-absent manner!*
- *If the food or supplement is "**natural**," it is 100% healthful, organic, & safe – with no side effects.*
- ***Absorption** of food doesn't matter – just taste.*
- *Healthful food can't **taste** delicious – only junk food tastes good.*
- *A food's health value should only be determined by the **macronutrients** it possesses as we're currently unaware of most of the **healthful micronutrients** they contain.*
- ***Iceberg Lettuce** has no nutritional value.*
- ***& Gluttony & Laziness** should be accepted & rewarded by society as it doesn't hurt your health (or anyone else – in any way) – as long as you enjoy your food & can un-button your pants!*

As mentioned previously, these are just some of the **myths** that will be "refuted" in greater detail in chapters 5 & 6.

Definition(s) of Obesity

The CDC (Centers for Disease Control & Prevention) **defines Obesity** as **BMI (Body Mass Index) 30 or higher**.[2]   For example, if a 5'4" adult is over 174 pounds (or a 5'9" adult is over 203 pounds), their BMI is 30 or higher & they are, therefore, considered by the CDC as "obese."[2]   Measuring one's body fat percentage is the best way to measure obesity.[3,4]   However, it would be too difficult (very expensive & time consuming) to measure **body fat percentage** of millions of Americans.   If body fat percentage is over 20% for a man – or over 30% for a woman: they are considered "obese."[3,4]

Surely a 5'9," 203 pound male athlete with 10% body fat (as muscle weighs more than fat) should in no way be considered obese.   However, the CDC's method for measuring obesity is probably the easiest way to collect large amounts of nation-wide data.   In addition (unfortunately), the average American adult with BMIs over 30 are NOT "athletes" or even athletic!   **Have**

we gone from the most athletic country to the most "pathetic" country?
America & the rest of the world are _"FULL OF"_ more Obesity than ever before

Obesity rates in the U.S. as a whole (as well as for all age groups usually – including children & adolescents to the elderly) have gone on **a steady incline from the 1950s to current**.[2]   Obesity rates in U.S. adults have gone from under 10% in the 1950s to approximately 35.7% in 2010.[2]   It is estimated that 50% of the U.S. population will be obese by 2030!   _Over 67% of all U.S. adults (measured in 2010) are considered (by the CDC) either over-weight or obese._[2]

In 2010, the CDC reported that the age group in the U.S. with the **highest rate of obesity** was "**60 & over**" (39.7%)![2]   This is just one of the major reasons why people over the age of 60 are at such risk for so many diseases (as well as chronic pain)!

Don't be fooled when you learn that obesity rates are "only" 15.5% of the Europe's population (as of 2010).[5]   Smaller portions, walking, & bike riding _has been_ (at least 20 years ago) more a part of their culture (perhaps like it was for Americans in the 1950s).   As we continue to "**Americanize**" **Europe** (& the rest of the world) with our **sugary soft drinks** & restaurant chain "**super-sizes**" (**full of toxic ingredients**), **European obesity rates have more than doubled in the last 20 years** in most EU countries.[5]

Aren't we proof that Charles Darwin was wrong?

I do NOT mention this to add to any controversy. This is simply a humorous observation.

Evolution by means of "**_natural selection_**" is the process by which **_genetic mutations that enhance survival & reproduction_** become & remain, more common in successive generations of a population.[6]   Compared to previous generations, **the human population has become**: **Less Fit (physically & mentally)**; **More Obese**; **More Diseased**; **More Disabled – especially with chronic pain (especially in America)**; & **More Toxic (in our bodies, minds, & souls)**!

Have we really evolved? ☺   I understand a chimpanzee may share over 98% of a human's genes.   However, I also understand that a banana may share 70% of a human's genes!? ☺   Don't mean to add fuel to the fire.

Many strong believers of Darwin's theories will simply state that Darwin's theory DOES explain how our population has become "less fit."
Are the following behaviors genetic mutations:

- Laziness (physically & intellectually)?
- Gluttony?
- A lack of discipline (in our diets & exercise regimens)?
- Choosing to bombard your body, mind & soul with toxins?
- Choosing to become "_**FULL OF**_" the body mind, & soul toxins (analyzed in the 1st 3 chapters of this book)
- Choosing to avoid all of the "10 Non-Dietary Cleansing Methods" (analyzed in Chapter 5)?
- Choosing to avoid all the super-cleansing foods & supplements (illustrated in Chapter 6)?

- &/or consistently choosing to break all "10 Dietary Commandments" (chapter 5)? Even _if there were_ genes for these, **do they really enhance survival & reproduction**?! I learned a long time ago from a brilliant mentor of mine (Dr. Stanley Paris, PhD P.T.) that you can never win or lose a debate or argument. You need to simply present your case in the best manner.

Keep in mind I am severely over-simplifying Darwin's theory of evolution. I consider myself a child of God (believer in Christ) – as well as a scientist. As I mentioned earlier: most, if not all scientific laws have been confirmed by the bible (& vice versa). Scientific laws & God's living word go hand in hand. I believe Darwin's theory is one of the most brilliant _theories_ to ever come to the scientific community in the past 300 years!

Remember: **_God created & gave Darwin (& Nietzsche_**) amazing gifts (even if they or their "followers" never acknowledge the Giver) of brilliance to be able to write such brilliant books. However, many well-respected scientists have shown that evolution fails to answer many scientific questions. I believe children should be taught this theory. I believe Christian adults should educate themselves on this theory & be open-minded & open-hearted when discussing this topic with atheistic "evolutionists."

Think about where we are in American culture. It is acceptable to label a believer in Jesus Christ: "narrow-minded" & even "arrogant!?" It is also acceptable to label a "**_confirmed atheist_**": open-minded & humble!? Would this be true in America 100 years ago?

I don't like labels. As I mentioned in chapter 2, I believe our 2 most important identities to God is whether you have already accepted Jesus Christ as your personal Lord & savoir – or you have not done so yet. Questions are the key to opening up the mind. We should allow questions to be asked by everyone about all things. That opens up our mind & soul. If you want to see me as the world sees me – you can label me. I am not a "Christian Scientist." Some label me as a "scientific Messianic Jew." However, my **_most important identity_** is a "scientific **_Christian_**!" ☺

The whole purpose of science is to ask questions & learn more. Christians should be open-minded (& open-hearted) to have evolution taught to children. Shouldn't "evolutionists" be open-minded to also have "creationism" taught to children?! Can't we all just get along? ☺

The rising cost of Obesity

Obesity has been cited as a contributing factor to approximately 100,000-400,000 deaths in the U.S. per year (as of 2005).[7] This approximate number is rising every year as obesity rates seem to be rising every year (for the past 50+ years) in the United States.[2,7] Obesity has increased health care use & expenditures costing society $117 Billion (estimated in 2006)[8] or $147 Billion (estimated in 2008)[2] in:[2,8]

- Direct costs: preventative, diagnostic, & treatment services for obesity-related medical problems. **Obesity-related medical problems include: disability, type II diabetes, hypertension, cardiovascular disease, ischemic stroke, & certain types of cancers** – some of the leading causes of death.
- & indirect costs: absenteeism & loss of future earnings due to premature death.

2 RECOGNIZED reasons WHY Obesity rates have been rising

Obesity (similar to cigarette smoking – including passive smoking) may be considered one of the most PREVENTABLE causes of DEATH in the western world![2,7,8]   There are many recognized reasons why we Obesity rates are rising.   They include social & cultural.   A sedentary lifestyle (lack of exercise) & over-eating (being a "glutton") are two major contributing factors of Obesity that have become "acceptable" *SINS* (see chapter 1) in our culture.

1.   **Sedentary Lifestyle (lack of exercise) or "Laziness"** has become an acceptable SIN (mentioned in chapter 1) in America's culture – contributing to our rise in Obesity (& diseases).

We are "***FULL OF***" Physical Laziness.   As mentioned in chapters 1 & 3, physical inactivity (a form of laziness) – not achieving 150 minutes of moderate exercise a week – is a major contributor of:[9,10]

- Major diseases like heart disease (including, but not limited to ischemic strokes, hypertension, etc.) Type 2 diabetes, & breast & colon cancer.
- The death of 5.3 million people in the world in 2008 (compared to 5 million from smoking).

This physical inactivity also predisposes you to obesity - which predisposes you to the abovementioned diseases!   This is a dangerous cycle of physical inactivity leading to obesity & obesity-related diseases – which makes it more difficult to exercise (which leads to more obesity & diseases)!

The expansion of technology may be a factor for this.   Every American I know uses a machine to wash their clothes & dishes.   As you read "About the Author" in this book, you will see I have invented robots in 1990 that can mow the lawn, vacuum, be converted into a motorized wheelchair, walker, & even type for disabled individuals!   Should we blame robotic inventors like I for our lack of exercising?! ☺   I think not!   My robotic inventions were designed to help people ***with disabilities*** become more Independent & "able."   They were NOT designed to help able-bodies people become lazy!

Americans in the 1950s (& Europeans – at least 20 years ago) led more active lifestyles – walking & bike riding more than we currently do.   Even Americans that go to fitness centers usually drive there!   We have replaced walking & bike riding with automobile driving.   We have replaced stair negotiating with elevators &/or escalators.   We used to get up from our couches to change the television channel.   Instead of playing sports with our friends & family, we get together at restaurants.   Events are planned around eating.

2.   **Being a "Glutton" (Eating Excessively)** has become another acceptable SIN (mentioned in chapter1) in America's culture – contributing to our rise in Obesity.

We are "***FULL OF***" Gluttony – a currently acceptable sin in America (as well as other parts of the world).   It is no coincidence that these two sins are grouped together in the bible.   Has America become a bunch of sinful "***lazy gluttons?***" (Titus 1:12)

American adults are consuming 20% more calories than 50 years ago![11]   One reason for this may be that portions in restaurants have **quadrupled since the 1950s!**[12]   The 400% increase in restaurant portion sizes since the 1950s may be analogous to the increase in size of our televisions.   Americans simply desire/demand larger televisions – as well as restaurant portions.   Many of us leave restaurants - or our own living/dining rooms (after over-eating) – waddling (with our belts & pant buttons un-done).   This puts excessive stress on our gastrointestinal, immune, musculoskeletal, & cardiovascular systems.   Remember your brain's satiating sensors (possibly located in the ventromedial nucleus of the hypothalamus – from my days in college psychology courses) have a delayed reaction (20 minutes or so) & will not tell you that "*YOU'RE FULL*" - immediately after swallowing your food! **If you become _full_ - while you are eating, you have eaten too much!**

Besides the delayed reaction time it takes your brain to feel satiated, there are some other under-recognized reasons WHY we over-eat - including:

- **Poor absorption of the foods/beverages we consume**.   Because we break all of the "10 Dietary Commandments" (mentioned in Chapter 5) on a daily (if not multiple times per day) basis, we are NOT optimally absorbing the food we consume.   Remember, you are what you ABSORB – not what you eat!   If the food/beverages you consume do not get digested/absorbed, they stay in your intestines (as intestinal putrefaction). Thus: you become "*FULL OF IT*!"   Because your body does not ABSORB the nutrients it needs (from even healthful foods & supplements), your brain tells you to continue to eat/"over-eat" in an attempt to receive them.   The end result = over-eating (gluttony)!

- **Avoiding "breaking-the-fast" (breakfast) &/or eating only a huge dinner**.   If you avoid breakfast or wait too long between small meals, you're probably depriving the body of necessary food/nutrients.   Your body may go into starvation mode & try to store your fat (become "*FULL OF*" fat). This slows down your metabolism even more! I believe this is a huge mistake Americans make!   Many Americans eat a very small (or no) breakfast & a huge dinner!   I believe this is diametrically opposed to good healthful sense!   We must flip that habit around.   A sensible breakfast rich with healthful protein, fat, fiber, enzymes, & nutrients will **give** you energy & help cleanse your body.   An *excessively large dinner (over-eating* to make up for starving your body for the past 24 hours) may be stored as mostly intestinal putrefaction or body fat!

- **Trying to "fill a void" in our lives, many have replaced GOD with an addiction for over-eating**!   *We are all like sheep have gone astray.*   When we have problems (sadness, anxiety, or any other kind of stress in our life), we will often "over-eat" as an "answer/solution."   Besides focusing on what, how, & when you are eating: we also should ask "*What's EATING YOU?*!"   In the Old Testament, they used to fast when mourning!   These days it is acceptable - & usually encouraged - to commit gluttony when mourning!

- **Lack of discipline to NOT "over-eat."**   This is another under-recognized SIN (analyzed in Chapter 1) that can lead to Obesity – as well as other diseases.   Our flesh is weak.   We should *not lead ourselves to temptation*.   I can go years without ever eating junk food.   However, if you put it in front of my face (& I see & smell it), I may be tempted to eat the junk food.   Try not to focus on the junk food.   Try to focus on healthful foods (which can be even more delicious than junk foods).   Try to focus on God & His temple – your body!

If you believe that avoiding physical laziness & gluttony (both part of "Dietary Commandment #1") are the only 2 causes of obesity, then "*YOU ARE FULL OF IT!*"

10   Under-recognized reasons WHY Obesity rates are rising

1.   The relationships between our nation's largest God-deficit leading to our largest:

a.   **Health, financial, & moral deficits** (discussed in chapter 2).

As explained in chapter 2, the 4 abovementioned "deficits" are all **psychological/physiological "stressors"** connected to each other (&,

123

unfortunately, rising every year). Our God-deficit is larger than ever in our nation's history (&, unfortunately, rising every year –as analyzed in chapter 2). Therefore: We are also more obese, diseased, & disabled with chronic pain –than ever before in our nation's history. Our anti-Godly tax & government policies (from 1997 to current) have created **large financial stress** to most Americans. The "poor" (& those not-so poor) eat fast foods. Fast foods usually cost less money & time (which in our fast-paced society: "time = money"). These fast foods are usually high in calories & low in nutrients. Your body doesn't receive the nutrients it needs, so it tells the body to over-eat (which predisposes one to obesity, diseases, & even chronic pain).

2. **The mind & soul toxins discussed in chapters 1 & 2 that create "stress" can increase the risk of obesity (as well as diseases & chronic pain)**

This **stress** (as mentioned in chapter 3) causes us to increase our cortisol production &, therefore, **store more body fat**.[13,14] Stress also stimulates the sympathetic nervous system (the "flight or fight" reaction). This creates poor digestion & absorption of the foods we consume. This poor absorption creates intestinal putrefaction (which slows down your metabolism) &, therefore, increases our risk for **obesity** (as well as diseases & even chronic pain). Remember, any SIN is a direct mind & soul toxin (a "stressor") & an indirect body toxin ("stressor") – which can, therefore, trigger the "physiological stress reaction" predisposing us to diseases (including obesity & even chronic pain).[13,14]

3. **The non-dietary toxins our bodies are bombarded & flooded with & "*FULL OF*" (mentioned in chapter 3).**

The non-dietary direct body toxins (mentioned in chapter 3) we're exposed to = **stressors** that have an accumulative negative effect on our health – as well as our weight. We can absorb these direct body toxins via inhalation & even our skin! Consider **how many pounds** of cigarette smoke, gasoline, pesticides, BPS, BPA, Volatile Organic Compounds (VOCs), toxic perfumes, soaps, shampoos, & other airborne &/or tactile toxins do we inhale, swallow, &/or absorb via our skin on an annual basis? **How many pounds** do we unfortunately absorb & store in all different parts of our body (not only our intestines, lungs, & brain –but everywhere – don't forget the skin is the largest organ)!

4. **Hypothyroidism** (mentioned in chapter 3) possibly due to:[15]
- The excess of fluoride, chlorine, & bromine;
- & the deficiency of iodide & iodine.

This "imbalance" may increase the risk of fatigue & hypothyroidism (as well as atherosclerosis, thyroid cancer, & breast cancer)![15,16] Increased fatigue will result in lethargy & a lack of exercise (a recognized cause of weight gain). Hypothyroidism may result in a decreased metabolism.[15] This decreased metabolism results in decreased digestion & absorption of our food (resulting in intestinal putrefaction). This may be why people with hypothyroidism may suffer with cold-intolerance, constipation, recurrent infections, & difficulty losing (or gaining) weight![15]

5. **Lumbar & Cervical Spinal Stenosis** (mentioned in chapter 3)

As mentioned in chapter 3, the dysfunctions associated with these can be treated by a qualified physical therapist (see chapter 3 for more details). Muscle cells burn calories (even when sleeping). Motor nerve compression (via Lumbar & Cervical spinal stenosis) is the number one reason (in my strong opinion) for muscle weakness as one gets over the age of 60. Disuse atrophy (AKA: physical laziness = "*if you don't use it = you lose it*") should be considered the number two reason. The muscle weakness caused by spinal stenosis can cause significant muscle atrophy &, in severe cases, partial or complete muscle paralysis. Thus, spinal stenosis **can decrease the**

calories you burn (which can lead to weight gain)!   Spinal stenosis also limits what fat & calorie-burning exercises you can & should do (see chapters 3 & 5 for what are "good" versus "bad" exercises based on the age of 55).   This may be one reason why the "over 60" age group has the highest rate of obesity in the U.S.A.![2]

6.   Breaking the "10 Dietary Commandments" shown in Chapter 5 & Avoiding "Super-Cleansing Foods/Supplements"(Chapter 6)

The poor quality of our foods –processed, dead, genetically-modified, & filled with ("***FULL OF***") sugar, high fructose corn syrup, antibiotics, hormones, pesticides, MSG, mercury, artificial coloring & flavoring, & other toxins is an under-recognized culprit of obesity (& other diseases).   Consider the fact that the average American consumes 53 gallons of soda & 24 pounds of artificial sweeteners (like aspartame, "Splenda," "Sweet N Low, & Saccharin) per year.[17]   ***The pounds of these man-made chemicals have a negative accumulative effect on our health,*** (see Chapter 3) ***as well as our waistlines (or hips & overall weight)!***   The weight alone of these substances (possibly hundreds of pounds consumed each year) has to have a negative impact on our weight!

All the sugars we eat - also feed yeast & fungus (like candida albicans) &, therefore, increase the risk of candidiasis.[18]   This can cause gastrointestinal bloating, constipation, & other gastrointestinal problems – as well as many other symptoms & disease(s).[18]   This yeast &/or fungus-induced bloating, gas, & constipation slows down your metabolism &, therefore, increases the risk of weight gain – as well as diseases.

The poor state of mind (with toxic minds & souls) in which we consume our foods under high-stress & arguing is also a culprit to poor absorption (&, therefore, intestinal putrefaction & a slower metabolism).

The poor manner in which we combine our foods is another culprit to poor absorption (&, therefore, intestinal putrefaction & a slower metabolism).

Breaking all "10 Dietary Commandments" will have an accumulative negative effect on our health - & our weight!

The hormones injected into many of our poultry & other animal products may be harmful to your health & your waistline.   The plastic containers & bottles we eat & drink out of (already mentioned in chapter 3) may contain Bisphenol A – an artificial hormone that acts like estrogen (& can increase body fat in men).[19]

7.   "You Are Not Fat" – But You Look it!

No – this is not a section on fashion –although clothes can make a huge difference. As mentioned in chapter 3, poor posture can cause serious diseases.   Poor posture can cause spinal stenosis – which (as analyzed in greater detail in chapter 3) can cause muscle weakness (& in severe cases, atrophy & even paralysis) &, therefore lead to weight gain (as previously mentioned).   In addition, poor posture (as mentioned in chapter 3) makes you look "heavier" than you actually are!   ***The sway back posture (mentioned in chapter 3) makes your belly & buttocks "stick out" & appear to be larger than they actually are!   The "hunched over" thoracic posture & forward head posture (mentioned in chapter 3) make you look decades older & less attractive to the opposite sex!***

Do I NOW have your attention?   Yes – good posture (discussed in chapter 3) makes you look thinner, younger, & more attractive.   To encourage/motivate my patients to improve their posture:

- I often imitate their poor postural habits as we both look in the mirror.

- Then I demonstrate good posture on myself & them (via the postural exercises mentioned in chapter 3).
- Then I ask them questions such as: "Which person do you want to dance with? Which person do you want to introduce to your friends & family members?" ☺

8. **Avoiding all "10 Non-Dietary Cleansing Methods"** shown in chapter 5. This can hurt your health & your belt!
9. **& 10. The fact that we are also "_FULL OF_" more chronic body pain & diseases than ever before**.

I do not believe that it is simply a coincidence that we are "**_FULL OF_**" more **obesity, diseases, & chronic pain** than ever before. Chronic body pain & diseases can interfere with your ability to perform fat-burning exercises –as well as your overall activity level. The strong correlation between diseases, obesity, & chronic pain is analyzed in greater detail in the next section of this chapter.

II.   The Answer = The "_FULL OF IT_ Level of Disease, Obesity, &/or Chronic Pain"

This is the "Level" at which the accumulation & compounding effect of the combination of all the body, mind, & soul toxins causes or exacerbates disease(s), obesity, &/or chronic pain in that individual.   This "Level" of toxicity creates an **inflammatory state** which adds to this "Level." Therefore, this "Level" can **cause, exacerbate, &/or even keep one** diseased, obese, &/or chronic pain!   **WHY or HOW someone developed diseases** (including acute diseases such as the common cold, influenza, acne, boils, etc. - & chronic diseases such as – cancer, multiple sclerosis, heart disease, arthritis, etc.), **obesity, &/or chronic pain** is best explained by this "**_FULL OF IT_ Level**" better than any other scientific principle I am familiar with!   This section of this chapter is perfectly placed here because it beautifully summarizes how:

- Being "**_FULL OF_**" all the body, mind, & soul toxins ("**_IT_**") – illustrated in Chapters 1-3 (as well as the 1st section of this chapter) – to this "**Level**" have led to our being "**_FULL OF_**" more diseases, obesity, & chronic pain than ever before.
- The next Chapters will show non-Dietary (Chapter 5) & Dietary (Chapters 5-7) cleansing methods to reduce &, theoretically, eliminate this "**Level**" of toxicity.   Said differently: God wants us to use the "natural" & the "super-natural" to maximally cleanse (& optimize the health of) our bodies, minds, & souls!

There is a **strong connection between** the fact that we are "_FULL OF_" more **disease, obesity, & chronic pain** than ever before. These are not simply coincidences.   There are physiological & psychological problems that accompany all of the three. These problems that are associated with one of the above can exacerbate or even cause the other two.   **Depression** is probably the best example of how

all three of the above are connected strongly together.   As mentioned previously, if you are in chronic pain:
- You may take toxic pain killers which can lead to diseases
- You may not exercise enough or effectively/properly which can lead to obesity & diseases
- & you may be depressed which may lead to more pain killers, less exercise, more diseases, weight gain, & even more chronic pain! Thus, the cycle continues.

As mentioned previously in this chapter, if you are obese:
- You may get diabetes, heart disease, stroke, & certain types of cancers – as well as become disabled.
- You may exacerbate or even cause body pains (discussed in chapter 3).
- & you may be depressed – which can lead to more diseases, chronic pain, & even more weight gain! Thus, the cycle continues.

If you are diseased (from cancer to the common cold):
- You may not be able to exercise enough or properly which may lead to weight gain &/or chronic body pains.
- You may become depressed which may lead to more chronic pain, weight gain, & diseases! Thus, the cycle continues.

As there is a strong connection between the body, mind, & soul – there is also a strong connection between diseases, obesity, & chronic pain.   The above connection creates the following questions:
- Is **depression** a body, mind, &/or soul toxin?   By now: you should realize the answer = "yes" = all three.
- Is **depression** a cause or a result of diseases, chronic pain, &/or obesity?   By now, you should realize the answer = "yes" = both.

Remember from chapter 3, the CDC reported that over 50% of American adults had at least one chronic disease.   The psychological & physiological **RESPONSES** to having a life-changing chronic disease = **depression**, anxiety, deconditioning, poor sleep, neuroendocrine changes, & **more STRESS** (which repeats the disease, obesity, & pain cycle)![14]   Consider the following relationships:
- "**Depression** (considered a psychological **disease**) may be a risk factor for the onset of **chronic pain**. Most patients with chronic pain are depressed, & most of the depressed patients had depression before the onset of **chronic pain**."[20]
- "The greater the severity of the **depression**: the more elevated **inflammatory markers** – such as C-reactive protein (CRP) - are."[20]
- Studies have shown that **high CRP levels** significantly increase the risk of death from a **heart attack or stroke**![14,21]

The "**FULL OF IT** Level of Disease, Obesity, &/or Chronic Pain" is the level at which the **accumulation** & **compounding** of the **combination** of all the **body, mind, & soul** toxins reach high enough to exacerbate or cause disease(s),

127

obesity, &/or chronic pain.   This is the "Level" of toxicity that puts the body in a state of **inflammation**.   Being at or above this "***FULL OF IT* Level**" for a prolonged period of time: puts the body in a state of "**chronic inflammation**" – *keeping you* **at or above** this "*Level*" ***chronically***.   Therefore, this state of "*chronic inflammation*" (as mentioned in chapter 3), can cause **chronic diseases** (&/or *keep one* "chronically diseased").   These chronic diseases (already mentioned in chapter 3) include: Diabetes; Heart disease; Stroke; Cancer; Arthritis; & Neurological Diseases like Parkinson's, Alzheimer's, Multiple Sclerosis, & ALS ("Lou Gehrig's Diseases").

These chronic diseases (as mentioned above) can also lead to obesity &/or chronic pain (which adds to the "toxic load"/stress even more).   Thus, the cycle continues.   The psychological & physiological **responses** (mentioned in Chapter 3) to having a chronic disease create more **stress** – elevating the "*Level*" of ***body, mind, & soul*** toxicity!   This added **stress** (as mentioned in chapter 3) can cause more diseases, weight gain, &/or chronic pain!   Therefore: reaching at or above this "***FULL OF IT*** Level" creates **a dangerous cycle of more disease(s), weight gain, &/or chronic pain**!

The word "**accumulation**" is underlined to emphasize that it is our "storing" (becoming "***FULL OF***") & adding of these toxins that is so detrimental to our health.   We can try our best to avoid body, mind, & soul toxins.   However, it is the fact that we are "holding on to"/saving & adding these toxins to each other that is so detrimental to our health.

The word "**compounding**" is underlined to emphasize that the accumulation of different toxins has a multiplying detrimental effect (a "toxic load") on our health.   For example, being exposed to & "storing" (becoming "***FULL OF***") lead with mercury makes the mercury 100 times more toxic.[14]   Combining drugs with each other usually makes them more toxic.   In addition, combining intellectual & spiritual toxins (sins) with each other also has a multiplying detrimental effect on our health.

The word "**combination**" is underlined to emphasize that the combining/mixing of all 3 different types of toxins is most responsible for destroying our health.   Because there is a strong connection between the body, mind, & soul:

- Every direct body toxin hurts the body – as well as the mind & soul to some extent.

- Every mind toxin hurts the mind – as well as the body & soul to some level.

- Every soul toxin hurts the soul – as well as the body & mind to some level.   Soul toxins can't hurt your spirit - if you're *filled with the Holy Spirit*.   However, they can destroy your soul.

- We should NOT blame diseases, obesity, or chronic pain on being "***FULL OF***" one body, mind, or soul toxin (or even one type/category of toxin).   It is the **combination** of all the different body, mind, & soul toxins that destroys our health the most!

As mentioned throughout this book, we are bombarded with (&, therefore, "***FULL OF***") more body, mind, & soul toxins than ever before!   Said differently, we are more "***FULL OF IT***" than ever before!   Therefore, **more people are at or above this "*FULL OF IT* Level of Disease, Obesity, &/or Chronic Pain**" than ever before in our world's history.   This is why more people are diseased, obese, & in chronic body pain than ever before in our nation/world!

Staying at or above this "***FULL OF IT* Level of Disease, Obesity, &/or Chronic Pain**" for a prolonged period of time puts the body in a state of **chronic inflammation** (creating continual "**physiological stress reactions**").   The more "***FULL OF IT***" we are: the more

128

stress & less healing our bodies can achieve. This is one detrimental cycle.   As mentioned in chapter 3, this "physiological stress reaction" causes more symptoms &, eventually, diseases (including obesity & chronic body pains).   Therefore, staying at or above this "***FULL OF IT*** **Level**" creates another **detrimental cycle** to our health where we get more **diseases, obesity, & chronic pain**!

This is the "**level**" (unfortunately) at which most Americans **begin** to get concerned for their health. This is when many Americans *finally* seek the help of health care providers. As our health care system is diseased-based (versus health based), **this is (unfortunately) the level** at which many Americans find out:

- They have diabetes – *then start* to try to reduce their sugar consumption.
- They have cancer or heart disease – *then start* to eat right & exercise.
- Their body pains are not going away after 12 weeks – & *then start* to seek the help of a health care provider.
- They are obese versus simply being "over-weight" - & *then try* seriously to lose the excess weight & body fat.

Since our health is mostly destroyed by the accumulation & compounding effect of the combination of these body, mind, & soul toxins: cleansing should be done using a combination of dietary & non-dietary methods (mentioned in chapters 5 & 6).   Cleansing should be done using the natural & "super-natural" (mentioned in chapters 5 &6).   We may cleanse ourselves so that we become **just below the** "***FULL OF IT*** **Level**." This does not mean we have achieved optimal health. Remember: optimal health is **NOT** the absence of disease.   People **just below** this "***FULL OF IT*** **Level**" may become bombarded with, & therefore, "***FULL OF***" some direct body toxins (such as pesticides, heavy toxic metals, industrial chemicals, poor posture, etc.), mind toxins (such as financial stressors due to our Anti-Godly tax & governmental policies), &/or soul toxins (such as fear, greed, hatred of others, etc.).   The addition/accumulation & compounding of the combination of these body, mind, & soul toxins can raise our toxicity to (or above) the "***FULL OF IT*** **Level of Disease, Obesity, &/or Chronic Pain**!"

The true cause of diseases, obesity, &/or chronic pain can be explained best by this "***FULL OF IT*** **Level**" better than any other law/theory I am familiar with. I consider this concept a "law" – but the scientist in me labels it a "theory, concept, or principal."   Consider the examples shown below.

Example # 1 = "Mr. Chronic Pain."   Regarding "this level" consider the following simplified example of Mr. Pain suffering with chronic right shoulder pain.   Mr. Pain is over 70 with degenerative disc disease in the neck leaving less space for the nerves in his neck. He has a poor "forward head postural habit" (more than a fist distance between chin & chest: AKA increased cervical lordotic posture) & a poor habit of tilting/side bending his neck to the right (possibly because his left eye sees better or he compensates for side bending the lower part of his spine to the left). The poor postural habits alone can cause right cervical radiculopathy. This can cause:

- nerve pain in the right shoulder (as well as anywhere from the right side of his head/neck to the right fingertips)
- abnormal sensations (numbness, absent sensation, pins & needles = AKA "paresthesias," &/or hypersensitivity to touch, etc.) from the right side of his head/neck to his right fingertips
- &/or muscle weakness in the right shoulder (as well as his entire right upper extremity). This weakness can be as severe as partial or even complete

129

paralysis.   This weakness can also lead to severe shoulder muscle strains. The more demand Mr. Pain puts on his shoulder muscles, the more likely he is to strain/partially tear his right shoulder muscles. Thus the pain cycle continues.

Realize this example simply blamed the poor postural habits - which can be changed if he has enough mobility to "get out" of this poor postural habit.   If Mr. Pain does not move out of this poor neck postural habit –he may develop a severe limitation in neck mobility (arthro-kinematic hypo-mobility & adaptive shortening of his neck muscles – especially on his right side).   This continues to encourage more right nerve compression – continuing the nerve compression (&, therefore the pain) cycle continues.

Mr. Pain's right shoulder **muscle strain** (as mentioned in chapter 3) can be described economically as **"demand"** on the muscle **greater than the "supply" (strength)** of that muscle/muscle group.   Right neck nerve compression will obviously lower his supply/strength.   A deficiency of healthful protein in the diet can lower his supply.   Taking some prescription antibiotics (such as levaquin-derivative antibiotics) may predispose Mr. Pain to muscle strains/tears – lowering his "supply." Taking other prescribed medications (such as statins to reduce cholesterol levels) may also predispose Mr. Pain to muscle strains/tears – lowering his supply/strength.   If he adds some resistive demand to that muscle (picking up an object, etc.), he may go above that "***FULL OF IT* Level**" & re-tear that muscle.   If he adds some other body toxins (like toxic heavy metals, industrial chemicals, pollutants, etc.) & some psychological stressors (mind & soul toxins mentioned in chapters 1 & 2) – the demand grows (raising the "level" even higher) - & the cycle of chronic pain (as well as obesity &/or disease) continues/worsens - & grows!

Mr. Pain's reaction to having this chronic right shoulder pain will probably be lack of active shoulder mobility (as well as an overall lack of exercise), fear/anxiety, & depression.   The lack of active shoulder mobility can lead to a "frozen shoulder" (arthrokinematic hypo-mobility of his right glenohumeral joint & possibly other shoulder complex articulations).   This will increase demand on the shoulder muscles leading to more strains/partial tears of his right shoulder muscles.   Thus the pain cycle continues.   The lack of overall exercise, fear, & depression (all "sins" discussed in chapter 1) can lead to more chronic pain (as well as obesity & other diseases). Adding more body, mind, & soul toxins (like those mentioned in chapters 1-3) elevates Mr. Pain's "***FULL OF IT* Level of chronic pain**" even higher!   Thus, the cycle of chronic pain (as well as diseases & possibly even obesity) continues!

So **what causes Mr. Pain's chronic pain**?   It is the <u>accumulation & compounding</u> effect of the <u>combination</u> of the <u>body mostly</u> (as well as the <u>mind & soul toxins</u>) reaching his "***FULL OF IT* Level of Chronic Pain**."

Example # 2 = John Doe wants to know **WHY** he developed **pancreatic cancer** at age 40?   He was born with a certain amount of toxicity (from the mother's womb – as mentioned in chapter 3).   He may or may not have a "genetic predisposition" for this cancer.   By age 40: the accumulation & compounding effect of the combination of all the body, mind, & soul toxins reached his "***FULL OF IT* Level**" of pancreatic cancer.   When he reaches this "Level" & develops this disease, then he becomes concerned about how to cleanse himself from this toxicity!

Example # 3 = Jane Doe wants to know **WHY** she developed **Multiple Sclerosis** at age 35 - or why her friend developed **Parkinson's** at age 65. This "**FULL OF IT** Level" concept is the answer to **why we get any chronic diseases** (as well as chronic pain &/ obesity) in my strong opinion.

Example # 4 = "Mr. **Acute Infection**" & "Mrs. **Acute communicable disease**" want to know **WHY** they developed these acute communicable diseases. Again, this "**FULL OF IT** Level" concept is the answer to **why we get any acute – or chronic diseases** (as well as chronic pain &/or obesity) in my strong opinion.

Example # 5 = Mr. & Mrs. America want to know WHY they are both obese. Again, this "**FULL OF IT** Level" is the answer to **why we become obese** (as well as diseases &/or in chronic pain) in my strong opinion.

Therefore, our traditional American "Health" Care system addresses disease(s), obesity, &/or chronic pain with the following limitations:

- We often evaluate & "treat" the abovementioned with more direct body toxins (toxic radiological exams, medications, &/or surgeries) that elevates our "**FULL OF IT** Level" even more! This is the **dangerous/harmful cycle** the majority of American adults are currently (unfortunately) faced with.
- We often mask the symptoms of chronic pain with more direct body toxins (oral, transdermal, &/or injectable analgesic &/or anti-inflammatory medications) versus addressing the arthrokinematic dysfunctions (& other direct body – as well as mind & soul – toxins) we are "**FULL OF**." These toxic meds elevate our "**FULL OF IT** Level" even more.
- We often treat Alzheimer's disease & other dementia-related illnesses with toxic meds that add to & elevate our "**FULL OF IT** Level" even more. This may be why these meds often worsen the dementia & the patient's overall physical & cognitive functions.
- We often treat cancer, osteoarthritis, & neurological diseases (like Parkinson's, Multiple Sclerosis, & ALS) with toxic meds that elevate our "**FULL OF IT** Level" even more.
- We often attempt to mask the symptoms of depression (often with toxic pharmaceutical anti-depressants) elevating our "**FULL OF IT** Level" even more! Depression (as discussed previously) may be considered a risk factor – as well as a result – of chronic pain, obesity, &/or diseases!

In summary, we have a symptom &/or disease-based "health" care system versus a health-based system. Until we choose to focus on a truly holistic approach & recognize how "**FULL OF IT**" we are:

- Our "Level" of toxicity will continue to grow like a ***flood*** of body, mind, & soul toxins in every town in America (if not the world) – ***drowning*** (destroying the health) of everyone!
- & our "Level" of ignorance &/or apathy about the abovementioned "toxic ***flood:***"
  - o Makes us no different from those who drowned/died during the days of Noah.
  - o & also allows the "Level" of toxicity to grow higher and higher elevating the "***FULL OF IT*** Level" for everyone in the world!

Consider Mr. Pain. He may see an allopathic or osteopathic physician specializing in one area of the body – but not looking at him "Holistically." Mr. Pain may see the following physicians:

- Rheumatologist, pain management physician (often an anesthesiologist specializing in pain management), physiatrist, orthopedic surgeon, neurologist, neurological surgeon, general practitioner, psychiatrist, etc.

Mr. Pain may also see a physical therapist (often referred to by the abovementioned physicians) – or a whole host of other health care providers (including "alternative" practitioners). Medicine/health care is very "territorial," & everyone wants a piece of the "chronic pain pie!"

Mr. Pain may receive a number of toxic radiological exams – none of which reveal his arthrokinematic dysfunction (the _major_ cause of his chronic pain in this example)! In other words, these wonderful pictures don't tell anyone the intimate motion of his joints (based on his age, sex, & body type). Some "health" care providers believe they can _assume_ how the joints move arthrokinematically based on these pictures. However, these providers should be considered (how can I say this without offending them?): "_**FULL OF IT**_!"

From the diverse group of health care providers, Mr. Pain may eventually receive the following diagnoses:

- Osteoarthritis right shoulder; strain/pain right shoulder; right rotator cuff tear; frozen shoulder; right cervical radiculopathy; cervical spinal stenosis; depression; &/or anxiety.

From the diverse group of allopathic & osteopathic physicians, Mr. Pain may (as already mentioned) receive toxic pain &/or anti-inflammatory meds (&, eventually, anti-depressant &/or anti-anxiety meds) which "mask" the symptoms caused by the arthro-kinematic dysfunctions. These meds also elevate his "_**FULL OF IT**_ Level of chronic pain" even more – continuing the cycle of chronic pain (& possibly helping to lead to more diseases &/or obesity). Many health care professionals simply try to treat the patient's pain because they do not have the: Time; Understanding; Education &/or qualifications to treat **ALL** the causes of the patient's pain. The best clinicians should realize that Mr. Pain has ALL of these diagnoses & utilize a team approach.

The best health care provider to address Mr. Pain's orthopedic arthrokinematic dysfunctions (in my humble opinion) is a physical therapist who continued their education after graduating as a physical therapist to become a certified specialist in orthopedics & manual therapy. This physical therapist should be able to look at Mr. Pain truly holistically to evaluate & treat all the above diagnoses (except for the depression & anxiety diagnoses of course – which may improve greatly or even be eliminated when the arthrokinematic dysfunctions are eliminated).

In defense of my humble opinion, consider the facts that Mr. Pain may need skilled physical therapy treatment consisting of:

- Manual therapy (often with the use of ultrasound as a preparatory deep heating modality) to increase the mobility of the hypo-mobile cervical joints not allowing Mr. Pain to change his posture to decrease the pressure on his right cervical nerves.
- Manual therapy to increase mobility of any arthrokinematic hypomobility in the glenohumeral joint (as well as any other shoulder "complex" articulations).
- Postural re-education training to decrease the pressure on the right cervical nerves when sitting, standing, lying down, etc.

- Self-passive range of motion (PROM) to maintain the ROM gains in his right shoulder in between & after therapy sessions.
- Motor nerve electrical stimulation to increase the strength of the right shoulder muscles (as well as any other muscles weakened from the right cervical radiculopathy).
- Other right upper extremity strengthening therapeutic exercises usually in a pain-free, low ROM zone.
- Home exercise program instructions to: Maintain the gains made in Range of motion neck & right shoulder; Preserve, & gradually improve his strength & posture on his own.   Remember: the person most responsible for Mr. Pain's health care = Mr. Pain.

The above treatment dramatically lowers Mr. Pain's "**_FULL OF IT_** Level of Chronic Pain."   But to what extent will the treatment lower it?   Besides the orthopedic arthrokinematic dysfunctions, Mr. Pain is "**_FULL OF_**" other body (as well as mind & soul) toxins that elevate his "**_FULL OF IT_** Level!"   The best health care should also involve **educating** Mr. Pain about all the non-dietary & dietary cleansing methods to optimize the health of his entire body, mind, & soul.   Besides following all "10 Dietary Commandments," Mr. Pain may also benefit from:
- Methylsulfonylmethane (MSM) 2 grams/day to possibly help repair the partial tears/muscle strains
- & anti-inflammatory foods such as organic turmeric, ginger, walnuts, & flaxseed.   Realize these anti-inflammatory foods have anticoagulant properties (&, therefore, a bleeding risk – analyzed further in "Dietary Commandment #6").   Mr. Pain may also benefit from other super-cleansing foods/supplements mentioned in chapter 6.

By looking at Mr. Pain holistically ("as a whole") – educating him on all the dietary & non-dietary cleansing methods – we are providing the best "health" care for Mr. Pain!   Then (& only then) are we providing the tools/education to helping Mr. Pain maximally lower his "_FULL OF IT_ Level of Chronic Pain (as well as diseases &/or obesity)!"

Regarding the "**_FULL OF IT_** Level," are you more at risk for disease(s) [& if so – which disease(s)], obesity, or chronic pain [& if so – what part(s) of the body will you "feel" the pain]?   This brings back the old debate "nurture versus nature" (of which, I attribute much more of the blame on nurture). Your risk for the above should be seen as some type of a combination of the following:
- **"Nature:" Genetic predispositions** to **diseases &/or obesity** seem obvious.   Certain people have a genetic advantage or disadvantage to absorbing certain super-cleansing foods/supplements versus absorbing certain toxic foods.   This is why **_nutrition is an artistic science_** in my opinion. Certain people possess superior genes to actually absorb & benefit from consuming "highly toxic mucus-forming foods" that are harmful to most (this is shown in "Dietary Commandment # 4")   Certain people have a genetic advantage or disadvantage for triggering a disease by being "**_FULL OF_**" certain

body toxins (like certain heavy metals).   If certain diseases &/or obesity are prevalent in your family, you are probably more at risk for these than most.
However, there may also be some **genetic predispositions for chronic pain!**? Consider the following:

- You may have genetic predispositions for your intervertebral discs shrinking more than most do (usually after age 55). This leaves less space for the nerve (narrows the intervertebral foramen) predisposing you to nerve compression (which can cause weakness, abnormal sensations, &/or **PAIN** where the nerve(s) travel to/from)!
- You may have genetic predispositions to increased osteoporotic compression fractures in the thoracic vertebra.   This creates an increased thoracic kyphosis – which can predispose you to:
    o Cervical nerve compression - which can be painful (as well as possibly cause muscle weakness &/or abnormal sensations) in the neck, same side of head to fingertips.   Any nerve compression-induced muscle weakness can also predispose you to muscle strains in that area – which can also be painful.
    o Thoracic muscle strains.
    o & even an increased lumbar lordosis (usually a risk factor for thoracic kyphosis as your body tries to compensate for the increased lumbar lordosis) as the lumbar spine can, theoretically compensate for the increased thoracic kyphosis. This increased lumbar lordosis can, theoretically, cause lumbar nerve compression - which can cause pain (as well as abnormal sensations &/or muscle weakness) from low back to toes. Any nerve compression-induced muscle weakness can also predispose you to muscle strains in that area – which can also be painful.
- "**Nurture**."   This can include the following:
    o The direct body toxins "***YOU'RE FULL OF***" you receive from when you're in **your mother's womb**. The "transferring" of the direct body toxins the biological mother is "***FULL OF***" to the fetus (as well as the toxins the biological father is "***FULL OF***" - which can damage the DNA of his sperm &, therefore harm the newborn) **should be blamed on "nurture**" – **not nature**!   Does the father have a genetic predisposition for smoking, spraying pesticides in his home, consuming man-made toxic foods?
    o The direct body, mind, & soul toxins you have been/are/& will be bombarded with & become "***FULL OF***."   This includes the above (which we have no control over – though the mother does before & during the pregnancy).   This also includes poor postural habits (an under-recognized body toxin analyzed in chapter 3) that we may have "learned" (AKA "mimicked") from our family members.   This also includes the food, water, & air we breathe in our homes, buildings, cities, etc.   This also includes the "sins" that our family, society, culture finds acceptable & bombards us with.
    o Choosing to avoid or become bombarded with (&, therefore) "***FULL OF***" all the body, mind, & soul toxins mentioned in chapters 1-3.

- Choosing to avoid or follow the "10 Non-Dietary Cleansing Methods" shown in chapter 5.
- Choosing to break or follow the "10 Dietary Commandments" shown in Chapter 5.
- Choosing to avoid or consume the "super-cleansing foods & supplements" illustrated in chapter 6.

As you can see, this book illustrates/demonstrates that we have much more control over our health than simply what our genes predispose us to.

As mentioned in the preface & in chapter 2: Society's apathy & acceptance of being "**_flooded_**" with body, mind, & soul toxins (to the abovementioned "**_FULL OF IT_** Level") is very analogous to those who drowned during the days of Noah. God gave those people 40 years to prepare. How much more time do you need? My goal is that everyone gets on the "**arc of salvation**" of cleansing (& optimizing the health of) their bodies, minds, & souls!

Since the beginning of man (God's creation – or Gods' creation depending on your interpretation of Genesis 1:26), we have all been born "**_FULL OF_**" a certain "level" of mind & soul toxins (AKA "_born into sin_" – due to the _fall of Adam_). However (in the past 100 years), we are also being born "**_FULL OF_**" a certain level of direct body toxins – due to the pollution of the earth (another one of God's creations). Due to the increased level of pollution by man of God's earth in the past 100 years, many humans reach this "**_FULL OF IT_** Level" before they leave the womb! Because we are "**_FULL OF_**" more body, mind, & soul toxins than ever before: more humans are reaching this "**_FULL OF IT_** Level" than ever before! I believe strongly (based on His word) that it is God's will for none of His children (all humans) to ever reach this "**_FULL OF IT_** Level!" I believe strongly that it is God's will for all of us to maximally cleanse (optimize the health of) our bodies, minds, & souls. This can only be achieved if we lower our "Levels" to zero (or as close to zero as possible)! I believe strongly that Chapters 5 & 6: show us "_the way!_" ☺

CHAPTER 5: "Natural" & "Super-Natural" _Cleansing_ Methods

Breaking all 10 of these "10 Dietary Commandments" & avoiding all of these "10 Non-Dietary Cleansing Methods" may be seen as **SINS** (mentioned in chapter 1) - as we are not treating our bodies like the _temple of the Holy Spirit_ that it truly is!   These dietary & non-dietary cleansing methods: lower our "**FULL OF IT** Levels" (analyzed in the last chapter).   Since the world is "**FULL OF**" more body, mind, & soul toxins than ever before in history, following these "10 Non-Dietary Cleansing Methods" & "10 Dietary Commandments" seem more important than ever before!

After reading the 1st 4 chapters, the following concepts have been proven (hopefully):

- We should not blame diseases, chronic pain, &/or obesity on just one body, mind, or soul toxin.   Nor should we blame them on just one type/category (body, mind, or soul) of toxin.
- The **accumulation** & **compounding** of the **combination** of these body, mind, & soul toxins we become "**FULL OF**" - destroys the health of our body, mind, & soul.
- The accumulating & compounding effect of the COMBINATION of all the different direct body, mind, & soul toxins to reach the "**FULL OF IT** Level of Disease, Obesity, &/or Chronic Pain**" causes &/or exacerbates diseases, obesity, &/or chronic pain!

The abovementioned body, mind, & soul destruction concepts are analogous to health & _cleansing_ concepts in this book (Which will be proven & demonstrated in chapters 5, & 6 –if they haven't been proven yet!).

Optimal health (maximal "CLEANSING") of your body, mind & soul reduces &, theoretically, eliminates the abovementioned "**Level**" of toxicity.   This is achieved by:

- Using **Dietary & Non-Dietary _CLEANSING_** Methods.   This means using the "**natural**" & the "**super-natural**" (via God's Love & Power).
- Avoiding all the body, mind, & soul toxins (mentioned in the 1st 4 chapters).
- Following some, if not all of the "10 Non-Dietary Cleansing Methods."
- Following ALL 10 of the "10 Dietary Commandments" as often as possible.
- Not relying on just one Healthful "Super-Cleansing food &/or Supplement." We must use a combination of many of these as they also have healthful synergistic properties (such as combining vitamins C & E; combining turmeric with cruciferous vegetables; etc.).

I.   The 10 Best Non-Dietary Cleansing Methods

Before discussing the "10 Dietary Commandments," it is only appropriate to show 10 non-dietary methods that reduce (& possibly eliminate) the "**FULL OF IT** Level" to maximally detox/cleanse (& optimize the health of) your body, mind, & soul.

1. **Become closer to God (& God's Love)** thanking Him for cleansing –
& optimizing the health of – your body, mind, & soul.

1a. Confess & Repent for the Body, Mind, & Soul Toxins we have become
"FULL OF!" Read chapters 1 & 2 (as well as 3 & 4) - & the Bible- to realize
that you need God's GRACE (& LOVE) to forgive & cleanse away your SINS.
Realize only the Messiah (Jesus Christ) was (& is) without sin. Jesus was
bombarded with many mind & soul toxins from His social environment.
One may argue that our society is more immoral (satanic) than Rome &
Jerusalem were 2,000 years ago. Our physical environment is definitely
more polluted with direct body toxins – than Rome & Jerusalem 2,000 years
ago. However, Jesus never became **"FULL OF"** any sin (mind or soul toxins)!
This is the key: just become you are bombarded with mind & soul (as well as
direct body) toxins from your environment, does NOT mean you have to
"absorb" or become **"FULL OF IT!"** Jesus Christ is the best role model in
the world to achieve optimal health of your body, mind, & soul. Thus,
trying to be more "Christ-like" helps you:

- **Maximally Cleanse the body, mind, & soul toxins ("IT") - you're already "FULL**
  OF"
- **& prevent from becoming "FULL OF IT" again or possibly in the first place!**
  Remember: "Lead me not into temptation!" This biblical phrase can apply
  to avoiding mind & soul toxins (like greed, hatred of others, lusting after your
  neighbor's wife, pornography, violence, etc.) as well as direct body toxins (like
  physical laziness, gluttony, lack of dietary discipline, binge-drinking, drug
  addiction, etc.).

1b. Worship & Praise the Lord always with ALL your heart, **mind, soul, &**
body! It is NOT a sacrifice to worship, pray, or tithe "half-heartedly."
"Rejoice in the Lord ALWAYS!"

1c. Pray to God as often as possible - to keep Him close to your mind, soul,
& body! Praying to God should NOT be the last thing we do when trying to
cleanse ourselves. Praying to God should be the 1st thing we do. Without
praying to God, you'll never achieve: **Optimal peace; Optimal happiness;**
Optimal patience; Optimal Love; & optimal cleansing & health of your
body, mind, & soul! This can also help you prevent from becoming **"FULL**
OF IT" in the first place. Remember: this concept of "absorption" is the key
to this book/diet/way of life. You have control over your environment.
What you choose to listen to, read, & watch can greatly affect whether you
become closer to God (& optimal health of your mind, soul, & body) or
become **"FULL OF IT!"** Just because your friends are going to the strip club,
doesn't mean you have to expose yourself to that. Just because your
friends want to watch violence & pornography on the television, doesn't
mean you have to. Your friends can *make you* or *break you* as peer-pressure
exists for everyone at every age. Certain sins we are bombarded with (like
those at our workplace, family, etc.) we may have less control over. Just
because you become bombarded with sins, doesn't mean you have to

137

become "**FULL OF**" them. Keeping yourself covered with the protective shield of the Holy Spirit can help you from becoming "**FULL OF IT**" in the first place!" Remember: *Lead me not into temptation*!

Therefore: Pray - preferably with another believer as "*if 2 of you agree on earth about anything that they may ask, it shall be done for them by My Father who is in heaven.*" (Matt 18:19) **Pray before each meal & before going to bed –something like this**:

"Thank you God for forgiving us of ALL our sins. We truly repent & will try with ALL our body, mind, & soul, NOT to repeat them. Thank you God for all the blessings – You have given us in the past & present – as well as those. You will give us in the future. Thank you God for: being with us eternally by giving the gift of Jesus. Thank you God for: eliminating our "*FULL OF IT* Level" of toxicity to maximally cleanse & optimize the health of our body, mind, & soul. Thank you God for: bringing us closer to You, Your love, – & the peace of the Holy Spirit. Thank you God for using us to do your will to bring us & others closer to God the Father, God the Son – Jesus, & the Holy Spirit. We ask that you bring everyone in the world closer to God the Father, God the Son – Jesus – the messiah, & the peace of the Holy Spirit. We thank you for any specific prayers we have. We love you so much – **more than anything or anyone**. Amen."

Be more cognizant of how God loves you - more than anyone will ever love you. Therefore, love God 1st & foremost with all your heart & might more than anything else. I have seen a bumper sticker that reads: "*God is my co-pilot.*" However, I prefer the bumper sticker that reads: "*If God is your co-pilot, you are in the wrong seat!*" REMEMBER: GOD'S WILL IS FOR YOU TO MAXIMALLY CLEANSE (& HAVE OPTIMAL HEALTH OF) YOUR BODY, MIND, & SOUL - TO BECOME CLOSER TO HIM!

2. **2a. Follow all the recommendations in chapter 3 trying your best to avoid direct body toxins** (such as from toxic heavy metals, industrial chemicals, poor posture, etc.) - **as we have become "FULL OF" Direct Body Toxins!**   The dietary toxins we are bombarded with are mentioned again in the second part of this chapter.   If you are going to cleanse your body, it doesn't make sense to get it dirty again & again. Would you clean your car or home (or "*temple*") & then throw dirt all over it?!

2b. Giving birth to a baby (as mentioned in chapter 3) is probably the most powerful/effective way for a woman to cleanse herself from all the harmful body toxins she was "**FULL OF**" before getting pregnant!   This may help women (who have given birth) live longer, look younger, &/or prevent diseases!   I mention this powerful *cleansing* technique for women NOT to offend, judge, or to make any woman (or man for that matter) feel guilty. I mention this powerful technique for women – as a way to **motivate women (& men) to: avoid the direct body toxins** mentioned in chapter 3; & maximally cleanse (& optimize the health of)

138

their bodies, minds, & souls – before attempting to become pregnant (as well as during the pregnancy & the breast-feeding).

2c. Raising the child can also help the father (as well as the mother & the rest of the family) – gain more happiness, become closer to God, & maximally cleanse (optimize the health of) their bodies, minds, & souls.

This is because babies are blessings from God in many ways.   Besides the "body cleanse" the biological mother receives, the parents that raise the child (the "real" dad & mom who <u>raise</u> the child) receive a spiritual & intellectual cleanse.   They realize what is important in life &, hopefully, learn to love God & (secondly) the rest of the people of the world as well.   The parents (& perhaps the rest of the family) may become more motivated ("for the baby/child") to maximally cleanse (& optimize the health of) their bodies, minds, & souls.   The parents (& perhaps the rest of the family that help raise the child) may become more motivated to read this book &:

- Avoid all the body, mind, & soul toxins shown in Chapters 1-4
- Follow these "10 non-Dietary Cleansing Methods"
- Follow the "10 Dietary Commandments"
- Consume some of the "super-cleansing foods/supplements"
- Be more aware of - & try to stop sinning.   In summary, these "real parents" (*as it takes a village to <u>raise a child</u>*) may become more motivated to be better role models for the child.   They may try to become more "*Christ-like*" (physically, intellectually, & spiritually)!

2d. Similar to raising a child, having a pet (especially a feline or canine), may increase the amount of:

- Love, happiness, & peace you **receive** from that pet.   This love & affection may reduce your blood pressure, anxiety, depression, lower overall stress levels (both psychological & physiological stress levels).   Thus, the pet helps lower one's "***FULL OF IT* Level**" of toxicity.
- Love, happiness, & peace you **give** to the pet.
- Love, happiness, & peace you give & receive to/from other humans.   This beneficial change in your mind & soul (which also benefits your body – obviously - as readers of this book are very aware of this connection) is "felt" by others.   Humans (& especially animals) sense this beneficial change.
- Love you give & receive to/from God.   God always loves you – no matter what you do. However, many people do not "receive" (AKA "absorb") His Love – as much as they should.   Remember God's greatest commandment of the new covenant: *Love God the most - & then love everyone else* (including yourself, family, friends, neighbors, strangers, enemies) *2nd most*!
- Cleansing (& health) of your body, mind, & soul.   When you adopt a pet from a shelter: who benefits more (you or the animal)? ☺   If you think an animal can't give you love, then "***YOU'RE FULL OF IT***!"

3.   Exercise via "Interval Training" regularly – as we have become "*FULL OF*" Laziness & ignorance about exercise.

There are many rules we should consider regarding exercising.

- Exercise when medically stable & only under the supervision of a qualified health care provider.

- You're cells are considered alive. For a cell to be considered "alive," movement (either intra- or extra-cellular) must exist (from my days of "Cell Biology" in college)! ☺ As the great theologian/physicist Isaac Newton taught us (via his Law of Momentum): "*An object at rest: stays at rest. An object in motion stays in motion!*"
- You are a dying breed (see chapter 4 for more details on this). As the percentage of Americans that identify themselves as atheists, the percentage of Americans that have become more sedentary has skyrocketed! As the percentage of Americans that identify themselves as Christians has decreased, the percentage of Americans that regularly exercise has decreased. Is this a "coincidence" or a "God-incidence?"
- Congratulations & Gratitude are in order. With more of a "universal health care system" approaching our nation, you will be saving us all money as you will decrease your likelihood of needing expensive health care! ☺
- Don't exercise EXCESSIVELY! Excessive, intense aerobic exercise may create more oxidation![1] A sedentary lifestyle can increase the risk of atherosclerosis, blood clots, obesity, chronic pain & a whole host of other diseases. However, intense (excessive) aerobic exercise may lower immune response & create more oxidation through stress than anaerobic exercise (strength training).[1] Marathon runners often struggle with decreased resistance to viruses & bacterial infections in peak training sessions.[1] They also battle chronic ligament & joint degeneration problems that worsen.[1] It is extremely important to rest in between exercise sets/programs.
- **Good quality & proper quantity Sleep** is usually facilitated by [& **needed - to** receive the maximal benefit of] regular exercise. As deep sleep includes the "delta cycle" of sleeping – which regenerates/heals/repairs the body: getting 7 to 9 hours of quality sleep is a very important component of the total body "*cleansing*" process to boost your immune system & achieve optimal health.[2] Therefore: exercise can help you get **better quality & quantity sleep** – reducing your risk of (as well as helping reverse) obesity, chronic pain, chronic diseases (like diabetes, cancer, heart disease, etc.), & becoming "*FULL OF IT*!"[3,4]
- Stretch properly before exercising. Stretching should be gentle, in "**good posture**" (see chapter 3), **never bounce**, & hold for a period of time (or until you don't feel the gentle stretch). Stretching can be considered **resistive training** as you're muscle's God-given "**stretch reflex**" (which resists the muscle from being elongated &/or torn for approximately the 1st 12 minutes – 30 minutes [for larger muscle groups] of a stretch)[5,6] provides your own internal resistance![5,6]
- "Warm up" before exercising. This usually includes performing the activity at a slower pace or with less resistance in the beginning to "prepare" your body for faster, more resistance exercising.
- Is stretching a form of exercising? Yes. Applying Wolf's Law in Physics, the repetitive stress (in the "elastic range") to the muscles (or any other structure) will result in the muscles becoming stronger.[6] As mentioned above, the "stretch reflex" exists as a protective mechanism to help prevent muscles from tearing.[5,6] This "stretch reflex" acts as resistance to the muscle(s) you are stretching.[5,6] Therefore, this resistance makes stretching into somewhat of a "resistance training" workout.[5,6] This may explain why Yoga (done regularly) may result in increased strength (& possibly a fit body).

140

- No Pain or pain increase allowed during stretching or exercising. Remember: *His pain = your gain.* Some exceptions to this rule may include burn victims & total knee replacements (if we don't get the joints moving – with or without pain, there is a risk of contractures).
- Exercise in good posture & age appropriate (see chapter 3 –section II). We must realize the positives of high compression/impact exercises for people over the age of 55 are outweighed by their negatives (worsening the degeneration of the shock absorbers of our skeletal system). As mentioned & referenced in chapter 3, the intervertebral discs begin to shrink at approximately age 55. Therefore, many social sports like tennis & running on concrete become very detrimental (degenerating) to the shock absorbers (menisci, discs, etc.) of our skeletal system.
- **VISUALIZE**. Visualize receiving the maximum health benefit of the exercise you are performing. This may include:

burning excess body fat; losing excess weight; increasing muscle strength; increasing muscle mass; improving your endurance; improving your appearance*; lowering our body's level of cortisol (the stress hormone); stimulating the production of endorphins (which improves your mood – reducing the symptoms of depression &/or decreasing your pain)*;[7] sweating out the toxins in your body; inhaling healthy oxygen & exhaling carbon dioxide; &/or achieving optimal health (of your body, mind, & soul).

Exercise is also considered one of the best ways to "*detox pesticides & other toxins from the body.*"[2,8] Therefore, exercise can directly & indirectly help with the 3 major killers Americans & the rest of the world faces today: **diseases, obesity, & chronic pain**. Exercise can help reverse the harmful "physiological stress reaction cycle" (mentioned in chapters 3 & 4) &, therefore, help prevent the multiple symptoms & diseases that go along with that harmful cycle. Exercise can, therefore, reduce your toxic load to keep us [or get us way below] the dangerous "***FULL OF IT*** Level!" Said differently: **exercise gets your body, mind, & soul into a positive health/cleansing cycle**!

- **Exercise should be a combination of aerobic, strength training, flexibility, & BALANCE*****.

Remember: gaining more muscle mass (predominantly via exercise-induced muscle hypertrophy) will burn more calories – even when you are sleeping. Therefore, **exercise increases your metabolism & reduces your risk of committing "gluttony!"** Exercise helps prevent obesity (&, therefore, obesity-related diseases). Regular exercise can improve your sleeping, appearance, & attitude. Regular exercise can also improve digestion (to help **prevent** becoming "***FULL OF***" intestinal putrefaction) & bowel mobility (to **reduce** your being "***FULL OF***" intestinal putrefaction).[9]

*****The best exercise (in my opinion as a Physical Therapist that specializes in vestibular rehabilitation) for **BALANCE** (if you can tolerate it) is:
- One legged standing with eyes closed for as many seconds as you can stand with eyes open - each leg three times per day. Five seconds may be considered "normal" for people over 65 years of age & 30 seconds may be considered normal for 30 year olds. However, every individual is different.

141

Some 80 year olds can easily stand on one leg with eyes open for 15 seconds (3 times greater than their peers). You should be **safe & avoid falling** – as well as challenging yourself. When you lift your foot off the ground – you should hold onto the kitchen countertop with your same side hand. If this is too easy – you can try 4, 3, 2, 1, or no fingertip(s).

By standing on one leg (without holding on) & closing your eyes – your **vestibular system** (considered responsible for 70% of your balance)[10] will be challenged. By challenging your vestibular system via the abovementioned exercise (taking only 1-2 minutes per day), your balance can improve greatly. Therefore, dizziness may be reduced & balance may be improved greatly. I & my patients have found the vestibular system to be a part of your brain that learns very quickly.

Keep in mind: vision is only supposed to be responsible for 10% of your balance.[10] Someone with a "normal" (100% functioning) vestibular system should, therefore, be able to stand 90% as long with eyes closed (when compared to eyes open).[10] Many of my patients start out in physical therapy on a balance "rocker" (tested front & back – as well as side to side) for only 5 seconds with eyes closed (compared to 100 seconds eyes open). This may represent an initial 5% functioning of their vestibular system. After weeks of "vestibular rehabilitation," the patient is often able to stand on the same rocker for 90+ seconds! Imagine if all parts of your brain can learn quickly.

For most of my patients with lumbar spinal stenosis, I educate them on:

- Always stretching (**gently** holding still in a low back "flat back" – forward bent posture [see chapter 3], & without any pain or pain increase) to prepare themselves for any exercise (remember: ***don't kvetch –just stretch***);
- Salt-water pool walking;
- Walking with a rolling walker may be used as an endurance exercise [It can also help them to re-educate themselves how to learn to stand/walk in a "flat back" posture – as well as cause less pressure to the low back nerves, joints, etc.];
- Walking on the sand at the beach (if able/safe enough) can be considered a strengthening (with less compression to the joints & nerves than hard concrete), balancing, & "grounding" exercise - possibly negating damage from EMF pollution;[11]
- Riding a stationary recumbent leg bicycle;
- & riding a stationary arm bicycle either sitting or standing (in a flat back posture with pelvis thrust forward) with resistance as tolerated.

All of the above are done "as tolerated" with deep breathing during the exercising. Vital signs are measured before & after. Alternating days of riding a recumbent leg bicycle versus salt-water pool walking & arm bicycling resembles "**interval training**" (so they don't plateau). Alternating between 1 minute fast & 2 minutes slower of cycling (with arms or legs) &/or pool walking can also be considered a form of "**interval training**" (considered superior to continuous slow, excessive aerobic exercise re: fat-burning & overall heart health).[1] All of the abovementioned exercises may offer the benefits of aerobic training & resistance/strengthening training (which may stimulate muscle hypertrophy – which helps burn calories even when sleeping).

Personal comment on "exercising as tolerated"

When I was 8 years old, I did (tolerated) 20 consecutive push-ups. Every day, I believe God told me to add one more push-up (so that I could defend myself against the so-called Christian kids who ignorantly hated me for being Jewish). After 3 years, I could do (tolerate) over 1,200 consecutive push-ups (& became abnormally strong & healthy for a thin young 11 year old). I was able to defend myself.

Many Americans suffer from a term I coined in the late 1990s (in attempt to create humor) **"LTS" ("Lazy Tushy Syndrome")**! LTS (exercising moderately less than 150 minutes per week) may be destroying the health of millions of Americans (& may kill as many people as smoking!)![12,13] No wonder **God considers laziness a SIN** (see chapter 1)! People get "used to" lying in bed or the on the couch & not exercising. Success of sticking to an exercise regimen may have most to do with creating a routine (as well as discipline, attitude, & motivation). If one develops a routine of exercising, their body may "demand" they continue to exercise as they will probably have so much energy.

Besides turning (or being turned & positioned) in bed every 2 hours (to prevent pressure soars), **"bed-ridden" & "chair-bound" individuals can & should still exercise**. They may be able to tolerate "bridges," arm & even leg bicycling with a pedal exerciser, active &/or passive range of motion exercises, etc.

3b. *Cleanse* your prostate - or renew your vaginal flora.

This is mentioned under "exercise" as you should ask your doctor if it is safe for you to participate in **sexual activity (*either via masturbation or in a committed relationship*)**. Sexual activity may demand physiological energy similar to that of climbing up 2 flights of stairs at a fast pace. Keep in mind: some spouses prefer their sexual activity to mimic more of a "marathon!"

Sexual activity involves the sympathetic nervous system (for the initial arousal phase & orgasmic phase –which may increase the heart rate & blood pressure) & the parasympathetic nervous system (to maintain the erection & after the male's orgasmic phase to relax them).

Many men over 50 may get an **enlarged prostate (AKA "BPH" = Benign Prostatic Hypertrophy)** possibly due to the following under-recognized reasons: Hormonal changes, &/or decreased orgasmic activity. They often decrease the frequency of their masturbating &/or sexual activity. The prostate is a fluid-filled sack. If the prostatic fluid is NOT "released," this fluid builds up in the prostate. Thus, you become: "*FULL OF*" prostatic fluid. The prostate may grow externally (increase in diameter) &/or internally (squeezing on the urethra). An enlarged prostate may lead to urinary incontinence & impotence (which of course will decrease your "activity" - & lead to a larger prostate). The "squeezing" on the urethra makes it difficult for a man to completely empty their bladder. Thus you become "*FULL OF*" urine.

This urinary retention may lead to: Nocturia (waking up at night multiple times to urinate – which interferes with your sleep/rejuvenation of your body, mind, & soul); Urinary tract infections; &/or Hypertension (which predisposes you to a whole host of other diseases).

Men should consider other factors regarding "cleansing their prostates." Before the act (an hour before or so), certain foods high in zinc (like organic raw pumpkin &/or sunflower seeds) & certain herbs (like saw palmetto berry extract with 80+ fatty acids & sterols) may allow a "greater cleansing" of prostatic fluid.   Zinc levels will fall after the act as zinc is usually found in good quantities in seminal & prostatic fluids.[7]   The toxic metal cadmium (similar in structure to zinc) often displaces zinc.[7]   The more deficient the zinc level, the easier it is to become "***FULL OF***" toxic cadmium.   Proper zinc levels can help prevent lung cancer caused by inhalation of cadmium.[14]   Therefore, it is important (in my strong opinion) for men to consume super-***cleansing*** foods high in zinc (like raw organic pumpkin seeds) after an orgasm (as well as before).[15]   Beats smoking a toxic cigarette!

My personal journey with BPH

At age 18, I developed an enlarged prostate. After 2 months of college (a dramatic change in lifestyle going from studying 5 hours/week in High School to 100 hours/week in college), I developed BPH.   When I started college, I did nothing but study. I stopped everything -including masturbation – despite my nick name in High School! ☺ I ate an extremely unhealthy diet of high-sugar (& caffeine) sodas & chocolate bars. Two urologists examined me & concluded I should masturbate more often.

From age 18 to approximately 27, I suffered with BPH. I will admit - the following did help shrink my enlarged prostate (mostly temporarily): Consistent masturbation; Zinc 30-50 mg/day (never take over 100 mg/day as it can actually weaken your immune system);[15] Saw Palmetto Berry Extract 320 mg/day (with 80%+ fatty acids & sterols).[15]

However, God finally "cured" it as I strictly followed the "10 Dietary Commandments" shown later in this chapter.   God wants us to use the supernatural & the natural.   He wants us to treat our bodies like *the temples of the Holy Spirit* they are!

Thus, consistent/regular masturbation &/or sex (with their wives) may benefit a man's prostate (& overall health).

Consistent masturbation &/or sex (with their committed partner) may also benefit a woman's vaginal flora (& overall health).   Besides reducing the risks of urinary retention (for a man), it can be a great psychological stress reducer for both sexes.   Since we are all "***FULL OF***" psychological & physical stressors, this stress reducer can help reduce the risk of diseases [as well as possibly obesity & chronic pain] - & boost our health.

If you believe you should never masturbate &/or have sex (in a committed relationship): "***YOU'RE FULL OF IT***!"

4. **Breathe DEEP with your diaphragm while you MEDITATE upon the LORD (praising & worshipping Him) daily – as we have become "*FULL OF*" Shallow breathing, stress, & distance from God!**

We should consider "*Meditating before Medicating*."   This can create the peace of the Holy Spirit to come over us.   Remember to praise Him – BEFORE you ask Him! You can **VISUALIZE** breathing in the "white" peaceful light of the Holy Spirit & breathing out any "black" mind & soul (as well as body) toxins/stressors. This great stress-reducer beats any anti-anxiety medication in the world (in my opinion).

Reducing stress can also improve your immune, digestive, neurological, & cardiopulmonary systems (as well as all other organ systems in your body)! The connection between the pulmonary & cardiovascular systems is under-recognized.

Belly Breathing or lower ribs? Infants are instinctive "belly breathers," but most of us have learned to breathe from our chest in short shallow breaths that resemble a pant more than a deep breath.[1] As the lungs are somewhat "cone shaped" (larger near the lower ribs), training yourself to breathe deep with the lower ribs will help one optimally utilize their lung capacity.

Percent Oxygen Saturation

My opinion (shared by many physicians) is that percent oxygen saturation is the MOST important vital sign (when compared to heart rate & blood pressure) – to give that person a "general sense of their overall health!" This is why over 90% of all trauma centers used pulse oximetry back in the late 1990s.[16] As a physical therapist, I have measured over 40,000 adult's (mostly) percent oxygen saturation since the early 1990s. Back in the early 1990s, many health care providers did not know what percent oxygen saturation even meant. Therefore (to gain more clarity for everyone), I developed my own grading/rating system for present oxygen saturation - as follows: 100% is perfect; 99% is excellent or an "A+;" 98% is an "A;" 97% is an "A-;" 96% is good or a "B;" 95% is a "C+;" 94% is average or a "C;" 93% is a "D;" 92% is a "D-;" 91% or lower is failing or an "F." Below 90% can cause hypoxemia (a deficiency or abnormally low concentration of oxygen in the blood) – which may be indicated by cyanosis (a blue or purple coloration of the skin due to the tissues near skin's surface being low in oxygen).[17,18] This failing oxygen saturation, hypoxemia, & cyanosis can be a warning sign of PAD (Peripheral Artery Disease: a type of atherosclerosis) – as well as anemia.[19]

Keep in mind: there are limitations to even the best pulse oximeter. Pulse oximetry is able to detect only oxyhemoglobin or reduced hemoglobin – but not the other types of hemoglobin (e.g., carboxyhemoglobin, methemoglobulin); those types are assumed to be oxyhemglobin & may falsely elevate the SpO2 measurement![19] The best brands of pulse oximeters should have a finger probe, wire sensor, & accuracy light (to tell you if/when the measurement is accurate).[19] I prefer the "Nonin PalmSAT 2500®" that has received U.S. Military approval for its effectiveness.[20] Nonin is the only company I have seen trusted by Medicare & health care providers when testing for sleep apnea.

Very often, one's percent oxygen saturation starts out poor (a "D" – 93% or lower). It usually takes less than one minute for the patient to "retrain/re-educate" their body to breathe deeply (& slowly 4 seconds in & 4 seconds out) & feeling their lower ribs & belly (where the belly & lower ribs move outward when you take a deep breath). Some of my patients benefit from the famous visualization: "*smell the roses & blow out the candles*." Many of my patients benefit from placing their hands on the lower ribs & belly to feel them move. They usually aren't (at first) – as most of us are "upper-respiratory breathers" (AKA "chest breathers").

After the abovementioned diaphragmatic breathing exercise(s), their percent oxygen saturation often goes up dramatically (sometimes from "Failing" = 91% or lower to an "A" or higher 98% or higher)! Every cell in every "system" of your entire body (especially the neurological – as well as the cardiovascular, & cardiopulmonary systems) *need oxygen* to thrive![1]

4b. **Hyperbaric Oxygen Therapy (HBOT) may be beneficial for people suffering from Anemia –as well as other diseases contributing to low oxygen saturation**. I mention this here because low oxygen saturation is a risk factor with anemia.[19,21] HBOT is the medical use of oxygen at a level higher than atmospheric pressure.[21] The use of HBOT is indicated - & shown to have a positive result – to treat exceptional blood loss (anemia) when oxygen delivery to tissue is not sufficient in patients who cannot receive blood transfusions for medical or religious reasons (ex: Jehovah's Witnesses).[21] HBOT may be used for medical reasons when there is a threat of blood incompatibility or concern for transmissible disease.[21]

5.   Remove direct body toxins from your largest organ (your skin).
5a. Sweat out the direct body toxins *"YOU'RE FULL OF"* through your skin & avoid antiperspirants.

The skin can be considered the largest organ. Toxins can enter – as well as exit – the skin. Antiperspirants can be replaced with chemical free (& toxic perfume & metal-free) crystal deodorants. Aim to sweat at least 15 minutes per day to remove excess Flouride – as well as the Bt-Toxin found in GMO crops - through the pores on the skin.[22,23] Sweating has been proven an extremely effective method for cleansing toxic heavy metals (like lead, mercury, arsenic, & cadmium) & other toxic elements.[24,25] Considering the fact that more toxic elements have been found in sweat (when compared to blood & urine), sweating deserves consideration as one of the most powerful methods for toxic element detoxification.[24,25]

The SAUNA (when used properly) may be considered one of **the most powerful & under-utilized tools one has to detox**!   The sauna is considered one of the 5 best ways to detox fluoride,[22] pesticides,[2,8,25] & other toxins.[24,25]   Mercury levels normalized with repeated saunas in a case report.[24]   One should be medically stable & approved by their physician(s) (& have no bruises, bleeding, swelling, *heart disease*, or heat allergies).   In many other countries, the sauna is actually recommended as a treatment for *heart disease*! I believe the Finnish people have been way ahead of us in their awareness (& use) of the powerful benefits of the sauna.

The proper use of a sauna (in my humble opinion) includes:
- Drinking a quart of filtered water right before entering.   Adults may benefit from adding fresh squeezed organic lemon (the juice), cayenne pepper, cinnamon, &/or raw honey into the water to increase the cleansing reaction.[2] However, this may be too spicy for many adults.
- Sitting on a white 100% cotton towel naked with bare feet on the white towel (including no shoes as the toxic material from shoes can "leach" into the healthy dry air one is inhaling).
- Continually drink filtered water from a glass container during the sauna.
- Sweat out the toxins & stroke them off your body.
- VISUALIZE the toxins in your entire body being removed (via the sweating process) to create a clean body, mind, & soul.
- Immediately shower after the sauna.
- & then rehydrate & replace electrolytes (like with one of the "super-cleansing beverages" such as: kombucha, kefir, or a "green powder-drink").

Again, ask your physician of this.

5b. & 5c. Mud wraps/packs & Detox pads (usually applied to the feet) are
other ways people MAY (or may not) be able to cleanse their bodies of toxins via the skin. I know people who claim these things changed their lives.

However, I am not familiar with any strong scientific evidence of this. "Buyer Beware" = the attitude I would take.

5d. Anoint your skin with essential oils! Certain "spice oils" – such as clove oil – are believed to possess some of the highest ORAC (Oxidative Radical Absorbance Capacity) scores in the world.[26] Therefore, they _may_ have the highest antioxidant capacity in the world.[26] However, the antioxidant effects in vivo (& internally) are still undefined & questioned.   This is discussed later in this chapter.   In addition, clove oil taken internally may act as a strong irritant (it is referred to as a "spice" for a reason) to the gastrointestinal system. Thus, applying oils (such as clove, oregano, tea tree, etc.) to your feet (& then put on socks), under your nose, &/or putting a drop or two in a "**DETOX BATH**" (see below) – may allow for direct absorption/benefit & bypass any gastrointestinal irritation.

When using essential oils, be aware that they are highly concentrated & very potent. Phyllis Balch (author of _Prescription for Nutritional Healing_, 5th Edition) recommends the following precautions regarding essential oils:[15]

- _Do not use oils' full strength. Always dilute them first (with extra-virgin olive or coconut oil). Do not use oils near the eyes. Do not touch your face, mucous membranes, or genitals if your hands have been in direct contact with the oils. Keep essential oils out of the reach of children or those mentally challenged. Be cautious using essential oils during pregnancy._

Besides clove oil, there are other essential oils (there are many –but here are some of my personal favorites) that have the following healthful properties:[15]

- **Eucalyptus oil** may act as a nasal decongestant, chest expectorant, antiseptic, & antiviral.
- **Frankincense oil** (yes – the same oil brought to Jesus!) may act as an anti-inflammatory, antiseptic, sedative, expectorant, & promote cellular regeneration!
- **Lavender oil** may be very **calming** & helpful for sleep disorders, burns, acne, eczema, skin healing, & stress. _One may benefit from (to "de-stress") bathing in water with a drop of lavender oil –as well as Epsom salt (magnesium sulfate – a "natural" muscle relaxant)._
- **Peppermint oil** may be helpful for **headaches**, congestion, fatigue, fever, indigestion, muscle soreness (analgesic properties), sinus problems, & stomach problems.
- **Tea Tree Oil** may act as an antiviral, antiseptic, expectorant, fungicide, & anti-parasitic. May be helpful for athlete's foot, bronchial congestion, dandruff, ringworm, & yeast infections.

5e. A "Detox Bath" can include a cup of Epsom salt (magnesium sulfate – a muscle relaxant); a couple drops of essential oil(s); &/or a teaspoon of apple cider vinegar (to soften the skin).[2,27]   Adding lavender oil to the bath can be calming - & citrus-based oils (like orange or lemon) may be energizing.[27]

Caution: Many of my patients have reported too great a laxative effect from applying Epsom salt to their skin (as the Epsom salt gets absorbed through the skin). Therefore, start out with a teaspoon of Epsom salt per bath & increase – as tolerated up to 2 cups per bath (if desiring a greater muscle

147

relaxing effect).   Again, ask your physician's opinion of this. In the end, the person most responsible for your health = YOU!

Extra-virgin coconut oil can also be applied to your feet. Extra-virgin coconut oil contains caprylic acid (an antifungal agent) & may, therefore, help prevent athlete's foot &/or toenail fungus.   This oil (due to its' lubricating properties) may also be helpful as a moisturizer for the skin, lips, & even the anus**!   Keep 1 bottle in the kitchen & 1 in the bathroom (don't interchange them)!

   ** However, if "*YOU ARE FULL OF*" hemorrhoids: the most effective natural treatment for hemorrhoids may be an ice cube inserted in the anus & 1 applied externally (as this can decrease pain & swelling of the anal veins)! Other effective natural (God-given) treatments for hemorrhoids include:[28]

- Sitz Bath (may have some apple cider vinegar added to it – as mentioned previously);
- Applying Witch Hazel;
- Squat, don't sit to avoid putting strain on the rectum & relax the anal muscles.
- & avoid constipation by following the "10 Dietary Commandments." This includes a high fiber diet filled with probiotics –as well as hydrating (all helpful in preventing hemorrhoids).[28]

Of course, ask your physician about all of this.

5f. "**Ground**" as much of your skin (as well as the rest of your body) as long as possible each day to "*CLEANSE*" your body of the **EMF pollution** (illustrated in chapter 3) "*YOU'RE FULL OF*."   As per Dr. L. Beck (an Acupuncturist & Doctor of Oriental Medicine specializing in homeopathy & electric body field studies):[11]
*When we become "**FULL OF**" EMF pollution, our body's voltage is raised (positively charged) & this can be very toxic to our body –triggering the harmful "stress response"* (mentioned in chapter 3). *The **earth is highly negatively** charged - so having your **bare feet** (or the skin on other body parts) touch the earth/ground, neutralizes our positively charged bodies.   Consuming **antioxidants** (like **vitamin C, glutathione**, etc. – mentioned in "Dietary Commandment # 7") also flood the body with "electron donors" to protect us from the toxic free radicals (electron thieves).* Therefore you may benefit from following the suggestions mentioned previously in "5d!"

The only definitive method to negate & neutralize the voltage is to ground ourselves as much & as long as possible each day.

   Dr. Beck recommends an extremely affordable "**grounding device**" (for about the same price as your EMF polluting lamp) *to be used **when sleeping or sitting still** (watching the television or on a computer).*   Walking, standing, &/or lying (with skin touching the sand) on the beach for 6 hours/day may also "ground" your skin/body to effectively cleanse the EMF pollution from your body for that 24 hour period.

6. **Avoid tight clothing, prolonged sitting, pressure on armpits, & crossing legs or arms – to avoid interfering with your circulation - & facilitate the other cleansing methods!**

Camisoles may be good substitutes for bras.   *"Burn your bras."*   Bras (& tight undershorts) should not be worn to bed.[1]   Crossing legs or wearing tight undershorts may impede the arterial supply "down" to the legs (possibly worsening peripheral artery disease or diabetic peripheral neuropathy). It may also impede the venous & lymphatic return back "up" from toes to the right atrium of the heart – possibly increasing the risk of edema, venous blood clots, & a whole host of other diseases! **Our circulation may be interfered with by wearing tight clothing, prolonged sitting, pressure on armpits, &/or crossing arms & legs**.   Wearing loose clothing (preferably made of 100% cotton) & avoiding the abovementioned activities/habits are **under-recognized** *cleansing* **methods** as they may **facilitate**:

- The "junk"/waste products of the circulatory system to be:
  - *Cleansed*/filtered via the lymphatic system
  - & returned to the lungs (via the right atrium to right ventricle) where the blood is "filled" with oxygen
- The oxygen-rich blood (from the lungs to the left atrium) to "fill" the entire body (except the lungs) with oxygen & nutrients!   Thus: avoiding these activities/habits can facilitate the "*circle*" of the circulatory system!
- & **the other cleansing methods – such as exercising, sweating, sleeping, etc.**

On a deeper (& possibly controversial) level, we have to ask ourselves: is wearing tight revealing clothing (or loose humble clothing) the will of God?   Discuss amongst yourselves. ☺

7. Get some sunshine to strengthen the immune system & activate/manufacture vitamin D – as we are "*FULL OF*" ignorance as to the benefits of sunshine!

The human skin uses the energy from the sun to manufacture vitamin D (to strengthen the immune system & improve absorptions of minerals).[1]   When sunlight activates the phytochemicals in healthful foods, consumption of these foods not only blocks the harmful effects of UV rays, but they also produce "antiviral, antibacterial, & anticancer components, as well as pest repellents!"[1,29]   We should **VISUALIZE** the abovementioned healthful benefits of sunshine (another miracle from God).

Most people in the U.S. can meet their vitamin D needs via exposure to sunlight - even though most people are deficient in vitamin D.[30]   Some vitamin D researchers suggest 5-30 minutes (depending on skin color/pigmentation - avoiding sunburn, of course) of sun exposure 2x/week may lead to sufficient vitamin D synthesis.[31]   There is a seasonal relationship between decreased sun exposure and an increased risk of:

- Death;[32,33] Cardiac arrest;[34] Atrial Fibrillation;[35] Hypertension;[36] Depression – especially Seasonal Affect Disorder (SAD);[37] &, of course, hypothermia![38]

Thus: getting sufficient amount of sunshine may help reduce your risk of the abovementioned diseases/death, boost your immune system, help reduce excess weight (via manufacturing sufficient vitamin D),[39] & (therefore) lower your overall "*FULL OF IT* **Level**" of toxicity.

8. Go to sleep before midnight[1] – as we are "*FULL OF*" Poor sleeping habits!
8a. Get 7-9 hours of quality sleep/day (for an adult & 8.5-9.25 hours/day for a teen) - as an under-recognized way to cleanse your body, mind, & soul.

Several sleep studies have shown a direct correlation between the habitual lack of inadequate sleep (poor quality &/or insufficient amount = 6 hours or less) &:[3,4]
- BMI (Body Mass Index) – increasing your risk of becoming overweight by 27%
- Increased risk of Diabetes,[1,3,4,40] heart disease (by 48%), & cancer (breast cancer in women by 62%) - by diminishing the immune system's primary organs
- Increased stress levels - &, therefore, increased "***FULL OF IT* Level**" of toxicity!
- & serious cognitive dullness resulting in:[3]
    o 20% of MVAs (Motor Vehicle Accidents)
    o 100% more surgical complications by sleepless surgeons
    o & symptoms mimicking the effects of aging & & memory loss![1,40] Adults need about 7-9 hours/night (& teens need about 8.5 to 9.25 hours/night) for optimal cognitive acuity. As 60% of adults don't get enough quality sleep: taking **a 20 minute nap** can increase cognitive functionality by 40% (more effective than 200mg of caffeine)!

Thus: getting adequate sleep on a regular basis can help you lose excess body fat, decrease your risk of diseases, increase your cognitive acuity, decrease your stress levels (&, therefore, reduce your "***FULL OF IT* Level**" of toxicity)![3,4]

       8b. **Nasal Irrigation (one hour+ before sleeping) may be the most direct way to cleanse the nasal sinuses**.   Nasal irrigation should be considered an *essential part of your daily hygiene – like brushing your teeth or taking a shower*.[41] There are "Neti Pots" (AKA "nasal washes" or "nose bidets").   However, one must always use distilled or filtered water. Add some iodized sea salt with some baking soda (to neutralize the acid-like irritation of the salt).   All of these: - bulb syringes, "neti pots," or turkey basters - must be put in the dishwasher after each use to assure proper cleansing.   However (as we learned in chapter 3), ***repetitive use of plastics increase our level of toxicity***. Thus: we should use a clear colorless glass neti pot (or a straw you throw out after each use).   Of course if you are blessed enough to live near the ocean, God has His own form of nasal irrigation. I mention nasal irrigation hear because it may be most convenient (& less messy) to perform this in the shower **at night before sleeping** (or in the morning). As per the *Ear Nose & Throat Institute of South Florida* (Dr. N. Goldhaber & Dr. S Raja), the benefits of hypertonic saline nasal irrigation are threefold:[42]
- *One = It is a solvent. It cleans mucus, crusting, & other debris from the nasal passage. Keep in mind, each para-nasal sinus may theoretically be able to hold 3 tablespoons of mucus. That is a potential 24 total tablespoons in all the nasal sinuses (4 para-nasal sinuses on each side of the nose = 8 x 3 potential tablespoons).*
- *Two = It decongests the nose. Because of the high salt content, fluid is pulled out of the mucous membrane (lining tissue of the nose). This shrinks the membrane, which improves nasal air-flow & open sinus passages.*
- *Three = It improves nasal drainage. Studies have shown that saltwater cleansing of the nasal cavity improves ciliary beating so that normal mucus is transported better from the sinuses through the nose & throat.*

Again, we should VISUALIZE the health benefits of this nasal cleansing when we perform it. As Dr. Raja (one of the most knowledgeable **& honest** physicians I've personally ever met) told me years ago, *"This nasal irrigation has helped prevent over 99% of my patients needing sinus surgery!"*

9. Chelation Therapy – as we are *"FULL OF"* Toxic Heavy Metals that may be removed via chelation!

Chelation Therapy is somewhat controversial.   As per the American Cancer Society (in 2008): *Chelation Therapy can be harmful (even fatal), & medical evidence does NOT support the effectiveness of chelation therapy for any other purpose than **the treatment of heavy metal poisoning**.*[43]   What is being overlooked here is the fact (shown in chapter 3) that toxic heavy metal poisoning increases the risk of diseases! Thus: toxic heavy metal poisoning adds to our *"**FULL OF IT** Level of Diseases"* (as well as possibly Obesity &/or Chronic Pain Levels - shown in Chapter 4).   This is why some scientists (including allopathic & osteopathic physicians) *believe* certain chelation agents may help prevent atherosclerosis[15,44] – as well as neurological & perhaps almost any other disease.[15,45]   This may also be why approximately 800,000 patient visits for chelation therapy were made in the U.S. in 1997.[44]

In the past 20 years, some U.S. physicians have become certified by the American Board of Chelation Therapy as approved chelation therapists.[15]   They have specialized in oral, intravenous &/or intramuscular injections of chelation agents – depending on the agent & type of poisoning.[15,46,47]   They introduce chelation agents (such as glutathione or the most common **EDTA** – ethylenediaminetetraacetic acid) as an attempt to get a (most likely) more pronounced & faster chelating effect of **removing excessive iron** (including cases of thalassemia**), lead, arsenic, mercury, uranium, plutonium, & other forms of toxic heavy metal poisoning**.[15,46,47] However, EDTA (as well as other common chelation agents like DMSA & DMPS) is a synthetic chemical & is NOT found naturally.[15,45]   Since EDTA, DMSA, & DMPS can deplete certain vitamins (including the antioxidant vitamins C & E) & minerals, chelation doctors often add (or instruct their clients to take) them after or during the chelation therapy.[15,48]   The level/strength of chelation (synthetic versus natural – mentioned in the "Dietary Commandment # 5") one needs may be directly related to the "***FULL OF IT** Level*" of toxicity [&/or stage of disease associated with the toxins]![15,46,47]

10. Colon Hydrotherapy may be the most effective way of removing intestinal putrefaction – as we are *"FULL OF"* Intestinal Toxins that may be removed via colonics![2,15,49]

When medically stable & approved by your physician(s), a "high-colonic" 1x/year may eliminate toxins that have been stored for decades in your entire large intestine (versus an enema which attempts to cleanse just the rectum).[2,15,49]   VISUALIZING a perfect colon cleanse during the colonic may enhance the benefits.   One may benefit/need colon hydrotherapy more than 1x/year if one has a "sluggish colon" – often caused by hypothyroidism[50] or an "UNDISCIPLINED DIET" (via breaking the "10 Dietary Commandments" shown in the next section).   Therefore: Following the "10 Dietary Commandments" may eliminate your need to receive colon hydrotherapy.

However, since most of us break (on a daily &/or multiple times per day basis) ALL ten of the "10 Dietary Commandments," most of us would benefit from colon hydrotherapy.   Personally, I lost 3 pant sizes after only 1 colonic!   This proves that even I was "***FULL OF IT***!"   Some "super colon hydro-therapists" add wheatgrass "implants" after the colonic!

II. "10 DIETARY COMMANDMENTS"

BECAUSE AMERICANS HAVE BEEN INCREASINGLY BREAKING ALL 10 OF THESE "10 DIETARY COMMANDMENTS" SINCE THE 1970S (IF NOT LONGER), WE HAVE BECOME:

I. MORE DISEASED
II. MORE OBESE
iii. & MORE DISABLED – ESPECIALLY WITH CHRONIC PAIN – than ever before in our nation's history!

As mentioned in the "Introduction" of this book, nutrition is a scientific <u>ART</u> because every human is different.   Every human has their own individual genetic predispositions for disease.   In addition, every human has their own individual preferences (which may change throughout their lifetime) for food &/or dietary supplements regarding: Tolerances; Allergies; Taste preferences or dislikes; Positive & negative reactions.   For example (part of "Dietary Commandment # 6"): every food or supplement that has anticoagulant properties (to possibly decrease your risk of a blood clot) can also increase your risk of bleeding.   The concept of a healthy balance repeats itself as it is fundamental in diet/nutrition & the entire health of our bodies.

However, every human adult (& most teenagers) may benefit from following all of these "10 Dietary Commandments" to maximally "***cleanse***" their entire **bodies** <u>(as well as their minds & souls)</u>.   This is because we are "***FULL OF***" more direct body (as well as mind & soul) toxins than ever before in the history of God's earth.   Considering the growing level of toxicity to our bodies (as well as our minds & souls), everyone needs to know these "***<u>10 Dietary Commandments</u>***!"

There has been a huge **failure to disclose the truth** about food/nutrition.   One may say: The food/diet/nutrition industry is "***FULL OF IT***!"   I have no issue with adults consuming "junk food."   I take umbrage when adults consume "junk food" – but are told it is healthful!   If your "meal" breaks all 10 of these Dietary Commandments – then you should know the truth (that it is harmful)!   If your meal follows all 10 Dietary Commandments – then it is healthful.   The truth shall set you free!

As mentioned throughout this book: If you believe simply avoiding gluttony (part of "Dietary Commandment # 1") is the only dietary rule needed to create optimal health of your body - then "***YOU ARE FULL OF IT***!" If you believe that simply avoiding gluttony & physical laziness are the only 2 factors involved in creating the optimal health of your body – then "***YOU ARE FULL OF IT!***"   You can exercise regularly & avoid gluttony - & still not achieve optimal health.   As shown in chapter 4: health & fitness are destroyed by the <u>accumulation & compounding effect of the combination</u> of all the different body, mind, & soul toxins.   As mentioned earlier in this chapter: **health, fitness, & _cleansing_ [of the body, mind, & soul] are maximized via the combination of**:

- Attempting to avoid all the body, mind, & soul toxins (mentioned in chapters 1-3)
- Performing most – if not all - of the non-Dietary cleansing methods shown in the 1st section of this chapter
- Certain "Super-Cleansing Foods & Supplements" (shown in Chapter 6)
- & following all 10 of these "10 Dietary Commandments."

I believe these are the best dietary rules to follow for every adult human to maximally cleanse (& "detox" - & optimize the health of) their entire body (as well as their mind & soul) - & keep it clean.

Try to focus on the positive.   Try to focus on the healthful, delicious foods you eat (versus the harmful foods you should avoid).   Do not focus on the foods (or SINS) you should avoid.   This is a major reason why most diets fail.   If you tell someone not to think of a purple cow: they will then start focusing on that purple cow.   Focus on healthful foods (& God).   Try to focus on the health benefits you may receive by following these rules ("commandments").

I do not enjoy telling any friend or family to avoid or eat any food (Remember: I have never told a single patient to start or stop putting anything in their mouth)!   We all have individual preferences & dislikes.   If you love to eat junk food: try to exchange it (or make it) with healthier alternatives.   As you will see in chapter 7, you can even have "dessert" (like pudding, chocolate shakes, cakes, & brownies –made by following these "10 Dietary Commandments") on this diet!

However, we have wandered throughout the nutritional & dietary wilderness for too long.   Americans have purchased so many diet books (often from "celebrities" –because they are famous) without much biblical or scientific sense.   There is no other diet book that includes all 10 of these "dietary commandments."

Do not put yourself down – or others down for breaking 1 or more of these dietary commandments (on a daily basis).   We must encourage one another (as the Bible says we should).   _**Most people (especially those suffering with diseases- including obesity & chronic pain) break ALL 10 of these Dietary Commandments every day – often multiple times per day**_! As society has strayed farther away from God & His _10 Commandments_, we have become more diseased & (not ironically) strayed farther away from these "10 Dietary Commandments!"   Said differently, WE are all "_**FULL OF**_" **Dietary SINS**!   Imagine how diseased your mind & soul (&, therefore, your body) would become if you broke ALL of God's 10 Commandments three times a day!   Imagine you:

- Stole 3 times a day!   Coveted your neighbor's spouse 3 times a day!   Murdered someone 3 times a day!

You "get" my point.   If a Satanist tried to convince you that breaking all of God's 10 Commandments will lead to optimal health of your mind & soul – you would know better. This is because the truth has been disclosed to you (regarding knowledge of God's word). However, knowledge of these 10 Dietary Commandments has not been disclosed in its' entirety (Until now)! Again: the truth shall set you free!

The Standard American Diet is "S.A.D." & SAD!   As mentioned throughout this book, the S.A.D. breaks ALL 10 of these "10 Dietary Commandments" every meal (&, therefore, 3 times per day –if not more via snacks)!

Despite the body of knowledge in nutrition doubling every 7 years, we have become "lost" wandering through the wilderness of diet & nutrition. We have become "slaves" to the toxins we store in our body – mostly from the quality & quantity of the foods we consume (as well as how & when we consume them).

GOD'S COMMANDMENTS = HIS "*EMPOWER-MENTS*"

When God **Commands** you to do something: *He will always help/enable/****empower*** *you to accomplish it.* (Isaiah 41:10)

By simply following ALL of these "10 Dietary Commandments," I (& thousands of my "family & friends" –which I include as fellow health care providers over the past 16 years) have received/reported **the following life-changing *empowered* benefits**:

- Achieved optimal health & even improved fitness levels.   However, the improved fitness & health levels reported may have been because the "diet" helped them *feel* cleaner, better, & more motivated to exercise more frequently (one of the non-dietary cleansing methods mentioned earlier).
- Reported optimal (dramatically improved) **ABSORPTION+++**/digestion of the foods they consume. Reported great reductions in colitis, heartburn, &/or other forms of acid-reflux.
- Lost intestinal putrefaction –reported optimal bowel elimination (in size &/or frequency).
- Lost hip &/or waist size, excess weight & body fat (if needed, to an optimum weight & body fat percentage).
- Reduced or eliminated allergy symptoms.
- Decongested their sinuses – with reports of improved air flow &, therefore, sense of smell.
- Improved cardiopulmonary vital signs. Improved oxygen saturation & blood pressure were noted in the people that had their vitals taken (before & after starting the diet). ***
- Improved neurological functioning. Patients with Parkinson's disease had less: resting tremors, of a masked face expression, shuffling gait, & difficulty initiating movements. ***
- Reported a sense of great "*detoxification*" or "*cleansing*" from the bombardment of toxins we are all "***FULL OF!***"
- *Felt better, cleaner, & younger than they had in decades.*
- Felt they looked younger & more attractive (confirmed by their friends/loved ones). However, beauty is in the eye of the beholder.

- Reported a *"cleaner mind & body."*
- Reported a *"cleaner soul."* Even my friends that were &/or are atheists reported feeling *"more spiritual."*

+++This concept of "**ABSORPTION**" is what makes this "diet book" superior (in my strong opinion) to all other diet books. This "diet" consists of delicious foods that are ABSORBED optimally. Consider the following analogy. If you open the gas cap to your automobile & pour the gas all over your car (near the gas cap), your automobile will only "absorb" a fraction of the fuel. You won't get very far. If you use the worst sludge to replace your car oil with, you won't get very far either. When you break these "10 Dietary Commandments," you will not optimally absorb the food you consume. You may eat & then feel tired soon after. Food should give you energy/fuel (not rob it from you)!

***As a scientist (not a "Christian Scientist" – but a scientific Christian), I must admit that the abovementioned great results were not tested via double-blind, placebo-controlled methods. In addition, only a small percentage (20% or so) of these individuals had there vital signs (or blood) measured/analyzed before & after going on the diet – since the diet's inception in 1997. These great results are mostly testimonials & case studies of the over 1,000 adults who went on this diet.

How do we know if a food or supplement is healthful or harmful? Answer = If the person consumed that food breaking all 10 of these "Dietary Commandments," then it was harmful. If the same person consumed that same food following all 10 of these "Dietary Commandments," then it was healthful. Of course some people have likes/dislikes, allergies, etc. to certain foods/supplements. However (for the most part), now there should be no confusion to whether or not you eat a "healthful diet" or a "harmful diet."

Are all of these "10 Dietary Commandments" based on the living word of God? Answer = Yes & no.
Some of these dietary commandments will not be found specifically in the bible. However, all 10 of these commandments (I strongly believe) are the best "diet" to achieve:
- **Optimal ABSORPTION** of the healthful foods you consume
- **Maximal *cleansing* & health of your body (as well as your mind & sou**l).

Using a biblical analogy: even if you were to eat the most healthful foods in the world – you will NOT optimally **ABSORB** them if:
- You're intestines are "***FULL OF***" waste matter;
- &/or if you break these "10 Dietary Commandments" when consuming them!

It would be like ***planting a seed on hard soil***! It is God's will for His creation to have perfect **absorption** of His living word (***via good soil***). It is also God's will for His creation to have optimal health [& maximally *cleanse*] your *body (the temple of the Holy Spirit)* – as well as your mind, & soul. *"I came that they may have life, & have it abundantly."* (John 10:10) Having optimal absorption of God's food is an important component of this. Therefore: **all 10 of these "Dietary**

155

Commandments" (in my humble opinion) are based on major _principles_ of the God's living word!

In summary, the uniqueness to these "10 Dietary Commandments" is that it is the best (in my humble opinion – based on experience, testimonials, scientific & scriptural principles) "diet" to achieve **OPTIMAL**:
- Digestion & **ABSORPTION** of the healthful nutrients you consume
- **Elimination** of the toxins in your intestines – as well as the rest of your body
- & health ("_CLEANSING_") of your **_body, mind, & soul_**!

This diet has a strict "**Cleansing Phase**" - & a less-strict **"Lifestyle Phase."** The diet starts with the _"Cleansing Phase"_ – which is somewhat strict & follows all of these "10 Dietary Commandments" - **without any exceptions**! The "Cleansing Phase" is _from one day to 2 weeks_ - depending on your will power, tolerance, & needs.   It helps to put some biblical reference to "sticking" to this "Cleansing Phase."   For example think of Jesus & His disciples fasting before they started their ministry &/or missionary journey. Think of the people of the Old Testament who fasted after funerals, for repentance, etc.

The _"Cleansing Phase"_ is –for the most part- a 100% raw, organic, vegan, mucus-free, **allergy-free**, antioxidant-rich, liver-cleansing, blood-cleansing, food-combining, balanced-diet, & overall cleansing & immune boosting phase.   It includes extremely healthful, raw, & Organic: Fruits, vegetables, sprouted beans, cocoa, nuts, seeds, etc.

This _"Cleansing Phase"_ is an optimal way to _**CLEANSE**_ your **gastrointestinal system** (as well as the rest of your body) to become "_**good soil**_" so you can better _**absorb**_ your nutrients.   Some may consider the "Cleansing Phase" as an "avoidance" or "elimination" phase as you are eliminating many foods – as well as supplements.   You are giving your digestive system a well-deserved "vacation."   Since your body is not "working so hard" to digest the food you are consuming, this may allow your entire body to heal/rejuvenate!   Many people report feeling more energetic, thinking clearer, looking more youthful (besides losing the excess body fat & intestinal waste matter)!

This was my original "2 Week **Allergy-Free** & Mucus-Free Diet" (which I originally created in 1997).   After the "Cleansing Phase:" you can gradually add the non-raw "super-cleansing foods & supplements" (mentioned in the next chapter) one day at a time. This may allow you to determine which foods/supplements you may have an allergic or adverse reaction to!

The "**Lifestyle Phase**" (follows the "Cleansing Phase") **INCLUDES the exceptions** listed in the "10 Dietary Commandments."   This phase adds cooked foods –like extremely healthful organic, free-range (hormone-free):
- Meats (like chicken, turkey, lamb, etc.); probiotic goat's milk; probiotic soybean food sources (like natto, tempeh, etc.).   However, one should

try to consume the majority of "your plate" as raw & alive as possible (for optimal **_absorption)_**.

Realize this "Lifestyle Phase" also possesses cleansing properties.   This "Lifestyle Phase" may not cleanse your gastrointestinal system as strong as the "Cleansing Phase."   However, the "**_Lifestyle Phase_**" may actually **_CLEANSE_** **other parts of your body** as well – if not better than the "Cleansing Phase" – due to the addition of certain "super-cleansing foods/supplements!"   Most people benefit from being on this phase for **at least 90% of the year as this phase is better suited to create long-term optimal health**.   Many people feel so amazing during the **initial** "Cleansing Phase," they don't want to leave it.   However, the wonderful benefits of these exceptions are too beneficial to exclude for life – or even for more than 2 weeks straight (in my humble opinion).

Realize you can return to the "Cleansing Phase" anytime.   You can **"return" (for even 1 or 3 days) to the "Cleansing Phase"** if you: Get sick, "cheat" (especially when you travel, go to parties, go out with friends), or truly need to lose more body fat (or intestinal waste matter).

However, I would not recommend any friend or family stay on the "Cleaning Phase" for more than 2 weeks at a time. Due to all the "super-cleansing foods/supplements" added to the "Lifestyle Phase," the "Lifestyle Phase" is what most people benefit from 90% of the year.   For example: if you did an initial (first time in your life) 2 week "Cleansing Phase" of this diet from January 1st to 14th.   Then, you would go on the "Lifestyle Phase."   In April –due to either cheating on the diet or catching a cold – you may benefit from going back on the "Cleaning Phase" for a day or so.   Some adults prefer to be on the "cleansing phase" every day until Dinner-time.   That's why they have menus at restaurants!

The thousands of people who received/reported the abovementioned benefits stayed on the "Cleansing Phase" & "Lifestyle Phase" for at least 2 weeks.   Many people stayed on the "Cleansing Phase" for 2 weeks.   Some people had to leave this "Cleansing Phase" (& go to the "Lifestyle Phase") before 2 weeks due to the following reasons:

-    A weak sense of will-power or discipline. We are not here to judge. We all have our weaknesses/sins (mentioned in chapter 1).
-    Too strong a "detox reaction."   They were having too many healthy bowel movements (some reported 15 times per day)! Despite the bowel movements being healthy, it was too strong a "shock" to their system. They lost too much weight (including body fat, waist &/or hip sizes) too quickly a pace (they felt).   They reported an initial fatigue - perhaps from all the toxins leaving their system too quickly (some refer to this as a "Herxheimer-type reaction"[1] – which is a temporary detox/cleansing reaction where you "feel" worse before feeling better).

- Too great a change in their dietary lifestyles. Some could not understand how to change from all their bad dietary habits to all these good dietary habits. Remember, even Jesus did NOT heal everyone! We have to understand the fact that some people (hope this does not sound judgmental) do not want to get better! The only person who likes change is a wet baby. We are all creatures of habit. We get into a habit of eating junk food (even though we may believe it is healthful food)! I have had many people tell me: "I'll start that diet - AFTER I finish eating all the – (junk food) that is in my fridge!"

Warning to Dietary Lifestyle "**Vegans**"
"He who is weak (in faith) eats vegetables only." (Romans 14:2)
Vegans (abstain from all food sources that have a face!) who follow these "10 Dietary Commandments" **for life** may unfortunately:
- Lose too much body fat & weight. Remember, not everyone has excess body fat or weight they need to lose!
- Lose muscle mass (especially if they avoid the organic "super-foods": raw nuts, raw edible seeds, raw nut butters & raw sprouted beans).
- Be or become deficient in vitamin K2 (a "super-supplement"). However, consuming natto (or taking a vitamin K2 supplement of 100mcg/day - or to a lesser degree consuming other cultured/fermented probiotic food sources) may prevent this vitamin K2 deficiency.
- Be or become deprived of essential nutrients available only from meat & animal food sources. As per Jordan Rubin (Author of *The Maker's Diet*):[1] *"These nutritional deficiencies pose potentially deadly consequences to long-term health."*

Remember, the person who is most responsible for your health care is you!

I. Thou shall consume foods in a God–pleasing manner.

"YOU'RE NOT FAT. YOU'RE FULL OF:"
- Poor Gratitude for the food/beverages you consume; Stress (before, during, & after) you consume the food; Gluttony; & consuming foods in an "Anti-Godly" manner!

The reasons Americans (as well as most others in the rest of the world) have been increasingly breaking "Dietary Commandment #1" (as well as the other 9) since the 1970s (if not longer) have been mentioned in Chapters 1 & 2. Some of these reasons may include:
- Our society is faster-paced
- Families are more spread across this country (if not the globe)
- There is less importance placed on the "family unit" & **daily** "family breakfasts/dinners" (especially those with prayers to God)
- We have become so "***FULL OF***" sin – that we have become apathetic to consuming foods in a God-pleasing manner.

- We have become so "**_FULL OF_**" mind & soul toxins – that we have become apathetic to doing anything else to please God or our **bodies** *(the temple of the Holy Spirit)*.
- We currently have the largest "God-deficit" our nation has ever experienced. We are more concerned about pleasing ourselves or others – than God.   As our nation as a whole has become **more apathetic towards God** (the growth of atheism, immorality, sin, mind & soul toxins, etc.), **eating** (or doing anything else for that matter) **in a God-pleasing manner has become less important**!

Eating in a God-pleasing manner is an important commandment to follow when attempting to receive greater peace, digestion, & maximally cleanse (optimize the health of) your body, mind, & soul.

Thou shall THANK God for sanctifying ALL the food you consume.

(Exodus 23:25; Psalm 145:15-16; 1 Corinthians 10:31; & 1Timothy 4:3-5)

You should do this <u>AFTER</u> – you praise & worship Him.   Remember: *"Love God (the most) with all your heart & mind."* <u>Before</u> consuming any & all foods, you should say a prayer *similar* to this (if you are alone, substitute "we" for "I"):

- "Dear God the Father, God the Son – Jesus Christ my Lord & savior, & the Holy Spirit,: We love you & praise you with all our hearts.   We thank you for all the blessings - You have given us in the past, present, & future.   We thank you for being with us eternally.   We thank you for forgiving us of our sins – as we forgive those who trespass against us.   We thank you for healing ALL of our diseases.   We thank you for the optimal health of every living cell in our bodies (this includes losing intestinal putrefaction & excess body fat).   *We thank you for sanctifying the food we are about to eat so that we receive optimal digestion/absorption & benefit from this food.*   We ask that everyone in the world –including ourselves- become closer to Christ.   We love you with all our hearts.   Amen."

Thou shall let the <u>Peace</u> of the Holy Spirit fill you when you eat!

Digestion is predominantly a "parasympathetic" (relaxation) nervous system activity.   You should be in a relaxed & peaceful state when you consume foods.   You should not be arguing, "stressing-out," or doing anything that excites the "flight or fight" (sympathetic) nervous system response.   Having the sympathetic nervous system "stimulated" (high stress to fight or flight), will predispose you to poor digestion & absorption of the foods you consume.

Try the deep breathing exercises mentioned in section I of this chapter before (& possibly during) food consumption.   Having the parasympathetic nervous system "stimulated" (i.e. being relaxed & peaceful) will create an environment for optimal digestion/absorption of the foods we consume.   This is achieved by:

- "**Breaking-The-Fast" (eating breakfast**).   You may have "fasted" for 11 hours (3 hours after you finished your last morsel of food + 8 hours of sleep) before you eat breakfast.   If you want a faster metabolism & "feed" the calorie-burning machine, you should eat breakfast. Everyone is unique & some may benefit from eating within 3 hours of sleeping as it may actually facilitate their sleep. However, others may benefit from avoiding food within 3 hours of sleeping as it may help them: Lose weight; Avoid heartburn/acid reflux; & sleep –as some people report having a "cleaner mind!" Thus, I leave this (when to eat the last meal of the day/night) up to the individual as God did not create any one person identically (even identical twins)!

- **Eating smaller portions throughout the day**. As mentioned in chapter 4, consuming too large (in calories) at one meal puts great stress on your gastrointestinal, endocrine, cardiovascular, & immune systems.
- **Chew Food thoroughly & SLOWLY**. This is one of the biggest mistakes I see many Americans make. We have a fast-paced ("fast food") culture. We can **enjoy the food so much better** if we take our time & enjoy all the amazing flavors in God's amazing foods. This includes shakes, soups, & even green juices (which can be swished & chewed in your mouth) – which are foods in a liquid state. Therefore, food should be chewed (or "swished") in your mouth so that the body releases the salivary enzyme ptyalin (a form of amylase) which begins to break down carbohydrates.[1,15] This will optimize absorption/digestion & reduce stress on the gastrointestinal system. This reduction in stress may help the cardiovascular, endocrine, neurological, & immune systems![1,7,15,49]

God did NOT put your taste buds in your esophagus, stomach, or intestines! In addition to enjoying all the amazing flavors of "God's food" (by chewing thoroughly & slowly), you can actually sublingually **ABSORB certain nutrients** (like vitamin B12). Most digestion occurs in the small intestine. However, digestion truly should begin in the mouth. If you chew food thoroughly & slowly, certain nutrients (like vitamin B12) contained in the food, may be absorbed sublingually (under the tongue)!

Thou shall Visualize Optimal Digestion/Absorption & Benefits of ALL the foods you consume. (Proverbs 29:18)

This includes visualizing all the delicious flavors, minerals, vitamins, fiber, & other beneficial nutrients (macro & micro) contained in the foods you are consuming.

Thou shall Avoid Gluttony (eating excessively)

This SIN has already been discussed in chapters 1-4. Consider the following analogy. God never gives you more than you can handle. (1 Corinthians 10:13) Therefore, you should NOT give your *body (the temple of the Holy Spirit)* more than it can handle! This can apply to every part of your life. However, I am *simply* applying this principle to the food we consume. If you are ***LAZY*** (also a sin discussed in chapters 1-4) & live a sedentary lifestyle: you are more at risk for committing gluttony (eating excessively). If you regularly perform moderate exercise, chances are you will have more muscle mass.

This increased muscle mass will burn more calories – even when you are asleep.

Remember: gluttony is eating in _excess of what you burn_. For example: the professional athlete who burns 5,000 calories per day is _NOT_ committing gluttony when they consume 5,000 calories throughout one day. However, you _are_ committing gluttony if you consume 2,500 calories per day – but only burn (possibly due to the sin **physical laziness**) 1500 calories per day. This also applies to meals. If you starve yourself all day long & then consume a large 1,800 calorie meal for dinner (while only burning 1,500 calories for the entire day) – then you have committed gluttony. This is just another reason why we should eat small meals throughout the day.

Gluttony creates stress to our gastrointestinal, endocrine, cardiovascular, & immune systems. Since eating an excess of food creates poor digestion & absorption: gluttony creates intestinal putrefaction (making you "**FULL OF IT**"). This intestinal putrefaction (as mentioned throughout this book) is a breeding ground for harmful viruses, microorganisms, drugs, & other toxins (making you more "**FULL OF IT**"). Thus, eating an excess of calories (even at only one of your meals during the day) increases your risk of disease(s) (including obesity &/or chronic pain).   Thus: Acting like a "Glutton" (even once a day) increases your "**FULL OF IT Level diseases, obesity, &/or chronic pain**" (analyzed in chapter 4).

EXCEPTIONS: There are no exceptions to this rule.   However, if you believe all calories are equal in their effect on our health & weight: then "**YOU ARE FULL OF IT!**"
NOT ALL CALORIES ARE CREATED EQUALLY!
I don't believe in counting calories. The over 1,000 people I know personally that have benefitted from following these dietary rules never counted calories. As long as you are following these "10 Dietary Commandments," I don't believe you ever need to count calories.
Regarding their effects on health & weight:
-   Calories from "super-foods" (organic, usually raw & alive, God-made, etc.) that allow you to consume them in compliance with these "10 Dietary Commandments" – are diametrically opposed to the calories from harmful junk foods that break all 10 of these "Commandments" (usually dead, cooked/roasted with hydrogenated oils & trans-fats – high in sugar, etc.)!
-   Food eaten in obedience/compliance with these "10 Dietary Commandments" are diametrically opposed (in healthfulness) to food eaten in disobedience with them!   This is analyzed further in Chapter 6.

2.   Thou shall eat foods 100% created by GOD.
"YOU'RE NOT FAT. YOU'RE FULL OF" Man-Made, non-organic foods/beverages/supplements!
This is where many Christians (I believe) misconceive 1 Tim 4: 3-5.   God created these organic healthful foods & man has destroyed them. I

161

interpret "Foods God has created" (in 1 Tim 4: 3-5) as being **free of the following "MAN-MADE" Toxins**:

- **Pesticides; Herbicides; Processed** (often you will see an extremely healthful God-created food – such as cocoa – include the man-made destruction of it via the ingredient: "processed with -!" This is why we must read ingredients).
- **Hormones** (most animals we consume as food in the U.S. have been treated with animal growth hormones to make the animal bigger – to sell more by the pound as *money has become our master*).
- **Antibiotics** (as mentioned in chapter 3, an estimated 29 million pounds of antibiotics are added to our animal feed every year!)
- **Hybridization; Irradiated; Genetically Modified Organisms (GMOs); Artificial preservatives; Artificial flavors; Artificial colors; Artificial sweeteners;** & anything else that is **NOT** "Free-range & 100% Organic" ("USDA Organic" is **supposed** to imply GMO-free also). In other words, anything else that is not 100% God-made!

If you believe the abovementioned man-made toxins are NOT harmful to our health, then "***YOU'RE FULL OF IT***!" As illustrated in chapter 3: The above mentioned toxins (such as pesticides & herbicides) have been linked to cancers, neurological diseases, atherosclerosis, & a whole host of other diseases. The **accumulation & compounding effect** of the hundreds (if not thousands) of pounds of man-made toxins the typical American consumes annually **adds to our weight** – as well as our **toxic load**! This is extremely under-recognized in our society today. In other words: these man-made creations add to our "***FULL OF IT*** Level of diseases, obesity, &/or chronic pain (often with accompanied disability)"!

Therefore, "***Foods God has created*** should be "***100% Organic/Free-Range***." This includes food, beverages, & even **supplements!** The abovementioned anti-Godly toxins that have found their way into our food represents another powerful example of how: our "God-deficit" has led to our health deficit. We have replaced God for money! It seems more important to make our animals larger & fatter ("***FULL OF***" hormones, antibiotics, & pesticide filled feed) - to make more money – than it does to keep "God's foods" healthful! It seems more important to make our fruits & vegetables larger (genetically modified, hybridized, etc.) – to make more money – than it does to keep "God's foods" healthful! It seems more important to make our food protected from pests (sprayed with pesticides & herbicides) – than it does to keep "God's foods" healthful!

God's earth (soil) has become man-made & man polluted.
The decades of pesticides sprayed –combined with the farming of crops in limited spaces – has led to a depletion of the minerals, vitamins, & nutrients found in our crops.[51] Therefore, the non-organic vegetables, fruit, & other crops we consume may possess:[51] An increased ability to harm you (compared to 50 years ago); & a decreased ability to help your health (compared to 50 years ago)!

The CCOF (California Certified Organic Farmers) have stated:[51] *In organic farming the soils are nurtured by adding organic matter, rotating crops and planting beneficial cover crops, unlike conventional farming where the soils are replenished with chemicals and synthetic additives. Organic farming works in harmony to sustain a healthy, fertile and biologically active (living) environment.* Therefore, having our food 100% God-made ("USDA Certified Organic") fulfills "Dietary Commandment #2" – as well as part of "Dietary Commandment #3!"

Shouldn't we COMPROMISE our standards?

Everyone in the Bible who compromised God's way for "the world's way" - suffered horrible consequences.   Because we have compromised "God's food" for "the world's" corruption/poisoning, our health has suffered.   It is inconceivable that our farms spray so much of these harmful toxins.   Many of these farms don't need nearly as much pesticides as they use!   It is inconceivable that costumers must pay so much more for "100% Organic/Free-Range."   Are consumers being punished for trying to get "closer to God?"

As our nation has turned far from God, our food has become more "man-made" (versus "God-made"). This is no coincidence. Farmers can sell more of the items as they claim "pests" don't destroy the food. Farmers can sell more of the food if it is larger (via hormone injections or genetically modified). Food distributers can sell more of these items also. Americans demand their food to be larger, "fresher," & more artificially colorful/flavorful (despite the potential health consequences). As *money has become the master of many Americans* (especially in "power"), our food has become less "God-made" (& more "man-made"). As "toxic food" has simply become accepted in our culture, our food has become less "God-made" (& more "man-made"). *What has man done to God's earth!?*

Pesticides consumed from our food have been linked to (but not limited to) the following health problems:[7,52-54]
-   Neurological problems/diseases (including Parkinson's – as well as Multiple Sclerosis, ALS, & Alzheimer's disease),
-   Cancer* (including breast, prostate, brain, bone, thyroid, colon, liver, lung, & leukemia), Autoimmune diseases, Hormonal disruption, Obesity,[7,53] Diabetes,[7,53] Depression, Fertility problems, Birth defects, Lower intelligence levels (including Autism & ADHD),[53] & skin, eye, & lung irritation.

* *"Parental exposures may act before the child's conception, during gestation, or after birth to increase the risk of cancer."*[7,53]

The Environmental Watch Group (EWG) has published (in 2012) the fruits & vegetables most contaminated with pesticides.[54]

17 of the most commonly pesticide-contaminated Fruits & Vegetables include ("non-organic" – obviously):[54]

1.   **Apples** – 98% tested positive for pesticides.

163

2. **Celery** – 96% tested positive for pesticides & pone sample tested positive for 13 different pesticides!
3. **Sweet bell peppers** – had 88 different pesticides as an entire category.
4. **Peaches** – 97% tested positive for pesticides, some with combinations of up to 57 different chemicals.
5. **Strawberries** – had 13 pesticides in a single sample.
6. **Nectarines** (imported) -100% tested positive for pesticides.
7. **Grapes** (should include **raisins** here also) – had 15 pesticides in a single sample & 64 different pesticides as an entire category. **Raisins** may contain 55 times more fluoride than tap water due to "Cryolite" – a sticky fluoride-based pesticide.[55]
8. **Spinach**
9. **Lettuce** – had 78 different pesticides as an entire category. Iceberg lettuce may have the most fluoride (180 times more than tap water) due to "Cryolite."[55]
10. **Cucumbers** – had 81 different pesticides as an entire category.
11. **Blueberries (domestic)** –had 13 pesticides in a single sample.
12. **Potatoes** - may have as much as 22 times more fluoride (on the outside; twice as much on the inside) than tap water due to "Cryolite."[55]
13. **Green beans** – often found in baby food. Almost 10% of green beans contained the pesticide *"methamidiphos"* in amounts that could easily increase the risk for brain & nervous system damage in infants consuming a 4-ounce serving of green beans on a regular basis.
14. **Kale/Collard Greens**
15. **Plums** (should include **prunes** here also) – 96% tested for pesticides.
16. **Cilantro** – 92.9% is contaminated, 70.1% of which is contaminated by more than one chemical.
17. **Pears –** 92% tested positive for pesticides, including *iprodione* –categorized by the EPA as a probable human carcinogen, & not registered for use on pears. Therefore, the *iprodione* was found in pears – & this represents a violation of FDA regulations!

We should NEVER compromise (no matter how less expensive they are) on purchasing/eating the abovementioned "NON-ORGANIC" foods. We should only purchase/eat them when they are certified "ORGANIC." Remember: you should still wash off (preferably with filtered sink water) all ORGANIC vegetables, fruits (even those with the inedible skins like organic bananas, melons, etc.), nuts, seeds, etc. Some claim vinegar (preferably apple cider vinegar) & water may help to remove more residue than just water alone. Either way, just rinse off with filtered water after you use this vinegar rinse.

Foods containing "Genetically-Modified Organisms (GMO)" or "GMO Foods" - have also shown to cause harm to animals, the environment, & possibly (probably) to humans.[56] Is America behind the times regarding the labeling of our poisoned foods? While food sold in America only labels "non-GMO" – as well as "organic" foods (leaving foods containing harmful GMOs & pesticides, etc. "**unlabeled**"), most countries either ban GMO foods or label foods that "***CONTAIN GMOs***" (as well as *containing pesticides*)!

Since GMO foods have shown an increase in mass tumors & damage to the liver & kidneys in **rats**: the French government is asking European authorities *to protect human health & abandon the use of GMO crops*.[57]   After Poland banned genetically modified maize, India has signed a mandatory law that all GMO food must be labeled as such by 1/1/2013.[58]

Scientists have found that the BT toxin (Bacillus thuringiensis – a bacterial toxin used as a pesticide) exhibit direct toxicity to human cells even in low doses.[59]   This Bt-Toxin (found in GMO crops) may elevate antibodies associated with allergies, infections, arthritis, inflammatory bowel disease, & cancer![59]   This Bt-Toxin is found in most North Americans – as well as their unborn fetuses![59]

Mercury has been found in approximately half of the highly popular (usually genetically modified) high fructose corn syrup – an ingredient found in over 90% of processed foods.[60]   Mercury may damage the neurological, digestive, & immune systems in humans –especially developing & unborn children.[7,60]

If produce is certified "USDA-organic," it's non-GMO (or supposed to be!).[56]   Perhaps we should all start our own organic gardening!

Here are the ***Top 10 worst GMO foods for your "do not eat" GMO foods list***:[56]

1. **Corn**: 50% of the U.S. farms growing corn (for "Montsano") are using GMO corn – which has been associated with weight gain & organ disruption. The Bt toxin used in GMO corn was recently detected in the blood or pregnant women & their babies.[59]
2. **Soy:** In 2006, there was over 96 million pounds of glyphosphate sprayed on soybeans alone.   90% of the soy grown is being genetically modified to *resist* herbicides!
3. **Sugar**: Should be avoided anyway! Sugar beets are being genetically modified to resist herbicides.
4. **Aspartame**: Is a toxic additive that should be avoided anyway – besides the fact that it is created with genetically modified bacteria.
5. **Papayas**: GMO papayas have been grown in Hawaii for consumption since 1999. They are banned in the European countries – but welcome with open arms in the U.S.!
6. **Canola**: One of the most chemically altered foods in the U.S. diet.
7. **Cotton Oil** (from India & China): have serious risks.
8. **Dairy**: 20% of all U.S. cows are pumped with growth hormones –like the health-hazardous rBGH (banned in 27 countries). "Probiotic-rich Organic goat's milk" is the best dairy source - after the "Initial Cleansing Phase."
9. & 10. **Zucchini & Yellow Squash**: are modified to resist viruses.

Three GMO foods likely in your Multi-Vitamins may include the following:[61]
- GM Corn in the form of Ascorbic Acid or Vitamin C & Maltodextrin
- GM Soy in the form of a "filler"
- & GM Sugar Beets in the form of HFCS (High-Fructose Corn Syrup) or sucrose.

As mentioned in chapter 3, there are many **man-made toxic ingredients allowed in the U.S. while banned in other countries.** These include (but are not limited to):[62]

- **Azodicarbonamide** (found in frozen dinners, boxed pastas, bread, & packaged baked goods) may increase the risk of asthma.
- **Brominated vegetable oil** (found in sodas & sports drinks) may increase the risk of schizophrenia, growth problems, hearing loss, birth defects, & major organ damage.
- **Potassium Bromate** (used in baked goods *to save time & money*) may increase the risk of cancer, nervous system damage, & kidney damage.
- **Olestra** (AKA "Olean") may cause vitamin depletion, cramping, & *anal leakage*!
- **Arsenic** (used in chicken to make it look pinker & prettier?) is a toxic poison analyzed in chapter 3.
- **Artificial colors** (ubiquitous in foods sold in the *"United Shame of America"*) may increase the risk of brain cancer, ADHD, nervous system damage, etc.

Fast Toxic-Food for a Fast-Paced Toxic society

As mentioned in chapter 2, families don't gather together every night for dinner anymore (for a whole host of reasons analyzed in the 1st 4 chapters). Fast, fried, & **processed foods** are considered the worst foods to consume while sick or battling a cold (as well as any other time!) as they:[63]

- Are usually void of nutritional value;
- Usually produce inflammation (which weakens the immune system);
- Are usually genetically modified & contain HFCS (High Fructose Corn Syrup), aspartame, artificial colors, flavors, preservatives, MSG, dimethhylpolysiloxane, etc. *Would you like kidney damage with your fries or extra pesticides with your salad?*

There's something "Fishy" about our FISH! Is Fish *still* a "God-created food?" Did God intend our seafood to be raised in farms consuming soybeans? Did God intend for man to poison His waters (where the fish live)?

One gram per day of the omega 3 fatty acids EPA (eicosapentaenoic acid) & DHA (docosahexaenoic acid) found mostly in fish &/or fish oil (originating from photosynthetic & heterotrophic microalgae the fish eat) may decrease the risk of: Blood clots;[64] Primary & secondary heart attacks;[65,66] Ischemic & thrombotic strokes;[64] Death, cardiovascular death, & sudden cardiac death by 20%, 30%, & 45% respectively;[67] & Coronary Heart Disease. The FDA has given a "qualified health claim" to the *EPA & DHA omega 3 fatty acids [that they may reduce the risk of coronary heart disease (CHD)].*[68]

However, consuming **over 3 grams per day** of the omega 3 fatty acids EPA & DHA increases the risk of: Bleeding;[64,69] Hemorrhagic strokes;[69] **Oxidation** of omega 3 fatty acids, forming biologically active oxidation products;[69] **Increased levels of low density lipoproteins (LDL) cholesterol** or apoproteins associated with LDL cholesterol among diabetics & hyperlipidemics (which, therefore, actually increases the risk of atherosclerosis!);[69] & reduced glycemic control among diabetics![69]

More importantly, man (humans) has polluted the waters (including the air & land-based foods). Consuming fish increases your risk of toxic heavy metal poisoning as fish contain mercury, lead, nickel, arsenic, & cadmium.[70,71] Other contaminants (PCBs – Polychlorinated biphenyls, furans, dioxins, & PBDEs) may also be found in fish.[70,71] As shown in chapter 3, these toxins increase the risk of many diseases.[7] However, heavy metal toxicity from consuming fish oil supplements is much less likely (as compared to consuming fish itself) because heavy metals seem to selectively bind with the protein in fish flesh rather than accumulate in the oil![70] The U.S. FDA has advised *pregnant & nursing women to stay away from (to help avoid mercury-induced brain & nerve damage to their baby): shark, tilefish, king mackerel, & swordfish, but says pregnant women can eat up to 12 ounces of a variety of other fish each week, as long as weekly intake of albacore tuna is limited to a single 6-ounce can.*[72] Based on the above, I would _educate_ all my **pregnant (as well as those planning to become pregnant) or nursing** "friends & family" to **avoid fish**! What about the rest of my "friends & family?"

In 2004, Physicians for Social Responsibility & the Association for Reproductive Health Professionals advised young women & children to eat no more than one or two servings each of salmon, sardines, herring or bluefish to reduce PCB exposure.[72] The groups added that orange roughy, marlin, & grouper should only be eaten once weekly.[72]

The "Smart Seafood Guide" printed (in 2007) by "Food & Water Watch"[73] (a nonprofit organization) printed their own extensive list of seafood that should be limited (or avoided) due to concerns about **excessively high levels of mercury or other contaminants**. This list included:[73]

-     Toothfish; Groupers; Orange Roughy; Rockfish Black; Rockfish Trawled (Trawled = *Conical net towed behind a boat – can cause habitat destruction*); Sharks; Red or Mutton Snapper; Bluefin or Canned Tuna; Bluefish; Oysters; Blue Crab; U.S. Swordfish; Croaker; Mackerel; & Striped Bass (also called "Rockfish" on the east coast of the U.S.A.).

This same organization has the following recommendations for consumers to make the following "green" seafood choices:[73]

-     **Buy Local.** *If you don't live near water, stick to U.S. fish.*
-     **Avoid imports.** *Less than 1% of imported seafood is tested for contaminants. Imported- shrimp is especially contaminated.*
-     **Eat fresh seafood.** *Avoid processed seafood, which travels farther, uses more fuel, & lacks country-of-origin labeling.*
-     **Avoid farm-raised marine finfish**, *especially salmon. They can threaten wild fish populations & are fed chemicals that can harm consumers.*
-     **& eat a variety of fish** *to reduce your exposure to possible seafood contaminants & to relieve pressure on wild populations.* **I disagree with this** last "green" seafood choice (for my "friends & family")! It seems inconceivable that we should bombard our bodies with a variety of CONTAMINANTS (toxins –mostly neurotoxins)! Remember: fish has changed -

& the environment in which fish live/come from has changed (for the worst) in the past 2,000 years (especially in the past 100 years)!

Fish versus Fish oil: Which is more harmful?!

- **Fish oil has a higher risk of bleeding** (& **other above mentioned side effects** that may be caused by consuming over the 3 grams of EPA + DHA omega 3 fatty acids).[64,69] "Un-concentrated" Fish oil by itself naturally contains approximately a 27.9% Omega 3 fatty acids EPA/DHA profile.[49,64,65] Some fish oil supplements are "concentrated" to increase the amount/percentage of EPA/DHA it contains (often to 1 gram of EPA/DHA per capsule). It is "easier" (faster) to reach above the dangerous 3 grams of EPA/DHA per day level by simply swallowing more than 3 of these "concentrated" fish oil capsules.[64,69] To reach above the dangerous 3 grams of EPA/DHA by consuming fish:[64,69] You would have to consume over 10 ounces (approximately 750+ calories) per day of certain fish high in these omega 3 fatty acids (like herring, sardines, Spanish mackerel, salmon, etc.)![74-76]
- Fish oil has a much **lower level of contaminants** than fish.[70-72,75] Toxic heavy metals selectively bind with protein in the fish flesh rather than accumulate in the oil.[70] The most stringent current standard is the International Fish Oils Standard.[71] Fish oils that are molecularly distilled under vacuum typically make this highest-grade, & have measurable levels of contaminants.[71]

What I would tell my "friends & family" is to avoid **all fish & fish oil products if** the following applies to you:

- You are taking pharmaceutical anticoagulants (unless your physician approves of this combination).
- You are scheduled for surgery (unless your physician/surgeon approves of this).
- You already have a bleeding disorder (unless your physician approves of this).
- You are pregnant, nursing, or planning on becoming pregnant.
- You have a Central Nervous System (CNS) Disease (such as Parkinson's, Multiple Sclerosis; ALS = "Loo Gehrig's Disease;" &/or Alzheimer's disease). Keep in mind, obsessive compulsive disorder (& other psychiatric tendencies/disorders) may be related to the toxic heavy metals &/or other pollutants found in fish (& to a much lesser degree in fish oil)!
- &/or you have a family history of any of the abovementioned CNS disorder(s)/disease(s).

Again, the person most responsible for your health is YOU! I have never told anyone to ever start or stop putting anything in their mouth. The ultimate decision is yours.

EXCEPTIONS: If you don't fall into the abovementioned categories, the benefits of consuming fish &/or fish oil (in small amounts & frequencies) *MAY* outweigh the negatives! However, these exceptions are done as part of the "Lifestyle Phase" (after the "Cleansing Phase").

If you can't find (or afford) "organic," there are **14 "non-organic" foods** that are *usually* NOT-GMO & have been considered (by the Environmental Watch Group = EWG) to be the 14 "cleanest" (*least* sprayed with pesticides). The "*clean 14*" include:[54]

1. **Onions**
2. **Pineapples** – fewer than 10% of samples contained pesticides
3. **Avocado**
4. **Cabbage**
5. **Sweet Peas**
6. **Asparagus**
7. **Mangoes** – fewer than 25% of samples contained pesticides
8. **Eggplant**
9. **Kiwi** - fewer than 25% of samples contained pesticides
10. **Cantaloupe (domestic)** – fewer than 40% of samples contained pesticides
11. **Sweet Potatoes**
12. **Grapefruit**
13. **Watermelon** –fewer than 40% of samples contained pesticides
14. **Mushrooms**

Remember: whether you eat "organic" or the above "close to organic" (despite not receiving the "certified USDA Organic" label), you should still wash (preferably with filtered sink water) ALL fruits (including the skin of the melons, avocados, etc.), vegetables, seeds, nuts, etc.! These "*clean 14*" foods may be why some studies may show very little difference in pesticide contamination between **certain** organic versus non-organic foods!

5. Thou shall consume foods 100% ALIVE – *restoring yourself like an EAGLE.*

"YOU'RE NOT FAT. YOU'RE FULL OF" Dead Foods!

God "*renews your youth like the eagle.*" (Psalm 103:5 & Isaiah 40:29-31)   Eagles (unless held in captivity) eat things that are **alive**.   The word of God is **alive**. God wants you to renew yourself by reading the bible (i.e. "feeding your mind & soul the **LIVING** word of God")!   God doesn't want you to renew yourself like a buzzard or chicken (they usually eat dead food)!

The abovementioned concept *may* apply to the foods we consume. Do you believe: "*You are what you eat*" (& absorb)?   Will you be "more alive" by eating (& absorbing) foods that are dead or alive? Think about that.   What I've said for decades: "*You are NOT what you eat – but what you absorb!*"   As mentioned throughout this book, this pertains to our mind & soul – as well as our body.   This pertains to dietary & non-dietary absorption of harmful toxins – as well as beneficial nutrients!   If you absorb (become "***FULL OF***") toxins: they can harm you.   Healthful Foods that are 100% alive are easier to absorb than when the healthful food is dead (see below)!   If you don't absorb all the healthful micronutrients in your food: are you truly getting all the benefits?

Realize forgiveness may happen instantaneously.   However, *restoration* usually takes time. Sampson's hair did not grow back instantly! It may take time to *restore* all the digestive enzymes you have "used up" throughout your life.

169

Adults have *a "bank" of digestive enzymes* (to help "break-down"/digest/absorb) the food we consume. By consuming enzyme-dead cooked &/or processed foods - & not replenishing our "bank" with enzyme-rich foods, we end up with a **"digestive enzyme deficit!"** This "deficit" may result in a whole host of digestive problems, including:[1,15,49]

- Mal-absorption, poor digestion, acid reflux, heartburn, constipation, gas, bloating, diarrhea, etc.

This may also result in a weakened immune system & inflammation – possibly increasing the risk of atherosclerosis![15,49]

Americans in the past 50 years are consuming fewer servings of enzyme rich foods, while *loading up on junk food virtually **devoid of all nutrients (& enzymes)**.*[1] This national eating pattern has produced widespread *nutrient & enzyme deficiencies*, thus leading to a number of health problems (like obesity).[1] Since your body desires/needs healthful nutrients (vitamins, minerals, phytonutrients, etc.): we end up over-eating high calorie, low nutrient "junk foods."

Therefore: <u>Thou shall consume only 100% living foods rich in ENZYMES</u>.

God put all the digestive enzymes you need to digest/absorb the 100% "living" food – in that living food. **Foods that are considered 100% "alive" & rich in digestive enzymes include ORGANIC RAW**:

- Fruits, Vegetables, Honey, Sprouted Beans (including Raw Sprouted Soybeans), Sprouted Lentils, Sprouted Quinoa (as well as other 100% Raw Sprouted Grains), Nuts & Raw Nut Butters, Seeds, Cocoa (often in the form of "Raw Cocoa Powder"), Almost any other "100% raw" vegan food,+++ & certain Probiotic Food Sources & Supplements. ***

+++Vegan foods that are 100% raw can be considered "100% alive." However, non-vegan raw foods [such as: raw eggs, fish (sushi), beef ("Steak Tartare"), etc.] are NOT considered alive - & may be very dangerous/harmful to consume.

***Unlike the abovementioned "digestive-enzyme rich" foods, many probiotic food sources (such as yogurt & cultured coconut milk) are not considered 100% alive. Some probiotic food sources (as well as supplements) are considered "100% alive." The probiotic food sources that may be considered **100% alive** (& usually eaten un-cooked) **include the following cultured/fermented food sources**:

- *Umeboshi* (AKA "Japanese Salty Pickled Plums");
- *Sauerkraut, pickled beets, pickled carrots, & pickled cucumbers* (AKA "Pickles").

However, even these "super-foods" – umeboshi, pickles, & sauerkraut- should be limited to due *(usually)* containing an **extremely high amount of sodium.** 1 cup (236 grams) of sauerkraut (or one large pickle) typically contains 1,560 mg of sodium.[74] Only 100 grams of umeboshi typically contains 8,700 mg of sodium (over 4x the U.S. RDA for a 150 pound adult)![77]

I define the term "Probiotics" as:

- **Live** microorganisms that BENEFIT our intestinal microbial balance;
- & consumed via dietary supplements &/or fermented foods with specially added active **LIVE** cultures.

170

I emphasize the term "**LIVE**" here. Most probiotic food sources &/or supplements recommend storing in the refrigerator before & after opening (to keep the probiotics "alive").   Probiotic supplements & probiotic food sources will be discussed further in Chapter 6.

Remember: these living raw foods are loaded with healthful **micronutrients** (such as "phytonutrients," etc.) – as well as healthful **macronutrients** (such as vitamins, minerals, etc.).   Many of these healthful micronutrients (which may help the cells of our body to fight cancer, heart disease, boost our overall immune system & health) have not been identified yet.   God only knows how many there are in these raw, living foods! When the scientific community discovers some of them, we often try to receive their benefits in the form of a dead capsule versus consuming the raw living food!

EXCEPTIONS: AFTER the "Cleansing Phase," one may benefit from consuming certain healthful foods that may not be considered "100% alive" during the "Lifestyle Phase."
There are many healthful foods that may NOT be considered "100% alive" – but are rich in enzymes. These healthful foods include ORGANIC:
- Greens powders (usually added to filtered water) that contain probiotics   as well as wheatgrass & barley juice powders (possibly 2 of God's highest sources of the powerful antioxidant enzyme **S.O.D.**).[15]
- **Probiotic _Goat's_ milk sources** - such as *acidophilus goat's milk, buttermilk, kefir, & yogurt.*
- Probiotic dairy-free beverages such as "*Cultured Coconut Milk*" & *kombucha.*
- Probiotic soybean sources such as *doenjang, miso, natto,* & *tempeh.*

*** **Super Oxide Dismutase (S.O.D.)** is an antioxidant enzyme that occurs naturally in a variety of "super-foods," including **broccoli, Brussels sprouts, sauerkraut, wheatgrass, barley grass, & most dark green leafy plants.**[15]   Perhaps this is why it is written in Genesis 1:29-30: "*I have given [to everything that moves on the earth] every GREEN PLANT for food.*" S.O.D. may be considered one of the most important antioxidants in the world as it may:[15]
- Decrease inflammation; Decrease oxidative stress; &, therefore, decrease the risk of atherosclerosis, immune diseases, - as well as boost the overall immune system!

There are many healthful foods that are not alive or rich in enzymes. These healthful foods include **ORGANIC**:
- "Super-oils" (such as extra-virgin coconut oil, extra-virgin olive oil, etc.) – mentioned under "super-cleansing fats" in Chapter 6.
- Un-sprouted wheat-free & gluten-free grains – such as: quinoa, oats, millet, brown rice, etc.
- "Super-cleansing meats" – mentioned in chapter 6 (must be raised on organic feed & without injections of hormones or antibiotics).
- Anything you desire to cook (such as the abovementioned "super-cleansing meats") *should* ONLY be **cooked with** either: **water or organic extra-virgin coconut oil.   Refined high-oleic (a monounsaturated fat) safflower oil** may also be a healthful oil to cook with (as it can tolerate high heat –even higher

perhaps than virgin coconut oil) IF it is **ORGANIC!** This is discussed further in chapter 6.

Jordan Rubin (in *The Maker's Diet*) lists many of the **benefits of extra-virgin coconut oil**:[1]

- Can tolerate extremely high heat, unlike polyunsaturated vegetable oils;
- Lowers the total cholesterol/HDL & LDL/HDL ratios to decrease the risk of atherosclerosis (see chapter 6 under "super-cleansing fats);
- Reduces the symptoms of digestive disorders;
- Supports overall immune functions;
- Helps prevent bacterial, viral, & fungal infections;
- Helps treat candida yeast infections, due to the presence of caprylic acid and antifungal fatty acids in the oil;
- & may help balance the thyroid & improve metabolic function, which may result in weight loss!

Digestive enzyme supplements

Most adults would benefit from taking a **digestive enzyme supplement**** when (during or immediately after) they eat "super-meats" to:[1,15,49]

- Enhance digestion & absorption of the food; Reduce inflammation; & boost the immune system.

Realize most adults do not "need" (in my strong opinion) these digestive enzyme supplements during the "Cleansing Phase" because God put (in all the raw living food) all the digestive enzymes we need to digest that raw living food!

The major types of digestive enzymes are:[1,15,49] **Proteases** – to digest/absorb proteins; **Amylases** – to digest/absorb carbohydrates; & **Lipases** – to digest & absorb fats.

Adults with a **HCL** (Hydrochloric acid) deficiency (common with people who have hypothyroidism &, ironically, acid reflux) – may benefit from taking a digestive enzyme supplement that also contains HCL.[15,49] Surprisingly, many adults with acid-reflux may actually be deficient in HCL.[15,49]

However, the addition of HCL may harm adults with gastrointestinal ulcers (including Crohn's disease).[15]

**However, digestive enzyme supplements should be avoided (or at least used with caution after consulting with your health care providers) if you are pregnant, nursing, or at risk for bleeding.[15]

Another ***EXCEPTION*** to consider is that some physicians (such as oncologists) advise their **patients with weakened immune systems** (such as those undergoing chemotherapy) to avoid all raw foods as they might have harmful microorganisms on/in them (that would be killed if cooked). These oncologists believe the negative risk of consuming these raw foods outweigh their benefits on patients with severely weakened/compromised immune systems. The abovementioned "***EXCEPTION***" is mentioned to remind the reader of the following:

- This book is 100% educational. I have never told or advised anyone to start or stop putting anything in their mouth ("CYA" = Cover Your Asset(s)☺). The person who is most responsible for your health is you!
- Everyone is different & *"that's why restaurants have menus!"* Most of us benefit greatly from 100% living raw vegan organic foods. However, other people may have allergies, drug interactions, &/or dislike the taste to those same living foods.
- & all raw fruits, vegetables, seeds, & nuts should be rinsed off (in a stainless steel strainer preferably) thoroughly with filtered water on the outside & inside (if applicable) of that food! Even raw organic bananas & melons should be rinsed with filtered water – before & after it has been peeled/cut open! Even the inside (& outside of course) of a pepper should be rinsed off thoroughly with filtered water! Most people forget these things.

4. Thou shall avoid "toxic mucus" foods & consume foods to cleanse "toxic mucus" from the body.

"You're Not FAT. You're FULL OF" Toxic Mucus!

"Toxic Mucus" is defined (by Robert Gray in *"The Colon Health Handbook"*) as:[78] - *Being caused predominantly by **"mucus-forming foods."***

- Producing harmful effects *from the constipated feces remaining stagnant in the colon.*
- *Polluting the gastrointestinal system, lymphatic system, **respiratory (including clogged nasal sinuses)** & /or urinary systems; uterus, vagina, connective tissue, or other body part. Toxic mucus may be present in - or exude from - any body tissue.*

Toxic mucus is diametrically opposed to healthful mucus. Healthful mucus provides beneficial mucus in our body – such as in the inner lining of our intestines, our joint surfaces, etc.[78]

The *"toxic-mucus response"* to airborne pollutants (such as cigarette smoke – via smoking or passive/"2nd hand" smoking) is more harmful to the respiratory system than in the stools.[78]

Thou shall avoid highly "toxic mucus forming" foods.

The Hebrews mentioned in Hebrews 5:12 were choosing to be *spiritually infantile*. *"You STILL need milk & not solid food!"* Are we choosing to be *nutritionally infantile*? Are adults eating too many foods that create "toxic mucus" (as adults)!? My intent of listing these highly "toxic mucus forming" foods is not to offend anyone. My intent is simply to educate adults in my opinion on how to cleanse (& optimize the health of) their bodies, minds, & souls. Consuming highly "toxic mucus forming" foods raises our *"**FULL OF IT** Level of Diseases, Obesity, &/or Chronic Pain."* Therefore: avoiding these foods can help us lower this "**level**."

Based on Dr. Grey's book, my own personal experience, & testimonials from over 1,000 of my "friends & family" members who tried my allergy/toxic-mucus free diet introduced in the mid-1990s, I created an estimated "**toxic mucus scoring system**."   This "toxic mucus scoring system" consists of the following:

- "**100% toxic mucus capability**."   This property may, therefore, potentially:
    - Block the absorption of 100% of the healthful nutrients of this food (as well as other foods you combine with it).
    - &/or create the maximum amount of harmful "clogging" (AKA "plugging up" or "sluggishness") in the gastrointestinal, respiratory, &/or lymphatic systems!   Cow's milk products may be appropriately labeled in this category.
- To "**0% toxic mucus capability**."   This would include most raw organic sprouts, most vegetables, fruits, seeds, & nuts.

The most "toxic-mucus forming" foods (to avoid) include:[78]

- ALL uncultured (probiotic-free) Dairy products from **COW'S milk should be given a "100% toxic mucus capability**!" Cow's milk products are considered one of the 5 worst foods (due to their potential to create toxic mucus in the respiratory tract) to consume while sick or battling a cold.[63]   It has been estimated that the average American annually consumes over 600 pounds of non-cheese cow's milk products (plus over 31 pounds of cheeses –mostly derived from cow's milk)![79]   Many adults consume cow's milk products for the calcium or protein.   However, are we really absorbing the calcium or protein in these *highly toxic-mucus* cow's milk products?   Goat's milk, however, is substantially less "mucus forming" than cow's.
- **Non-Sprouted** uncultured ***SOYBEANS*** *are the MOST "mucus forming" of all plant foods*. Their toxic *mucus-forming activity comes close to that of cow's milk products*!   Therefore, these soy-based foods (usually processed like soymilk, soy cheese, soy burgers, soy ice cream, etc.) should be given a "**95% toxic mucus capability**!"   Soy-based foods that contain a large amount of probiotics (such as Natto & tempeh) have a very low toxic mucus capability (due to the "counter-mucus" effect of probiotics) & are, therefore, considered "Super-Cleansing Soy" foods.   "Super-Cleansing Soy" versus "Harmful Soy" is analyzed in greater detail in chapter 6.

Most store bought **protein powders & shakes** are "***FULL OF***" the highly toxic-mucus of the abovementioned un-cultured cow's milk (sometimes labeled as "whey protein," etc.) &/or soybeans (sometimes labeled as "isolated soy protein," etc.). **Cultured/Probiotic cow's milk products (like cow's milk yogurt, kefir, etc.) should be given a "0-100% toxic mucus capability" range –depending on the amount of live probiotic cells per serving (as probiotics possess a "counter-mucus" effect –see later).**   If the product has **1 billion live probiotic cells/cup** –then it should have a "50% toxic-mucus capability."   Any amount less than 1 billion per cup should have a greater than 50% - & any amount **over 50 billion per cup should have less than "10% toxic mucus capability**."   Yogurt mixed with any fruit besides an apple actually increases its' toxic mucus capability due to poor food-combining (which will be shown in greater detail in "Commandment # 10").

- Other **Non-Sprouted Beans** possess considerable mucus forming activity.   However, there is a considerable gap between non-sprouted soybeans & other non-sprouted beans.   Therefore, these non-sprouted beans should be given a "**50% toxic mucus capability**."   **Coffee** (liquid non-sprouted beans), & **peanuts/peanut butter** (even raw organic – without the sugar & salt additives as *peanuts are a legume* versus a "nut") should also be categorized as a "**50% toxic mucus capability**" food.   This may be why adults may experience feeling "gaseous" or "bloated" when consuming the above.   Are we really absorbing all the healthful nutrients in these foods?

- **Wheat Gluten &/or Wheat Bran should also be given a 50% toxic mucus capability**. *******   *Wheat (dramatically more than any other grain) is believed to actually "bloat" your intestines* & create (what Dr. William Davis, M.D.) a *"Wheat Belly."*[80]
- Gas-ripened bananas (many **non-organic bananas** sold in the U.S.) & "**sulphured" fruits** may be rare examples of mucus forming fruit & should be given a "**33% toxic mucus capability**."   This is mostly due to the *man-made processes to which they may have been subjected*.   Many people have witnessed non-organic bananas ability to "stop diarrhea" via their potential constipating effect.   All dried fruit –except for figs, dates, raisins, & prunes – may be "sulphured" unless specifically labeled otherwise.
- **Eucalyptus Honey** is a *rare type of honey noted for its' relatively high mucus-forming activity*.   Therefore, eucalyptus honey should be given a "**25% toxic mucus capability**."
- **Un-cultured goat's milk products should be given a low "20% toxic mucus capability."**   However, highly cultured probiotic goat's milk products (like goat's milk yogurt, kefir, etc. –with 1 billion live probiotic cells/cup) should be given a "**5% or less toxic mucus capability**."

*** Robert Grey (in *The Colon Health Handbook*) has 3 **objections to the ingestion of wheat bran**:[78]

- One: *commercially available wheat bran typically contains over 80% of all the phytates in the whole grain.   These phytates can block the absorption of minerals such as: iron, zinc, calcium, & magnesium.*
- Two: although wheat **bran** may possibly reduce mucus in the stools – *it can create mucus in other parts of the body (such as our joints, lymphatic system, & possibly our sinuses –affecting our respiratory system)*!
- Three: *wheat bran may not lower blood cholesterol levels, as do many of the vegetable & fruit fibers.*

***Dr. William Davis, M.D. (in his book "Wheat Belly") also has **objections to the ingestion of ALL wheat products**:[80]

- Wheat has become ***genetically altered*** (breaking "Dietary Commandment # 2") *into a nutritionally bankrupt yet ubiquitous ingredient*
- *Wheat causes **blood sugar to spike** more rapidly than eating pure table sugar* (breaking "Dietary Commandment # 8")
- Wheat causes us to *ride a roller coaster of hunger, **overeating**, & fatigue* (breaking "Dietary Commandment # 1")
- Americans – since the 1970s – have been told by "dietary experts" to avoid healthful fats & consume more "healthful whole grains."   *Americans* (even those that are *health-conscious – since the 1970s) have been consuming approximately 75% of their carbohydrate calories from wheat products.*   The above facts & trends have led to ***Americans becoming heavier & more diseased*** - *especially intestinal diseases –like celiac disease, ulcerative colitis, & constipation (as well as type II diabetes, metabolic syndrome, heart disease, & a whole host of other diseases).*

The overconsumption of high-carbohydrate grain based foods such as bran, fibrous breakfast cereals, & whole wheat bread (non-sprouted), which all contain high amounts of mineral blocking phytates (just like non-fermented soy), is a primary cause of intestinal disease (like constipation, ulcerative colitis, & celiac disease) & other diseases![1,78,80]   It has been estimated that the average American annually consumes over 192 pounds of flour & cereal products (134 pounds of which being wheat flour)![79]

Certain individuals are much more resistant to the effect of consuming high toxic mucus forming foods than the average person. These people may decrease the toxic mucus capability of some of these foods & increase their absorption capability.   These "more resistant" (hyposensitive) people include the following:

- Those who **regularly perform exercises** – especially strength training exercises. The increase in muscle mass allows their metabolism to speed up & improve the digestion & assimilation of even highly toxic mucus forming foods. This may be why certain professional body builders (who strength train/"body-build" for 4 hours/day) may actually benefit from the cow's milk & soy protein sources. However (in my strong opinion), most adults (including most people who exercise regularly) would still benefit from replacing these highly toxic mucus forming protein sources with low/no toxic mucus forming foods.
- Humans **under the age of 20** typically have a superior ability to absorb & utilize the nutrients in even these highly toxic mucus forming foods – when compared to when they are over age 20.   This has to do with the fact that they are still growing & their bodies have a greater demand for more protein, calories, & other nutrients from any source the body receives it.   Are you still growing when you are 30, 40, 50, or 90 years old?   If you are, it's probably NOT vertically!
- & people **possessing the genes to better absorb** these foods than the average person.   For example, people with northern European descent may possess a superior capability to absorb cow's milk products.

Certain individuals are much less resistant to the effect of consuming high toxic mucus-forming foods than the average person. These "less resistant" (hypersensitive) people include those with:

- **Sedentary lifestyles**.
- & **hypothyroidism** which may cause a sluggishness of bowel motility.   This hypothyroidism-induced constipation may lead to weight gain (or difficulty gaining weight) – as well as diseases from the storing of (being "*FULL OF*") toxins in the intestines.   Hypothyroidism (as mentioned in chapter 3) may be the result of years of *EXCESS chlorine, fluoride, &/or bromine* – as well as a *DEFICIENCY in iodine/iodide*![15,50]   Besides constipation, **hypothyroidism** may lead to the following problems (as illustrated beautifully in Dr. Brownstein's book Iodine: *Why You Need It – Why You Can't Live Without It*):[50]
    o Cold Intolerance (including cold extremities & lower body temperature). Armpit temperature 15 minutes in bed when you awaken in the morning should be tested.[15]   A temperature of 97.6 degrees Fahrenheit or lower may indicate an underactive thyroid (keep temperature log for 5 days & report to your endocrinologist).[15]

- - - - o Dry skin; Fatigue; Recurrent infections; possibly impaired memory (& irritability); Thyroid cancer – mostly due to an iodine deficiency; & breast cancer – mostly due to an iodine deficiency. When there is an iodine deficiency, the breasts, like the thyroid gland, enlarge to compensate for that deficiency (to increase their ability to absorb & store iodine). Remember: *"if thyroid hormone is given to an iodine-deficient patient, the increased metabolic rate due to thyroid hormone will actually increase the body's need for iodine as well as decreasing the ability of the cells to concentrate iodine."* Dr. Brownstein, M.D. recommended (in his abovementioned book) people with the above symptoms get an "Iodine-Loading Test" (from FFP Labs 1-877-900-5556) – as it is considered the best way to determine how much iodine one should take.
- Those who break all "10 Dietary Commandments" (often on a daily – if not multiple times per day basis), will also become "***FULL OF IT***" & be "less resistant" to the effect of mucus forming foods.
-

Thou shall consume foods containing little or no "mucus forming" activity.

These foods with a "**5% toxic mucus capability or less**" include ORGANIC:[78]
- **Raw seeds** (edible seeds - like sunflower, pumpkin, etc.)
- **Raw nuts** (including raw nut butters – make sure no other ingredients exist)
- **Raw Sprouts** (sprouting usually eliminates the "mucus forming" activity of almost any food –including **sprouted lentils, peas, beans (including sprouted cocoa beans & soybeans), & sprouted wheat-free grains**. If the grains are sprouted, they become: easier to absorb & digest as they are considered a *"vegetable"* versus a grain.   Sprouted grains are also much lower in simple sugars (usually).[74]
- **Raw Vegetables**. Raw & cooked vegetables have no or little "mucus forming" activity. However, must be eaten raw during the "Cleansing Phase" –*may* be cooked during the "Lifestyle Phase."   However (if you can tolerate it), try to eat all vegetables as raw as possible (in all phases). Remember: God created organic raw vegetables & man has added toxic salad dressings with artificial colors, flavors, pesticides, & toxic mucus from the cow or soy milk.
- **Raw Fruits** (except for most non-organic bananas & "sulphured" fruit) – should be eaten raw during any phase.
- **& Raw Honey** (except for "Eucalyptus Honey").

Thou shall eat foods (at least once/day) with "Counter–Mucus" influences (to "cleanse" toxic mucus from the body).

These **4 *food categories*** with **"Counter-Mucus" influences** can actually lower your "***FULL OF IT* Level of Diseases, Obesity, &/or Chronic Pain**."
These foods with counter-mucus influences include ORGANIC:[78]
- **One: Probiotic** food sources & supplements. Probiotics should be consumed twice daily. The word: "Probiotics" means "For Life" (from the Latin word "pro" = "for" & the Greek word "biotic" = "life").[81]   Having a healthy population of **Lactobacilli** (the most prevalent beneficial bacteria in the small intestine)[49] & **Bifidobacteria** (the most prevalent beneficial bacteria in the

177

large intestine)[49] is *considered the most powerful way to control/reduce the toxic mucus content of one's stool.*[78] *Probiotics promote bulky, well-lubricated stools – as well as more frequent bowel movements.*[49,78]

The best probiotic supplements are a non-cow's milk probiotic blend (of Lactobacilli & Bifidobacteria) of over 1 billion active/live cells.   The only low or "mucus-free" forming Probiotic food sources (that may be considered "raw" to be consumed during the "Cleansing Phase") include the following **cultured/fermented food sources** –such as ORGANIC:

- **Kombucha; Pickled beets; & pickled carrots** (as these are usually low in sodium. **Sauerkraut** is another healthful probiotic food source if it is made with little or no salt!   Sauerkraut is much easier to digest than non-fermented/uncultured cabbage.[1]

Probiotics are mentioned again in chapter 6.

- **Two: Fiber**. The best "live" (or "raw" to be eaten during the "Cleansing Phase") sources of Fiber are ***found in*** most of the previously mentioned ***foods "that have little or no mucus forming activity"*** (except for honey & millet). Soluble fiber "absorbs" the toxins from the body & puts it into the large intestine. Insoluble fiber mostly acts as an intestinal broom.   Neither should be considered useless.   They are both valuable.

- **Three: Inulin & FOS** (Fructooligosaccharides). Inulin & FOS (which can be produced by degradation of inulin)[82] are "**prebiotics**" – meaning that they are scientifically proven to increase the activity of the beneficial bacteria (such as Bifidobacteria) as well as help prevent the growth of harmful bacteria in the digestive tract.[82] Inulin & FOS – present in common fruits & vegetables such as *artichokes, asparagus, raisins, oatmeal, & oat bran (most of these are not raw/100% alive &, therefore, should be eaten AFTER the "Cleansing Phase")* – are good sources of natural soluble fiber dietary fiber, and fine for diabetics because they don't increase the glucose or insulin in the blood.[82]

The only abovementioned **Inulin & FOS food-sources** that *can* be eaten (by most people – some may be able to digest raw artichokes or asparagus –but I would not try!) **during the "Cleansing Phase" include: raw organic raisins**.   The consumption of large quantities of Inulin or FOS (or even 1 gram of FOS – in particular by sensitive or unaccustomed individuals) can lead to gaseous discomfort![82]   However, these people may not get this side effect when ingesting the FOS (1 gram or less per day) in a probiotic supplement (which may actually help eliminate gaseous discomfort)![82] Supplemental Inulin & FOS found in these probiotic supplements must be consumed in the "Lifestyle Phase" (not the "Cleansing Phase" –as they are not 100% alive).

- **Four: Iceberg Lettuce** – the "*Rodney Dangerfield*" of Green Vegetables!   The myth/misunderstanding about iceberg lettuce having "*no nutritional value*" is a falsehood!

According to Robert Grey (in his book *The Colon Health Handbook*), iceberg lettuce is extremely unique & valuable as it is the ONLY food (this author is aware of) that has ALL of the following 5 properties:[78]

- 1, "**Anti-mucus agent**." Thus, *iceberg lettuce can loosen, soften, or dissolve hardened, stagnant, or impacted toxic mucus in the gastrointestinal tract – as well as the lymphatic system, the joints, &/or anyplace else "toxic mucus" may be in the body!*

178

- 2, **Powerful *lymph-purifying agent*.** *Lymph-purifying agents (like iceberg lettuce) can lessen the amount of toxic mucus present in the lymphatic system. Thus, iceberg lettuce insures the watery (rather than the thick & sticky toxic mucus) consistency of the lymph fluid*!
- 3, Lymph-purifying agent that uniquely **does NOT increase the toxicity of the blood**! Iceberg lettuce is one of the rare examples of a *lymph-purifying agent that does NOT increase the toxicity of the blood*!
- 4, **Lymph-purifying agent** that **ALSO** (uniquely) has "**anti-mucus**" properties! Iceberg lettuce is an extremely rare example of a *lymph-purifying agent* that is also an "*anti-mucus agent*!"
- 5, Anti-mucus agent that uniquely is **free of "*mucus-aggressive activity*.**" Most anti-mucus agents soften hardened or impacted toxic mucus without removing it from its location in the body. *In the process of being softened, the hardened toxic mucus swell (up with water). This creates a pressure among the tissues which are experienced as pain, stiffness, or swelling in a joint or muscle or as stabbing sensation among the body tissues.* Iceberg lettuce is a rare example of an anti-mucus agent free of this "mucus-aggressive activity." *Iceberg lettuce loosens, softens, &/or dissolves the toxic mucus – as well as removes the toxic mucus from where it was located in the body!*

The powerful ability of iceberg lettuce to cleanse toxic mucus from our bodies has been severely under-recognized for the past 40 years! Perhaps now – iceberg lettuce will finally "get some respect!"

EXCEPTIONS: After the "Cleansing Phase," one may benefit from certain **extremely healthful foods (in the "Lifestyle Phase") that either have "5% or less toxic mucus capabilities" or have "counter-mucus capabilities."** These include the following ORGANIC:

- **Fermented/Cultured Goat's Milk-probiotic (at least 1 billion live cells per cup) food sources**: yogurt, "acidophilus goat's milk," buttermilk, & kefir.
- **Fermented/Cultured Soybean-based probiotic (at least 1 billion living cells/cup) food sources** such as: natto, tempeh, & doenjang.
- **Fermented/Cultured Coconut-based probiotic food sources** such as: "cultured coconut milk yogurt (dairy-free & soy-free)."

Probiotic food sources are usually much easier to digest than their uncultured/non-fermented food sources.[78]

- **Wheat-free & gluten-free un-sprouted cooked grains** *may* include: *millet*, oats, amaranth, spelt, quinoa, &/or brown rice.[78]   *Millet has only about 25% the mucus-forming ability of other grains.*[78] Even if these grains are cooked, they usually won't cause the "bloating" of our intestines (or other toxic mucus side effects) that may occur with wheat consumption in certain adults. For example some people have "Celiac Sprue disease" where they must avoid all wheat products. Other adults may have under-recognized sensitivities to wheat. However, even these un-sprouted "healthful grains" should be eaten in moderation if you need to lose weight.
- **Slippery Elm Bark & Marshmallow Root** are both soothing (& gently cleansing) to the GI tract –from mouth/throat to anus.[15]   Marshmallow helps to **eliminate excess mucus** & is believed to possess the following additional benefits:[15] *Soothe & heal skin, mucous membranes, & other tissues, externally*

& internally.   Good for bladder infections, digestive upsets, fluid retention, headache, intestinal disorders, kidney problems, sinusitis, & sore throat.
Slippery elm bark is also believed to soothe inflamed mucous membranes of the bowels, stomach, & urinary tract – as well as possess the following additional benefits:[15] *"Good for diarrhea, ulcers, & for treatment of colds, flu, & sore throat. Slippery elm bark is also believed to be beneficial for Crohn's disease, ulcerative colitis, diverticulosis, diverticulitis, & gastritis."*
Their similarities (& most likely their synergistic combination) make it easy to see why I combine them together.   They can be in a powdered form (either in bulk or in capsules which can be opened) & added to filtered water & sipped throughout the day.

- **Fenugreek (seeds) & Thyme (leaves)** help **remove toxic mucus** from - the nasal sinuses (mostly as a nasal decongestant) – as well as the intestines (secondarily).[15]   They can be in a powdered form & added to a delicious "super-cleansing shake."

5.   Thou shall eat chelation agents created by God to CLEANSE your body from toxic heavy metals [&possibly other direct body toxins].

**"YOU'RE NOT FAT. YOU'RE FULL OF" TOXIC heavy metals** - that may be removed via chelation!"
As previously mentioned earlier in this chapter (section I.9), chelation therapy has become of greater recognition in the past 20 years.   The United States FDA considers *over-the-counter (OTC) chelation products to be "unapproved," & thus it is a violation of the U.S. federal law to make unproven claims about them.*[83]   As per The American Cancer Society (in 2008 – already mentioned previously): *Medical evidence does NOT support the effectiveness of chelation therapy for any other purpose than **the treatment of heavy metal poisoning**."*[43]   As mentioned in this chapter's first section – as well as chapter 3 - is the fact that this "heavy metal poisoning" increases our risk of diseases.   Thus: this accumulation of toxic heavy metals increases our "_**FULL OF IT** Level of Diseases_" (as well as possibly Obesity &/or Chronic Pain - shown in chapter 4).   Besides intravenous or intramuscular injections of chelation agents (mentioned in the first section of this chapter), there are powerful "**God-created" foods that possess a chelating effect** of removing excessive lead, mercury, & other toxic heavy metal poisoning.[15,45]   How much & how often one should eat these chelating **FOODS** may be directly related to the level of toxicity &/or stage of disease (associated with the toxins)![15,45-47]
Therefore: consuming "God-created" chelation agent foods may actually lower your "_**FULL OF IT** Level of Diseases_ [as well as **Obesity, &/or Chronic Pain]!**"
Thou shall eat at least one of these chelation agent foods daily (some may benefit most from alternating them from one day to another):

180

Raw, Organic Cilantro (AKA "**Coriander LEAVES**" or "**Chinese Parsley**") is considered to possess **the most powerful "chelation" properties** (of all the foods) in the world to: effectively <u>bind & remove (CLEANSE the body from) mercury, lead, aluminum, & other heavy metal toxins</u> from our nervous system – as well as other parts of our body.[45,84]   Cilantro is also considered to possess the most **powerful chelation properties** (of all the foods in the world) **to remove bacterial infections** – *as the infectious organisms may use the **metal toxins** to protect themselves from antibiotics!*[84]   Cilantro is mentioned again in chapter 6.

  Raw, Organic Garlic may be considered the 2nd best plant chelation agent in the world.[45]   However, raw garlic may be too irritating to most people's gastrointestinal systems. Cooked or Garlic capsules can be taken after the "Cleansing Phase." Garlic is mentioned again in chapter 6.

  Raw Organic: Sprouted Lentils & Sprouted Beans & Raw Onions produce **L-Methionine** in good quantities.[45]   L-Methionine is an amino acid, antioxidant,[15] & is also one of the most powerful natural dietary chelation agents.[45]   However, raw onions may be too irritating to most people's GI systems.   **You should NEVER eat a raw onion after it has been cut over a day old**.   Cut raw onions are great at absorbing direct body airborne toxins. Thus: a cut raw onion in your refrigerator, bathroom, &/or bedroom may help *cleanse the air* in these areas of harmful airborne toxins.   However, eating these day-old (or longer) sliced onion(s) may contain these airborne toxins.   Thus, consuming these day-old sliced onions can be extremely irritating to your gastrointestinal system – as well as toxic to your entire body. Cooked onions can be eaten after the "Cleansing Phase."

  Raw Organic Vitamin C – rich Foods have a natural chelation effect.[15,45] Vitamin C is discussed further in chapter 6.

  Pectin – found in **Raw, Organic**: **apples** (best source), **beets,** cabbage (low sodium **sauerkraut** – a probiotic food source - is the most healthful source of cabbage pectin), **carrots, citrus fruits, & sprouted peas (& pea pods)**.[15]   Pectin is a type of fiber healthful for diabetes.   It removes unwanted metals & toxins, reduces the side effects of radiation therapy, may help lower cholesterol, & may decrease the risk of heart disease & gallstones.[15]

  Raw Organic Avocados are naturally high in **glutathione** (a powerful chelation agent – mentioned below in "Exceptions"). Avocados are a "super-cleansing food" analyzed in great detail in chapter 6.

EXCEPTIONS: After the "Cleansing Phase" (during the "Lifestyle Phase"), you may benefit from the following chelation agents (that are not 100% raw/alive):

- **Powdered Cilantro**. However, I do not see why one would choose dead over alive cilantro. Raw cilantro tastes great. Raw cilantro can be used on tacos, salads, & even juiced with wheatgrass.
- **Cooked garlic & onions** (as mentioned above).
- **Buffered or Acid-Free Vitamin C** 500 mg twice/day with meals.
- **Greens Powders** (usually added to filtered water for a drink/shake) should possess vitamin C & apple pectin to bind with unwanted toxic metals (& other toxins) & remove them from the body.
- **Vitamin K2** (AKA "Menaquinones") help to prevent -& possibly reverse – calcification of the arteries & heart valves (especially the aortic valve)!

Vitamin K2 – found in abundance in Natto (a probiotic food source) – has been claimed to *remove the calcium from the arteries (& heart valves) & put them in the bones where it belongs!*[85,86]   Vitamin K2 & Natto are analyzed further in chapter 6.

- **Co Enzyme Q10** (One mg per pound of body weight per day) may improve oxygenation to all cells & act as a chelation agent.[15,87]   CoQ10 is mentioned again in chapter 6.
- **Glutathione** (500mg/day) is considered one of the most powerful, God-given chelation agents in the world.[15,45]   Many chelation physicians use glutathione intravenously to remove toxic metals (& other toxins) when treating (& possibly reversing) Parkinson's & Multiple Sclerosis!   **Avocados** (discussed in chapter 6 & the next "commandment") are a food naturally high in glutathione.[88]   Glutathione is mentioned again in chapter 6.

6.   Thou shall create an optimal healthy balance between preventing blood clots & bleeding!

This is the longest dietary commandment due to the fact that:
"YOU'RE NOT FAT. YOU'RE FULL OF:"
- **Toxins stored in the liver & blood;**
- **Trans-Fats & Hydrogenated Oils;**
- **& an imbalance between preventing blood clots & bleeding!**

It is crucial to "Cleanse" the liver for the following reasons:[88]
- *The liver's main job is to aid the lipase enzymes to digest fats.   If your liver or gallbladder (where bile is stored) is not working properly, fats & toxins will not be broken down correctly & will start building up, thereby causing weight gain.*
- *The liver is the largest internal detoxification ("CLEANSING") organ. When we eat poorly, the liver actually stores more fat (to store the toxins) & keeps us overweight.   Consuming herbs/foods that support overall liver cleansing helps us to eliminate the toxins instead of hold onto them.*
- *When the liver is cleansed & working better, it frees up energy to motivate us to exercise more –leading to the loss of more toxins & excess body fat.*

6a.Thou shall eat at least one of these Liver– &/or blood– cleansing foods daily (some may benefit from alternating them from one day to another):
- **Raw Organic Wheatgrass Juice** (drink within 30 minutes of juicing) is a powerful source of chlorophyll (which molecularly resembles that of hemoglobin, the oxygen-carrying protein of red blood cells).[15]   Anemic animals have had their blood counts returned to normal after 4-5 days of receiving chlorophyll.[15]   Perhaps this is why wheatgrass juice may be considered "God's chemotherapy!" Wheatgrass juice is discussed again in chapter 6.

- **Raw Organic Cilantro** (can be juiced with wheatgrass) to cleanse the blood stream – as well as bind to & remove metal toxins from the liver, brain, & possibly other parts of the body.[45,84]
- Raw Organic **Probiotic** Food sources (such as **kombucha, - & no/low salt** cultured/fermented vegetables including **sauerkraut, pickled beets, pickled carrots, & pickled cucumbers**) may decrease atherosclerotic risk.[85] Probiotics &, therefore, probiotic food sources may decrease atherosclerotic risk by decreasing LDL & total cholesterol levels in patients with high & normal cholesterol levels.[89] Also: Probiotics in the intestines help convert vitamin K1 into K2 – which (unlike vitamin K1) is inversely associated with atherosclerosis in humans![85]
- **Raw Organic Avocados** (discussed further in chapter 6) are considered one of the best liver cleansers God has given us.[90] Avocados are naturally full of **glutathione** – which helps the liver detox toxic chemicals.[88]
- **Raw Organic Apples** are full of pectin - which supports detoxification through the bowels – making the liver's job easier as it lessens the toxic burden.[88]
- **Raw Organic Lemons & Limes** are considered one of the best liver cleansers God has given us.[90] However, some people can't tolerate (in their gastrointestinal system) the "acidity" of these citrus fruits.
- **Raw Organic Garlic & Turmeric** are considered one of the best liver cleansers God has given us.[90] Garlic has allicin & selenium, which both help the liver to detoxify.[88] However, some people find these raw foods to be too spicy or irritating to the GI system. These are both mentioned again in chapter 6.
- **Raw Organic Red, Yellow, & Orange Peppers** are Rich in Vitamin C to help prevent atherosclerosis. The different phytonutrients in these peppers may protect us from some liver diseases as well. Vitamin C & its' food sources are mentioned again in chapter 6.

EXCEPTIONS to 6a: After the "Cleansing Phase," you may benefit from the following Liver &/or Blood Cleansing Foods/Supplements (that are not 100% raw/alive):

- **Menaquinone-7 ("MK7") is a type of Vitamin K2** found highest in natto (a probiotic food from fermented soybeans) & "produced" (converted from vitamin K1) by probiotics in your intestines.[15] MK7 (100mcg/day) can reduce the risk (& possibly reverse) the arterial calcification of atherosclerosis – to "***CLEANSE***" the arterial walls![85] MK7 may also reduce the risk of cancer, bone loss, & even aging! Vitamin K2 & Natto are analyzed & referenced in greater detail in Chapter 6.
- **Green Powders/Drinks** should contain: 1 billion live cells of probiotics; apple pectin; & the following sources of chlorophyll:[15]
    - **Wheatgrass, Barley Grass, Spirulina, &/or Chlorella.** As mentioned previously, chlorophyll is a powerful blood cleanser & may be beneficial for people with anemia.
- **Organic Apple Cider Vinegar** (a teaspoon/day may be added to your drinking water if desired). With its' vitamins, minerals, & alkalinity-restoring capabilities, ACV is wonderful for supporting the liver.[88] Many adults (including those with acid reflux problems) may actually be deficient in HCL (Hydrochloric Acid) & benefit from consuming 1 - 3 tablespoons of ACV with

their cooked foods.[15,49,74]   However, some individuals may actually have an excess of HCL –in which ACV may be detrimental.[15,49,74]

- **Oats** contain avenanthramides: compounds that have been found to reduce arterial wall inflammation &, thereby, help prevent atherosclerosis.[91] Oatmeal & Oat Bran have a type of fiber that:[15]

> iv.   Regulates blood glucose levels; aids in lowering cholesterol; & helps in the removal of toxins.

- **Milk Thistle** has been used for over 2,000 years *("B.C.")* to **support the liver** – as well as the gallbladder & kidneys.[88]   Milk Thistle (best in concentrated capsule form) protects the liver from toxins & pollutants by preventing free radical damage & stimulates the production of new liver cells.[15,82]   May be useful for a weakened immune system & all liver disorders.[15,82]   Long term use (in rats) has shown to reduce the risk of certain cancers.[92]   Consuming Milk Thistle is considered one of the best ways to detoxify from toxic chemical exposure.[8]
- **Glutathione** (mentioned above in "avocados") helps the liver to detoxify toxins such as alcohol, chemicals, & other poisons.[15]   Glutathione is a "super-cleansing supplement" illustrated in greater detail in chapter 6.
- **Green Tea** contains catechins –which support liver detoxification.[88]

6b.Thou shall avoid any processed foods containing "trans-fats" or "hydrogenated" oils.

They are both known to increase the risk of coronary heart disease. Trans-fats **increase the risk of CHD (Coronary Heart Disease) more than any other macronutrient**, conferring a substantially increased risk at even low levels (1-3% of total energy intake).[93]   The trace amounts of trans-fats present naturally in animal foods (2-5% of the total fat in the milk & body fat of cattle & sheep) are a different type than those of hydrogenated oils, and don't appear to exhibit the same negative effects.[93,94]

There is absolutely NO controversy over the increased risk of CHD from consuming hydrogenated oils &/or trans-fats (unsaturated fats with trans-isomer fatty acids).[95]   Trans-fats from partially hydrogenated oils (despite being inexpensive, increasing product shelf-life, & decreasing refrigerator requirements) are more harmful than trans-fats from naturally occurring oils.[94,96]   Trans-fats have shown to **raise LDL cholesterol** (the "bad") & **lower HDL** (the "good") cholesterol levels![97]   Replacing only 2% of food energy from trans-fats with non-trans unsaturated fats decreases the risk of CHD by 53%![93]   The topic of "super-cleansing fats" is analyzed in greater detail in Chapter 6.

In the U.S. in 2006, 100,000 cardiac deaths (up from 30,000 in 1994)[93] were suggested to be attributable to the consumption of trans-fats![95] One may say: we are "***FULL OF***" trans-fats & hydrogenated oils!   Replacing "Super-Cleansing Fats" (like those mentioned in Chapter 6 –section II) in our diets in the past 60 years – with refined carbohydrates, trans-fats, &/or hydrogenated oils (all strongly correlated with an increased risk of atherosclerosis) is definitely a factor in why Americans have become "***FULL OF***" heart disease!

Based on decades of research, 2 of the strongest predictors of atherosclerosis (& atherosclerotic events/diseases – such as: coronary heart/artery disease, ischemic & thrombic strokes, primary & secondary heart attacks, etc.) were found to be:

- **High LDL/HDL ratio** (the strongest predictor);[98] & High Total/HDL cholesterol ratio.[99]

While high total cholesterol levels (alone) are *somewhat* associated with atherosclerosis,[99] the above ***ratios*** were found to be the strongest predictors.[98,99] Avoiding "trans-fats" & hydrogenated oils - & replacing grain-based carbs with healthful fats ("super-cleansing fats" - mentioned in chapter 6) have shown to significantly reduce the LDL/HDL & total cholesterol/HDL ratio levels[100] (therefore, reducing the risk of atherosclerosis & atherosclerotic disease/events).[98,99]   See Chapter 6 for "super-cleansing fats."

EXCEPTIONS to 6b: There are **no exceptions** to avoiding processed foods containing trans-fats &/or hydrogenated oils.

6c.Thou shall create the healthiest (most optimal) *BALANCE* between preventing blood clots versus bleeding.

Americans have become "***FULL OF***" **the entire spectrum of cardiovascular diseases**:[101,102] from **blood clots** causing heart attacks, strokes, pulmonary emboli, etc. – to **bleeding** causing bruising, anemia, hemorrhagic strokes, gastrointestinal bleeding, etc.

Thus : **Bleeding & blood clots** can be seen as representing the **two major "poles"** amongst the spectrum of cardiovascular diseases (a general term encompassing heart attacks, strokes, & other diseases of the heart & blood vessels).[49,102]   For example, one can get a **stroke** (Cerebrovascular Accident = CVA) from a **hemorrhage (bleed)** or a **thrombus (blood clot)**.[101]   Since cardiovascular diseases are considered the number one cause of death in the western world,[49,102] we need to create an optimal healthy balance between preventing blood clots versus bleeding.

If you believe we should be paranoid of **blood clots** & negligent of **bleeding**, then: "***YOU ARE FULL OF IT!***"   The abovementioned concept of the healthiest *balance* is the goal.

Some ways to help reduce our risk of getting a blood clot include:
- Following the *"10 non-dietary cleansing methods"* such as: add more peace in your life (& **avoid stress**),[19,102,103] **exercising on a regular basis**[19,102,103] (to avoid physical laziness & **prolonged sitting**),[19,102,103] *avoid all the direct body toxins* mentioned in chapter 3 (especially **cigarette smoke**[19,102,103] – as well as avoiding the poor low back sway back posture which predisposes you to deep vein thrombi – analyzed in chapter 3)

185

- Following all these *"10 Dietary Commandments"* – especially **avoiding the**:[93,103] **Refined carbohydrates, high glycemic load meals, trans-fats, &/or hydrogenated oils** Americans have become *"**FULL OF**"* in the past 40 years!
- **Losing *excess* weight**[19,102,103] & *excess* **body fat percentage**[104]
- Consuming **Natural Anticoagulants &/or Pharmaceutical Anticoagulants** (via consumption or injection/Intravenous)
- Consuming the following **non-anticoagulant foods/supplements**:
    - **Carnitine** (500mg 2x/day with water) – in its L-Carnitine form or N-Acetyl Carnitine form – is an amino acid (mentioned again in chapter 6) that may reduce the risk of atherosclerosis (&, therefore, reduce the risk of arterial blood clots) by: Protecting against lipid peroxidation;[49] Improve exercise ability of those with angina;[105,106] & decrease body fat mass (if needed) & decrease fatigue.[107]
    - **Coenzyme Q10** (mg/pound of body weight per day) has shown to suppress LDL oxidation to help prevent atherosclerosis (&, therefore, arterial blood clots).[108,109] CoQ10 is mentioned again in Chapter 6.
    - **Oats** contain aventhramides that have been found to reduce arterial wall inflammation & thereby help prevent atherosclerosis (&, therefore, arterial blood clots).[91] Of course: raw organic sprouted oats would be the most healthful (if available)!
    - **High-fiber foods** (such as the "super-cleansing fiber" foods mentioned in chapter 6) help to lower blood cholesterol levels & stabilize blood sugar levels.[15,82] Thus, high-fiber foods may help reduce the risk of atherosclerosis (&, therefore, arterial blood clots).[15,82,103]
    - **Natural chelation foods/supplements** (like those listed in "Dietary Commandment #5") are believed to remove toxic heavy metals believed to impair arterial wall function (&, therefore, help reduce the risk of atherosclerosis & arterial blood clots).[15,49]
    - **Vitamin C &/or foods high in vitamin C** may actually help prevent blood clots – as well as bleeding. These – as well as other amazing qualities of this "super-cleansing supplement/food" are shown in chapter 6.
    - **Probiotics, Menaquinones (vitamin K2), & probiotic food sources** are also capable of indirectly preventing *arterial* blood clots – as well as preventing bleeding! These – as well as other amazing qualities of this "super supplement/food" are shown in chapter 6.

Because Americans (in the past 40 years) have been mostly avoiding the *"10 non-Dietary Cleansing Methods"* & the *"10 Dietary Commandments,"* we have become *"**FULL OF**"* more:
- Blood clots (venous & arterial)
- Diseases caused by these blood clots (like heart attacks, strokes due to blood clots, pulmonary emboli, etc.)
- & diseases that increase our risk of these clots (like atherosclerosis, obesity, diabetes, etc.).

This has caused our society as a whole to stray (in my opinion) to one side of the cardiovascular disease spectrum becoming "blood clot paranoid." Our blood clot paranoia has caused us (in my humble opinion) to become *"**FULL**"*

OF" more anticoagulants (**both pharmaceutical & "natural"**) than ever before!

I define the term "**anticoagulant**" as: Any substance that directly interferes with the coagulation (clotting) process.

Therapeutic uses of anticoagulants include potentially improving your health/save your life (in different ways) by **preventing the occurrence or growth of blood clots.** Anticoagulants possessing "**thrombolytic**" (AKA "Fibrinolytic") characteristics: may actually help **dissolve blood clots.** Thus, anticoagulants may help:[110]

- **Prevent the occurrence of blood clots** in patients with atrial fibrillation, cardiac stents, mechanical heart valve replacements, congestive heart failure, etc. – to help prevent: A myocardial infarction (heart attack) or re-infarction (subsequent heart attack); A stroke or transient ischemic attack from a blood clot going to the brain; &/or an obstruction of a blood vessel from a blood clot anywhere else in the body.
- **Prevent the growth or possibly dissolve** (when the anticoagulant possesses "thrombolytic" properties) deep vein thrombi (DVTs), pulmonary emboli, a blood clot in the brain (causing an ischemic stroke or transient ischemic attack), or a clot in a blood vessel anywhere else in the body.

However, anticoagulants (**especially when combined with each other**) may potentially harm your health/kill you by **increasing your bleeding risk (&/or anemia).** Our being "*FULL OF*" more anticoagulants than ever before has us more at risk for bleeding &/or anemia. Realize **bleeding** may occur anywhere in the body where blood vessels travel including, but not limited to, the brain (via a **hemorrhagic stroke or TIA**), the gastrointestinal system (such as "**gastrointestinal bleeding**"), eyes, nose, mouth (including the gums), & anywhere just under the skin (via **bruises**).

Some of the **pharmaceutical anticoagulant categories** (that all **decrease the risk of blood clots** – in different manners –as well as **increase the risk of bleeding**) we have become "*FULL OF*" (in the past 40 years) include:

- **Vitamin K antagonists** such as the well-known **Warfarin**[110-112] (brand names include "*Coumadin*," "*Jantoven*," etc.) & lesser-recognized **antibiotics**! Antibiotics often kill the healthy intestinal bacteria that "produce" vitamin K2 (via converting vitamin K1 to K2) &, therefore can increase the risk of bleeding (by causing a vitamin K-deficient hypothrombinemia)![113,114] Vitamin K2 is listed (& analyzed in great detail in chapter 6 as one of the most important vitamins as it helps reduce the risk of atherosclerosis (&, therefore, arterial blood clots) as well as helping to stop bleeding![85,114] Thus: there is recent evidence that *these vitamin K antagonists actually worsen arterial calcification in the long term* even though they help prevent blood clots (& increase the risk of bleeding – like all anticoagulants) in the short term!![85] Any drug that is linked to liver damage – such as **long-term alcohol consumption** – depletes the body of vitamin K (as well as vitamin C, B6, B12, & folic acid) &, therefore increases the risk of bleeding![115]

- **Indirect Thrombin Inhibitors: AKA "Antithrombin III Activators"** (antithrombin III blocks thrombin from clotting blood) such as the well-known Heparin.[110-112]
- **Direct Clotting Factor Xa Inhibitors** such as the well-known Rivaroxaban (brand name "*Xarelto*").[110,111]
- **Direct Thrombin Inhibitors** such as Dabigatran (brand name "*Predaxa*").[110,111]
- **Thrombolytic Drugs (AKA "Fibrinolytic Drugs")** such as Alteplase (brand names "*Activase*" & "*Cathflo Activase*") & Streptokinase ("*Kabinase*" & "*Streptase*").[110,111]
- **Antiplatelet Drugs** such as the well-known Clopidogrel (brand name "*Plavix*").[110-112] This category also includes:
   o All **aspirin** (brand names include "Ecotrin," "Bayer," "Bufferin," & over 100 more)[110,112]
   o 100+ **other NSAIDs** (Non-Steroidal Anti-inflammatory Drugs).[116] Other well-known NSAIDs include Celecoxib (brand name "*Celebrex*"),[116] Ibuprofen (brand names include "*Advil*," "*Motrin*," etc.),[112,116] & Naproxen (brand names include "*Aleve*," "*Naprosen*," etc.).[116]
   o Certain Antidepressants – Selective Serotonin Reuptake Inhibitors (SSRIs) & Serotonin Norepinephrine Reuptake inhibitors (SNRIs) have a mild inhibiting effect on platelets by themselves.[116] However, these SSRIs & SNRIs have an increased bleeding risk when combined with pharmaceutical anticoagulants (like warfarin, aspirin, & other NSAIDs).[116] Well-known brand names include:[117] "*Celexa*," "*Lexapro*," "*Luvox*," "*Prozac*," "*Paxil*," "*Zoloft*," "*Cymbalta*,"[116] "*Wellbutrin*," & even "*Valium*!"[118]

Some of these antiplatelet drugs can inhibit platelet aggregation (as assessed by aggregometry) for days and, therefore, may have a **long-lived bleeding risk for days** (up to 7 days for aspirin & 4 days for clopidogrel)[110] after swallowing these meds. Other NSAIDs (like ibuprofen) are reversible &, therefore, the effect on platelets is not as long lived.[110]

Natural anticoagulants (similar to pharmaceutical anticoagulants - in this respect) can have great health benefits – including, but not limited to, the **prevention of the occurrence of blood clots** & the **prevention of the growth of blood clots** (some anticoagulants like "nattukinase" may actually help to **prevent & even dissolve current blood clots**).   As beneficial as these natural anticoagulants are to possibly "*CLEANSE*" the blood of clots, they may also increase the risk of bleeding.   Society has gone to the extreme to prevent blood clots by consuming excessive amounts of natural anticoagulants that the *bleeding risk from natural anticoagulants has become an extremely under-recognized public health problem!*   Natural anticoagulants **may increase the risk of bleeding &/or anemia when taken:**

- *In excess*; with each other; with prescribed &/or over-the-counter pharmaceutical anticoagulants; near the time of surgery or trauma; &/or by someone who already has a bleeding/hemorrhagic disorder. **The horror is that patients on prescribed anticoagulant meds are NOT INFORMING their physicians that they are also consuming anticoagulant: foods, herbs, supplements, vitamins, &/or over-the-counter (OTC) meds!!**

Some of the "**natural**" **foods, herbs, &/or dietary supplements** that possess **anticoagulant** properties (that *may* be useful in **decreasing the risk of blood clots** – as well as possibly **increasing the risk of bleeding &/or anemia**) include, but are not limited to:

- Arnica (*Arnica Montana L.*): Despite commonly used to reduce bruises, the plant can cause GI bleeding & even the homeopathic form has shown to have antiplatelet properties![119]
- Bilberry (*Vaccinium myrtillus*)[110,120]
- Borage seed oil (*Borage officinalis*)[121]
- Bromelain (a protease enzyme found in pineapples)[82,120,122,123]
- Burdock (*Arctium lappa*)[124]
- Cayenne (*capsicum frutescens* or *C. annum* – AKA "Hot Pepper")[112,125]
- Celery Seed Herb (*Apium Graveolens*)[82,126]
- Chinese black tree fungus (*Auricularia auricular-judae* – AKA "Jew's Ear," "Jelly Ear," or "Tree Ear")[127]
- Clove (*Syzygium aromaticum*)[82,128]
- Curcumin (active ingredient in Turmeric)
- Devil's Claw (*Harpagophytum procumbens* – AKA "Grapple Plant" or "Wood Spider")[82,123,129]
- Dong Quai (Angelica sinensis)[110,123]
- Evening Primrose oil[121]
- Extra Virgin Olive Oil[130,131]
- Feverfew (Tanacetum parthenium)[15,110,117,123,129]
- Fish & Fish oil (discussed previously in "Commandment #2"): Over 3 grams of the omega 3 fatty acids EPA ((eicosapentaenoic acid) & DHA (docosahexaenoic acid) increases bleeding risk[64,69,110,120] – including hemorrhagic stroke![69] You would need to consume over 10 ounces/day (approximately 283 grams & 750 calories) of the following fish sources (rich in these omega 3 fatty acids) to reach this dangerous 3 grams+ of EPA/DHA:[74-76] Herring, sardines, Spanish mackerel, salmon, halibut, un-canned tuna, swordfish, & tile fish.
- Garlic (*Allium sativum*)[110,117,132,133]
- Ginger (*Zingiber officinale*)[117,122,123]
- Gingko (*Gingko Biloba L.*)[15,110,112,133]
- Ginseng[82,117,134]
- Grape juice (from purple grapes)[135]
- Grape seed & grape skin extracts[135-137]
- Guarana (*Paullinia cupana*): Despite possessing caffeine (a vasoconstrictor), shown to possess antiplatelet properties.[138]
- Kudzu root (*Pueraria lobata* – AKA "Fengen")[134,139]
- Lumbrokinase[140]
- Motherwort (*Leonurus cardiac*)[15,141]
- MSM (Methylsulfonylmethane)[122]

189

- Nattukinase[15,142]
- Omega 3 Fatty Acids which include:[112,120,143]
    - EPA & DHA: found predominantly in fish/fish oil (see "Fish/Fish oil" above)
    - & Alpha Linolenic Acid (ALA) found in the following vegan oils (from highest to lowest ALA %age profile):[112,120,143,144] Kiwifruit seed (62%), perilla seed (61%), chia seed (57%), flaxseed (57%), lignonberry seed (49%), camelina seed (36%), purslane seed (35%), black raspberry seed (33%), sea buckthorn seed (32%),[145] hemp seed (19%), walnut (10.4%), canola (9%), soybean (8%), & wheat germ (6.9%).

ALA's anti-platelet properties (& bleeding risks) have not been shown to be *as strong as that of EPA/DHA*.[82,146,147] However, ALA (&, therefore, its' food source) has antiplatelet properties[76,143] & can increase bleeding time.[120] In addition, ALA is converted to the stronger anticoagulants EPA/DHA in the human body-albeit with an efficiency below 5% in men,[148] & at a greater percentage in women.[149] ALA is considered an omega 3 "**essential**" fatty acid because the body can't produce it (& it, therefore, needs to be consumed). Note: The above information is about "Alpha Linolenic Acid" (an omega 3 Essential fatty acid) – NOT Alpha lipoic acid (a supplement also sometimes abbreviated "ALA")!

- Peony (*Paeonia lactiflora* – AKA "White Peony" or "Chinese Peony")[150]
- Pinokinase (A proprietary blend of Nattokinase – already mentioned - & Pycnogenol)[142,151]
- Procyanidins from cocoa (a type of proanthocyanidin)[152]
- Pycnogenol (U.S. registered tradename for a product derived from the pine bark of a tree known as *Pinus pinaster*)[151,153]
- Quercitin[120,154]
- Reishi mushroom (*Ganoderma lucidum* – AKA "Linzhi mushroom")[155]
- Resveratrol (found in the skin of red grapes; sources include Red Wine, Grape Juice & Pomegranate juice; & 70%+ cocoa)[156,157]
- Saw Palmetto Berry (*Serenoa Repens*)[117,128,158]
- Skullcap Root (*Scutellaria laterfolia*)[15]
- Turmeric (*Circuma longa*)[15,110,112,159]
- Vitamin E[15,82,110,120]
- & White Willow Bark (*Salix spp.*)[160]

There are also **foods & supplements** (not mentioned in the above list) **that may increase the risk of bleeding** &/or anemia –despite possessing **NO** known anticoagulant properties - **when combined with certain pharmaceutical anticoagulants**. This may be because these foods/supplements may decrease the speed at which the liver breaks down the pharmaceutical anticoagulants (thus: keeping more of the drug in your body longer). This below list should probably be avoided when someone is: already taking pharmaceutical anticoagulants; near surgery; &/or already has a bleeding disorder. These foods &/or supplements include:

- Birthwort (Aristolochia clematis L.): Can cause bleeding, anemia, lower platelet count[161] & has aristolochic acid – which is toxic & banned in most countries.[162]
- Boldo (*Peumus boldus*): When combined with the herb fenugreek - can increase risk of bleeding of warfarin.[163]
- Chondroitin sulfate[15,120]

- Cranberry juice: Has shown to increase warfarin activity[120,164]
- Cuckoo-Pint: Plant or root has strong internal irritant effects & may lead to (by itself) bloody vomiting & diarrhea.[134]
- Danshen (Salvia miltiorrhiza – AKA "Red Sage," "Chinese Sage," "Tan Shen")[123,163]
- Eucalyptus oil[129]
- European Mistletoe (*Viscum album L.*): May be highly toxic & linked with GI bleeding even when taken alone.[123]
- Fenugreek (*Trigonella foenumgraecum L.*): When combined with the herb boldo – can increase the bleeding risk of warfarin[163]
- Fo-Ti Root (*Polygonum multiflorum*)[129]
- Goji berry (*Lycium barbarum L.* – AKA "Wolfberry")[163]
- Grapefruit juice[129,163]
- Kava Kava root (*Piper methysticum*)[129]
- Magnesium: When combined with ibuprofen for a prolonged period of time, may increase ibuprofen's activity & bleeding risks.[15,120]
- Mango: May potentiate - & increase bleeding risk – of warfarin.[163]
- Meadow Saffron (*Colchicum autumnale* – AKA "Naked Lady" or "Autumn Crocus"): Can be very poisonous & toxic – causing anemia, GI bleeding, & low platelet counts.[134]
- Melatonin: Increased risk of bleeding when taken with warfarin.[120]
- Mugwort Leaf (Artemesia vulgaris – AKA "Ai Ye"): Can damage the walls of blood vessels & cause bleeding – especially menstrual/uterine bleeding.[122,161]
- Papaya Extract (AKA "Papain"): May potentiate - & increase bleeding risk (especially purpura) when taken with warfarin.[123]
- Peppermint (*Mentha piperita*)[129]
- Quilinggao (AKA "Turtle Jelly"): Shown to increase warfarin activity.[163]
- Quinine (Found in Cinchona Bark & available as a drug): The U.S. FDA has ordered unapproved quinine drugs to be removed from the market due to the risk of severe bleeding & low platelet counts.[134]
- Red Clover (*Trifolium pretense*)[82,110,129]
- Vervain (Verbena officinalis – AKA "Common Verbena"): Stimulates menstruation &, therefore, should be avoided when pregnant.[15]
- Vitamin A: Men taking over 3,000 I.U.s/day (or women taking over 2,310 I.U.s/day) have an increased bleeding risk when taking pharmaceutical anticoagulants.[120]
- & White Sandalwood (Santalum album – AKA "Sandalwood"): Intake may lead to hematuria (blood in the urine).[134]

The Lamb of God shed His blood for ALL of us. However, we currently shed too much of our own blood (often hurting our body = "*The Temple of the Holy Spirit*") by consuming an excess of the 2 abovementioned "natural" lists!

Other spiritual notes: As our nation's "***God deficit***" has grown larger than before, so has (by no coincidence) our "***blood deficit***!" As our nation has become more deficient in the ***blood of the Lamb of God***, our bodies have (by no coincidence) also become more deficient in **our own blood**!

As the world has become more integrated, the abovementioned pharmaceutical list & 2 "natural" lists have skyrocketed in the past 40 years! In the same time, the percentage of people who regularly consume the members of these lists has increased dramatically!   We have become "**_FULL OF_**" more anticoagulants (pharmaceutical & natural) –as well as foods/herbs/supplements that may increase our risk of bleeding in other ways!

The bleeding &/or anemia potential side effects of pharmaceutical & natural anticoagulants may be greatly reduced by:

- **Avoiding the <u>excessive </u>intake or combination** (unless prescribed by your physician, pharmacist, nutritionist, &/or other health care professionals) **of the 2 abovementioned "natural" list' members;**
- **Limiting or avoiding the combination** (unless prescribed by your physicians) **of pharmaceutical anticoagulants with the 2 "natural" list' members.**
- **Consuming enough probiotics** (1 billion+ live cells/day) **&/or Menaquinone-7** (100mcgs/day via its' food sources &/or supplements) **daily** – which may actually help prevent atherosclerosis (a risk associated with the long term use of vitamin K antagonists - like warfarin);[85,114]
- **Consuming foods high in vitamin C or taking buffered or acid–free vitamin C 500mg twice daily with meals;**
- **Consuming certain "Super-Cleansing Foods"** (like 1-2 ounces of freshly made wheatgrass juice; raw nuts; raw sprouted lentils & beans; &/or "**super-meats**") naturally high in iron - to help prevent the iron deficiency anemia the iron lost.   **<u>Wheatgrass juice</u>** is high in chlorophyll - which (as mentioned earlier in this "commandment") may help return blood counts to normal in humans who had anemia.[15] The "**super-meats**" mentioned in chapter 6 are a "heme" form of iron – making them the **best foods** to quickly **restore iron** in the blood to normal (lost from the anemia/bleeding).[15]

The need for a **_BALANCE_** – between preventing blood clots versus preventing bleeding – exists in many other aspects of our health.   We need a balance between rest & exercise.   We need a balance between foods that create an acidic environment versus foods that create an alkaline environment.   We even need a balance in the minerals we consume - such as copper & zinc.   In fact, every joint in your body needs a certain amount of stability – as well as mobility (based on your age, sex, & body type).

The **<u>BALANCE between iron deficiency & excess iron</u>** is also extremely important in achieving optimal health.   A **<u>deficiency in iron</u>** may increase the risk of:[15,74,82] **<u>Bleeding &/or anemia</u>.**   If you are at risk for &/or currently have a deficiency in iron (confirmed via blood tests), you may benefit (with approval from a physician) from consuming the following organic foods **<u>high in iron</u>**:[15,74]

- Meats, lentils, raw liver extract (from organically raised beef or goose); beans (kidney, pinto, & lima); nettle (an herb); blackstrap molasses; raw beet greens; mustard greens; prunes; spinach; & peas.   When sprouted: lentils, beans, & peas are much easier to digest/absorb. Sprouting the lentils, beans, & peas reduces the iron they contain by over 100%[74] - when measured by cups, etc. - &, therefore, makes them superior & "safer" – see below.

An **excess of iron** can:[15] **Damage the liver, heart, pancreas, & overall immune system -& has even been linked to cancer**! If you are at risk for &/or currently have an excess of iron (confirmed by a physician), you may benefit (with approval from a physician) from consuming the following **foods that interfere with iron absorption**:[15]

- Coffee (which contains polyphenols); Tea (which contains tannins); *cow's milk****; bilberry; burdock; damiana; juniper; "lady's mantle;" peppermint; chocolate; cocoa; spinach; & most nuts & beans. Notice **beans & spinach are on both lists** as they contain iron – but also contain oxalic acid which interferes with iron absorption. Again: sprouted beans are superior in healthfulness than non-sprouted beans for reasons already mentioned.

*** The AAP (American Academy of Pediatrics) recommends that **children under one year old NOT** drink unfortified **cow's milk** as it has been found to interfere with iron absorption & cause **gastrointestinal bleeding** in about 40% of otherwise healthy infants![165] The AAP published the results of a U. of Iowa study that found that the blood content in the stool of infants fed cow's milk was five times higher than children fed infant formula.[165] In addition, most "non-organic" cow's milk products (ice cream, cheeses, etc.) contain additives that interfere with iron absorption.[15]

Remember, optimal health is NOT simply the absence of disease. Optimal health is the optimal functioning of all your cells in your body! To repeat, the #1 goal of this book is to optimize your health & bring you closer to God!

7. Thou shall consume antioxidant–rich foods to cleanse your cells from free radicals.

"YOU'RE NOT FAT. YOU'RE FULL OF" Free Radicals!

Free radicals are atoms or groups of atoms that can cause damage to cells, impairing the immune system & leading to infections & various degenerative diseases such as heart disease & cancer.[15,82] **Antioxidants** are natural compounds that help protect the body from harmful free radicals &, therefore, lower our "***FULL OF IT*** Level of Diseases (as well as possibly obesity &/or chronic pain)."

Oxygen radical Absorbance Capacity (ORAC) is a method of measuring antioxidant capacities in biological samples in vivo.[166] There has been a lot of ***controversy*** as to WHY these foods with high ORAC scores reduce the risk of cardiovascular disease & cancer. Although research *in vitro* indicates that **polyphenols** may be good antioxidants & probably influence the ORAC value, their antioxidant effects *in vivo* are probably negligent or absent.[167] The U.S. FDA & the EFSA (European Food Safety Authority) have established that it *is illegal to imply potential health benefits* *on package labels of **products** with high ORAC.*[167,168]   These 2 regulatory agencies have valid reason for this in my opinion for the following reasons:

- Many of these products have been sitting in bottles & should not be considered 100% living (breaking "Dietary Commandment # 3"). They may contain healthful fruits or vegetables – but they may be considered 100% dead, oxidized, &/or have lost most of its antioxidant capabilities.
- Many of these products are loaded with sugar (added or even naturally occurring – without any fiber to slow down the spike in blood sugar levels) raising our "***FULL OF IT* Level of**" Diseases (especially diabetes, cancer, & heart disease), Obesity, Chronic Pain (as well as aging)!   This breaks "Dietary Commandment # 8."
- & many of these products break most of the other "Dietary Commandments" &, therefore, should NOT be considered "healthful!"   Many foods &/or food products contain pesticides, man-made chemicals, etc. To reiterate if the person consumes a food breaking all 10 of these "Dietary Commandments," that food should be viewed as harmful. If the same person consumes the same food following all 10 of these "Dietary Commandments," that food should be considered healthful.

However, consuming a variety of organic foods that have been given "high ORAC scores" seem to lower (for reasons we may - or may not have identified yet) our "***FULL OF IT* Level of**" cancer, heart disease, & aging!

Too often, society judges a food by the amount of healthful **macronutrients (**such as vitamins, minerals, fiber, etc.) they contain. However, it may be the powerfully healthful **micronutrients** (currently known – as well as unknown) that give these foods such great antioxidant benefits!

Antioxidants & antioxidant-rich foods **may lower our "FULL OF IT Level of" cardiovascular disease &/or cancer**.[15,26,49,82]   I will be referencing some of the peer-review studies of specific antioxidant-rich foods in chapter 6.   There **IS genetic evidence** that high antioxidant foods may reduce the risk of cancer – as well as slow the aging process[15] & even help improve memory![26]   The truth is that many of these cancer-fighting foods have extremely healthful **micronutrients** that have not even been identified. Macronutrients (as mentioned above) like vitamins, minerals, etc. have been identified & analyzed in most foods.   However, the hundreds – if not thousands – of powerful healthful micronutrients may never be identified. Only God knows.

Thou shall eat at least one of these high antioxidant foods daily:

- **Organic Raw Wheatgrass Juice** (should drink within 30 minutes of juicing). Wheatgrass juice (as previously mentioned) is one of the best sources of chlorophyll to cleanse the blood.   Wheatgrass is one of the highest sources of superoxide dismutase (S.O.D.). S.O.D. (as mentioned earlier) is an antioxidant enzyme (AKA *free radical scavenger*) that may:[15] Decrease Inflammation; Decrease Oxidative Stress; &, therefore, may decrease the risk of atherosclerosis & cancers. Other healthful **Raw S.O.D.** food sources include ORGANIC: **Barley Grass** (possibly the highest source of S.O.D. in the world –

194

may be juiced with wheatgrass), **Broccoli, Sauerkraut, & most dark green leafy plants**. *"I have given [to everything that moves on the earth which has LIFE] every GREEN PLANT for food."* If we want to live, eat greens!?

- **Raw Organic Probiotic food sources** – such as: **kombucha,** low/no sodium cultured/fermented: **sauerkraut**, **pickled beets, & carrots** – may create more probiotics in your intestines to "produce" (convert from vitamin K1) more **Menaquinone-7 ("MK-7")**. MK-7 (a type of vitamin K2) may protect us against cancer (as well as atherosclerosis, bone loss, & bleeding to death)! Probiotics & Menaquinone-7 (a type of vitamin K2) will be discussed & referenced in chapter 6.
- **Organic raw Apples** (Red Delicious, Granny Smith, & Gala) had 3 of the top 24 "Food ORAC scores" originally published by the USDA in May of 2010 (as mentioned earlier, the USDA has closed this site mostly due to the abovementioned *controversy*).[166]   Numerous research studies have shown that consuming apples help prevent cancer, & even fight cancerous tumors![169] Apples are mentioned again in chapter 6.

Other healthful foods that had (in 2010) the top 24 "Food ORAC scores" included **Raw Organic**:[166]

- **Sprouted Beans** (including the Small Red, Red Kidney, Pinto, & Black). As mentioned in "Dietary Commandment #4," sprouting these beans improves the absorption of all the healthful macro- & micro-nutrients contained in these beans. In defense of the 2 abovementioned regulatory agencies,[167,168] most humans probably absorb less than 50% of the healthful nutrients in these un-sprouted beans with high ORAC scores.
- **Unprocessed Cocoa** (had the highest ORAC score of all "beans"). Unsweetened raw, unprocessed cocoa powder (can be sweetened with organic raw honey & mixed with virgin coconut oil in the "Lifestyle Phase") can have an ORAC value of 50,000![26] However, most "cocoa" sold in the stores is harmful as it usually: processed, contains cow's milk &/or sugar!   Thus, we probably do not absorb the healthful nutrients in this "processed cocoa."
- **Berries** - the highest ORAC scores were found in Acai & Himalayan Gogi berries.[26] Other berries in the top 24 included: blueberries, cranberries, blackberries, raspberries, & strawberries.[26]
- **Pecans**.
- **Prunes**.
- **Spices**.   By weight, spices may possess the highest concentration of antioxidant "power" of all of God's foods.[26]   However, these raw spices should be used in moderation as they may be very irritating to the gastrointestinal system when used in excess. Perhaps these powerful antioxidant rich spices should simply be "sprinkled" onto more soothing/bland foods (like apples, avocados, etc.)   These powerful antioxidant spices include:[26]
  - **Raw, organic cloves** have an ORAC of about 300,000 units per 100 grams (the highest of all "foods"). Cloves contain high levels of phenolic compounds – which have antioxidant, anti-inflammatory, & anti-clotting properties.[170]
  - **Ginger root** contains some phenols that have stronger antioxidant activity than vitamin E.[7]   Ginger root may kill ovarian & prostate cancer cells better than chemotherapy![171]   Ginger root is considered to have strong antioxidant & anti-inflammatory properties.[15,170]   Ginger root is a "super-cleansing food" shown in greater detail in chapter 6.

- Oregano is rich in *antioxidants & phytonutrients*.[172]   Oregano has anti-bacterial, anti-fungal, **anti-inflammatory** properties - & has been linked with helping weight loss, digestive health, combating foodborne pathogens, & relieving pain![172]
- **Rosemary & vanilla** are two spices that may possess powerful antioxidants.[26]
- **Cinnamon** is another spice that has **anti-inflammatory** properties and **cancer-fighting** abilities.[26,170]   Cinnamon may help patients with leukemia & lymphoma cancer.[170]   Cinnamon is known mostly for its ability to help lower blood sugar levels (to help diabetes) & is, therefore, mentioned again in "Dietary Commandment #9."
- **Turmeric ("king of the herbs")** can reduce inflammation & has been researched extensively for its ability to beat cancer.[170,172]   Turmeric has antibiotic, *anticancer, anti-inflammatory properties - & fights free radicals*.[15]   Turmeric is a "super-cleansing food" also shown in greater detail in Chapter 6.

Combining turmeric spice with certain cruciferous vegetables containing sulforaphane (SFN) & PEITC (phenethyl isothiocyanate) increases their cancer-prevention/fighting properties.[173]   SFN has been found to prevent & suppress the growing of colon cancer in mice & humans with colon cancer.[173] The cruciferous vegetables possessing the natural cancer fighters SFN & PEITC include organic:[173] **Cauliflower** – combined with turmeric may *prevent or eradicate prostate cancer totally*; **Broccoli & broccoli sprouts***; **Brussels sprouts & cabbage; Watercress & winter cress; Kale, Kohlrabi & turnips ***Broccoli Sprouts have been found to possess 20-50 times the cancer fighting indole sulforaphane** than fully grown broccoli.[7]

- Go **NUTS**! Besides **raw pecans** having a high ORAC score (possibly 18,000), other raw nuts (such as walnuts & almonds) have great health benefits.[26] **Raw Brazil nuts** are a good source of selenium – a powerful antioxidant.[15] These "Super Nuts" are mentioned again in chapter 6.
- **Raw Organic Garlic** is a versatile herb that also has antioxidant properties. Garlic has compounds that protect against oxidation & free radicals.   Garlic also contains antioxidant nutrients such as vitamins A & C & selenium.[15,74] Garlic is believed to protect against:[15] Radiation & sunlight damage; DNA damage; Liver damage caused by carbon tetrachloride, a common indoor pollutant & free radical generator.   However, most people can't tolerate raw garlic's irritating effects on the GI system. In addition, Aged Garlic Extract ("AGE" – eaten during the "Lifestyle Phase") has shown to boost garlic's antioxidant potential![15]
- **Organic Tomatoes, red grapefruit, & red peppers contain lycopenes** – which may be cancer fighting.[7]   **Tomatoes (as well as carrots & strawberries)** contain **coumarins** that may help prevent intestinal cancer.[7]
- **Organic Red Grapes contain phenols that may inhibit stomach & esophageal cancer**.[7] These phenols (also found in green tea) may also protect against atherosclerosis & heart disease.[7]

EXCEPTIONS: Individuals with organ transplants may have to limit or avoid antioxidants due to fear of the immune system strengthening &, then, attacking the transplanted organ!   Thus, like everything else that goes in your mouth, ask your physician(s)' opinions of this.

   After the "Cleansing Phase," one may benefit (if desiring/"allowed" to strengthen their immune system) from the following (non-raw) food/supplements believed to possess antioxidant abilities:[15]

-   Cinnamon (see above);[26,170] Clove oil (see above) – some may benefit from adding a drop to their tea or home-made mouthwash (1 drop of clove oil with filtered water);[15,26,170] Cocoa unprocessed (see above);[26,166] Coenzyme Q10 (1 mg per pound of body weight/day); Coffee (without sugar or cow's milk or "soy milk" added) may have an ORAC value of up to 17,000 units & (in moderate amounts) may help protect against atherosclerosis, type II diabetes, depression, & even dementia;[26] Curcumin (found in the spice Turmeric);[170,172,173] Aged Garlic Extract; Ginger root – mentioned above;[7,170,171] Glutathione (see chapter 6 for more details); Grape Seed Extract; Green Tea (contains phenols that inhibit stomach & esophageal cancer, atherosclerosis, & heart disease);[7] Maitake Mushroom; Menaquinone-7 (a type of vitamin K2 found mostly in Natto) about 100 mcgs/day (see chapter 6 for more details on the amazing benefits of MK7); Methionine; Methylsulfonylmethane (MSM) (about 1 gram twice per day); N-Acetyl Cysteine (no more than 600mg/day – see chapter 6 under glutathione for more details); Oregano oil may add 1 -3 drops in your filtered water to add antioxidant - & possibly anti-fungal (anti - Candida albicans) benefits;[172] Probiotics – 1 billion+ live cells per day (see chapter 6 for more details); Resveratrol; Selenium (200 micrograms/day); S.O.D. (available in enteric pill form); Turmeric – mentioned above;[170,172,173] Vitamin C - Buffered (500 mg 1-3 times/day = a water soluble antioxidant working in both intra- & extracellular water soluble places);[7] & Vitamin E (100-800 International units/day = fat soluble antioxidant working in the lipid places of our body. This is one reason why it should be taken with vitamin C as they work synergistically as antioxidants.[7]

Many of the above will be mentioned in greater details in chapter 6.

8.   Thou shall avoid sugar & High Glycemic LOAD Meals.

"YOU'RE NOT FAT. YOU'RE FULL OF:" High Glycemic Load Meals/Foods – like dead fruit juices, sodas, sugars, & excess grains!

      As Americans have been increasingly breaking this commandment – becoming "*FULL OF*" more high Glycemic Load Meals/foods/beverages, we have become progressively more:

-   Diseased (especially type 2 diabetes & metabolic syndrome – as well as heart disease, cancer, etc.); Obese; & in chronic pain

Said differently, breaking this commandment: raises all of our "*FULL OF IT* Levels!"   Thus: following this commandment lowers all of our "*FULL OF IT* Levels!"   As you can figure out by now, this diet (as well as this entire book) is **NOT "SUGAR COATED**!" ☺

      Consider what "man" has done to God's food.   God created the organic potato - & man peeled off the nutrient-rich skin & sliced the starchy center into chips & deep-fried them!   God created organic wheat & cane -

& man turned it into white refined flour & sugar (& combined them) to please Satan to destroy your health (& waistline)!

Should SUGAR be considered a drug – or just another TOXIN?

As mentioned in "commandment 2," sugar beets are being genetically modified (to resist herbicides) since 2009 (in the U.S.).[56] With little regulation & safety tests performed by the companies doing the modifications themselves, it is unclear what risks these "man-made/modified" foods pose to us outside of what we already know. If a meal contains a lot of sugar, then it is a *"High Glycemic Load Meal"* (analyzed further later on).

We do know that consuming an excess of sugar(s) or "High Glycemic Load Meals" (analyzed later) increases the risk of (&/or worsens):

- Atherosclerosis;[103] Type II Diabetes;[174,175] Age-related macular degeneration;[174,175] Iron deficiency anemia & other bleeding disorders - as sugar consumption interferes with iron (& vitamin C) absorption;[15,82] Cancer & other Immune disorders - as sugar consumption can interfere with vitamin C absorption (& can reduce the ability of white blood cells to fight illnesses).[15,63,176]

Sugar consumption destroys our immune system by:[7,176]
- Increasing oxidative damage
- & produces free radicals in excess
- Stress, stress-related disorders, & the damaging "physiological (& psychological) stress response" mentioned in chapters 3 & 4 – which creates a whole host of other symptoms/diseases. This is probably because sugar consumption causes the abovementioned immune system damages as well as the following:[7,176]
  - Stresses our adrenal glands
  - & robs our body of minerals such as magnesium (a known muscle "relaxer") & the B vitamins (known for their ability to help us deal with "stress").
- & Candidiasis – as the *Candida albicans* yeast "feed" on sugar).[15]   As per Phyllis Balch (in her book *Prescription for Nutritional Healing*), Candidiasis can affect various parts of the body, including the following wide array of symptoms:[15]
  - Constipation, diarrhea, colitis, abdominal pain, headaches, bad breath, rectal itching, impotence, memory loss, mood swings, prostatitis, canker sores, persistent heartburn, muscle & joint pain, sore throat, congestion, nagging cough, numbness in the face or extremities, tingling sensations, acne, night sweats, severe itching, clogged sinuses, PMS, burning tongue, white spots on the tongue & in the mouth (*"thrush"*), extreme fatigue, vaginitis, kidney & bladder infections, arthritis, depression, hyperactivity, hypothyroidism, adrenal problems, & even diabetes.

There is no coincidence that sugar consumption & obesity (which may be caused by consuming an excess of sugars/high Glycemic Load meals) BOTH increase the risk of type II diabetes & cardiovascular disease![174,175]

Even if "cane sugar" is "organic," it is still extremely unhealthy.   It is (currently) usually refined & stripped of all its' fiber & minerals.   "Cane sugar (Organic or not)" & glucose have the highest Glycemic index (GI) of all foods.[177]

The **Glycemic index** or **GI** estimates how much each gram of available carbohydrate (AKA "**Net carbs**" = total carbohydrate minus fiber) in a food ***raises a person's blood glucose level*** following consumption of the food, relative to consumption of glucose.[177]   The limitation(s) to the Glycemic Index - such as the variety in scores for each food - is discussed in "EXCEPTIONS" of this commandment.

The average GI of 62 common foods derived from multiple studies by different laboratories was published in "Diabetes Care" in 2008 - & includes the following information:[177]

-   **A low GI** is 55 or less. Healthful examples allowed during any "Phase" include **raw & Organic**: Most fruits & vegetables, nuts,[178,179] **edible seeds (like pumpkin & sunflower seeds);**[178,179] **unprocessed cocoa; & practically all sprouts - like: sprouted beans (including sprouted soybeans), pea sprouts, sprouted lentils, & barley**. The healthy low GI foods allowed after the "Cleansing Phase" include Organic: cooked vegetables, beans, cooked peas, cooked lentils, brown rice noodles (gluten free); chickpeas, barley grass powder, probiotic based soybean-based foods (like natto, tempeh, & doenjang); probiotic goat's milk-based foods (like yogurt, etc.); & *oatmeal from rolled oats*.***

-   **A medium GI** is 56-69. Healthful examples allowed during any "Phase" include **Organic**: **Raw Honey (except eucalyptus honey)**.   The healthful medium GI foods allowed after the "Cleansing Phase" include Organic: Sweet potato; basmati rice; brown rice (boiled); & cooked millet porridge.

-   **A high GI** is 70 & above. Glucose has a GI of approximately 100.[178,179] Healthful examples allowed during any "Phase" include **raw & organic**: **Watermelon** (eaten alone –as will be discussed in "Commandment # 10). **High GI foods not allowed during either phase include**: white bread; whole wheat bread; & of course sugar.   High GI foods "allowed" (**in very small amounts**) during the "Lifestyle Phase" include organic: white rice; corn-based cereals; rice-based porridge; white potato (boiled or instant mash); rice milk; rice crackers/crisps; & *instant oatmeal (not from rolled oats)*.***   Despite the fact that these high GI foods *may* be organic, wheat-free, gluten free, & possess very low toxic-mucus capability: they should be **limited** as these **high GI foods have** the potential to become *high "GL" (Glycemic Load) meals*! "Glycemic Load" is much more important than GI (see below).

***Note: *oatmeal from rolled oats* has a low/medium GI of approximately 55.[177]   However, *instant oatmeal (not from rolled oats)* has a high GI of approximately 79.[177]   This is just another example of how one food (like "oatmeal") can be either healthful or harmful.   However, the GL is a better indicator than GI regarding whether a "meal" is healthful or harmful (see below).

Glycemic Load of **GL** is a better indicator than GI because your body's ***glycemic response is dependent on the type AND the amount of carbohydrate consumed*.**[177-179]

The **GL** is calculated as the GI (%) x grams of "**net carbs**" (net carbs = total carbs minus dietary fiber) per serving.[177-179]   Consuming high GL foods such as sugar & white, refined, fiber-less flour products (as well as processed cooked foods full of toxins) puts great stress on your waistline – as well as your pancreas, liver, & overall gastrointestinal, cardiovascular, & immune systems!   **A "GL meal" above 20 is considered "High."**[178,179]   A "**GL meal**" **below 10 is considered "Low."**[178,179]   Consider the following examples:

- 1 cup of watermelon (high GI of approximately 76)[177] has only:[74] 50 calories; 160 total grams & 12 grams of total carbohydrates (due to its high water content); 11.5 grams of "net carbs" due to containing 0.5 grams of dietary fiber; &, therefore, a "low GL meal" of **8.74** (76% multiplied by 11.5)![177-179] Thus: 1 cup of watermelon (consumed alone) is a **healthful "low GL meal."**[177-179] However, consuming over 2.3 cups of watermelon creates a **harmful "high GL (20+) meal!"**[177-179]
- 1 cup of lentil sprouts (low GI of approximately 32)[177] has only:[74] 81 calories, 77 total grams & 17 grams of total carbohydrates; 14.65 grams "net carbs" due to containing 2.35 grams of dietary fiber; &, therefore, a **healthful "low GL meal"** of only **4.7** (32% multiplied by 14.65).[177-179]
- 1 cup of instant mashed potatoes (high GI of approximately 87)[177] contains:[74] 222 calories, 35.4 grams "net carbs" (36 g of total carbs – 0.6 g dietary fiber); &, therefore, a **harmful "high GL meal"** of **30.8** (87% multiplied by 35.4).[177-179]

The abovementioned examples provide further evidence that **all calories are NOT equal in their effect on our bodies**.   Realize that the above examples are simply examples of individual foods eaten alone as a "meal."   In the real world, we combine foods together (see "Commandment #10" how to best combine foods). Thus 1 cup of lentil sprouts combined with only half a cup of instant mashed potatoes creates a **harmful "high GL meal" of 20+**.[74,177-179]

   A low GL diet (for example 100/day or less) has shown the following health benefits:

- May decrease body fat & weight in humans[178] & animals.[180]
- May increase lean muscle mass in humans[178] & animals.[180]
- Has shown (in humans who followed a low GL diet over many years) to significantly lower the risk of type II Diabetes, **atherosclerosis, **** & age-related macular degeneration.[174,175]
- Has shown to dramatically lower plasma triglyceride levels & significantly **decrease post-meal blood sugar**** & insulin levels in animals[180] & humans.[174]

   High post-meal plasma glucose levels & repeated glycemic "spikes" – may increase oxidative stress to the vasculature &, therefore, are more strongly associated with **atherosclerosis than fasting glucose or HbA1c levels![181]   I, personally, do not believe we have to count the GL (or even calories –for that matter!) for the entire day (just follow all 10 "Dietary Commandments").   Even if you avoided any GL from awakening to "dinner-time" (not recommended & probably not possible – unless you fast: drinking filtered water throughout the day) & then ate one very high GL dinner (that day): you may get a **harmful** high post-meal plasma glucose level (with a glycemic spike)![181]

For example: Orange juice may have a low GI (50).[177]   However, it is predominantly sugar (most store brands have almost no fiber, fat, or protein).[74]   Drinking over 13 ounces of orange juice alone - creates a **harmful "high GL meal"** of 20+.[74,177-179]   In addition, it is dead (versus alive). Most "juices" sold in the store are considered one of the 5 worst foods to consume while sick or battling a cold (<u>due to the excess sugar</u> that can reduce the ability of white blood cells to fight illness).[63]

We are "FULL OF" Harmful "High GL foods/meals"

It has been estimated that the average American consumes (on a yearly basis):[79]

- 29 pounds of **French fries**;
- 55 pounds of Corn Syrup – usually in the form of "**High Fructose Corn Syrup**" or "**HFCS**" (one of the cheapest & most health-hazardous forms of sugar that can be used.[182] May be filled with mercury, genetically modified, & increase the risk of **_diabetes, weight gain, & decreased memory/learning ability_**);[182]
- & 53 gallons of **soda**. This equates to about 18 ounces per day of soda. This amount of soda often contains over 60 grams of sugar – an amount that exceeds the recommended daily intake of approximately 15 grams![183]

Of the 100 plus pounds of sugar Americans eat in a year, 70 pounds are added to foods during processing.[176,182]   In addition, many chefs add sugar to their sauces, soups, etc. to satisfy the sweet cravings of the customers.   Therefore, our sugar consumption is not 100% voluntary![176,182] No matter whom you blame, the fact = the _average American consumes 3x more sugar daily than recommended_![183]   Since many "health conscience people" (like myself & my friends/family) almost NEVER consume the abovementioned foods (such as French fries, sodas, etc.), the amount consumed by those who do is actually much higher!   Thus, these Americans are consuming a lot of "**_High Glycemic LOAD meals!_**"   This is killing our nation!

We are "FULL OF" sugar - such as sugary drinks & sodas.

Sugary sodas are often sweetened in the U.S. with GMO corn-derived & mercury-containing high fructose corn syrup.[182-184]   The 7 trillion calories of sugar consumed annually (by the average American kid) just from sodas has predisposed this generation to diabetes, cancer, obesity, etc.[183]   Sodas often contain "_caramel food coloring_" – which <u>may</u> also increase the risk of **lung, liver, & thyroid cancer**.[184] Individuals with greater genetic predisposition to **obesity** appear to be more susceptible to the harmful effects of sugar-sweetened beverages.[183] Researchers have found men drinking one or more sugared soda cans/bottles saw a 66% increase in **non-Hodgkin lymphoma**.[182]

We are "FULL OF" too many grains (dead = un-sprouted)

The average American consumes 192.3 pounds of flour & cereal products - usually full of wheat (&/or other sources of gluten).[79]   Because of the "toxic mucus" of wheat (mentioned in "Commandment # 4") bloating your intestines – your appetite will be stimulated to eat more!   This is a very dangerous cycle![78,80]   White bread, wheat bread, _whole wheat/whole grain wheat bread; unleavened wheat bread_; corn flakes; & white rice (boiled) are all considered "**high GI**" foods.[177]   We should learn from the animals.   **Animals grain-fed are fatter** (as compared to animals grass-fed).   This will be mentioned (& referenced in Chapter 6) re: "super-cleansing meats."   If we want to lose excess body fat (& achieve optimal health), we should limit/avoid these grains (especially wheat).   Some of the "Super-Grains" mentioned in chapter 6 are organic, raw: sprouted quinoa; sprouted oats; sprouted millet, etc.

We are "**_FULL OF_**" **too much WHEAT** = the most harmful grain to our health![78,80]   **Is wheat (like sugar) a drug – or just another under-recognized toxin?**   As per Dr. William David, M.D. (in his book "*Wheat Belly*"):[80]

- *Today's wheat has been **genetically altered** to provide processed-food manufacturers the greatest yield at the lowest cost; consequently, this once benign grain has been transformed into a **nutritionally bankrupt** yet ubiquitous ingredient that **causes blood sugar to spike** more rapidly than eating pure table sugar and has __addictive properties__ that cause us to ride a roller coaster of hunger, **overeating, & fatigue**.*
- *Two slices of whole wheat bread can **increase blood sugar** more than 2 tablespoons of pure cane sugar!* This may be explained by wheat bread's **high GL meal factor**.
- *Health conscience Americans have been told by "dietary experts" since the 1970s to **reduce fat & eat more "healthful whole grains"** (consuming approximately **75% of their carbohydrate intake from wheat product**s). This (as well as breaking the other "10 Dietary Commandments") has led to Americans steadily becoming more obese, more diseased, & in more chronic pain.   These diseases include: **type 2 diabetes & the metabolic syndrome** – as well as heart disease, neurological diseases, inflammation, rheumatoid arthritis, osteopenia/osteoporosis, intestinal diseases (like ulcerative colitis & celiac disease), skin conditions (from psoriasis to oral ulcers & hair loss),& dementia.*

If we want to lose excess body fat (& achieve optimal health), we should limit/avoid this dead, *genetically altered, addictive, & nutritionally bankrupt grain*.[80] Replacing grain-based carbs (like those found in wheat products) with healthful fats ("super-cleansing fats" – mentioned in chapter 6) has shown to significantly reduce total cholesterol/HDL & LDL/HDL ratios[100] (&, therefore, reduce the risks of atherosclerosis & atherosclerotic events/diseases).[98,99]

A low-GL diet is not necessarily a "low-carb" diet.   Avoiding carbs may deprive you of extremely healthful fruits (rich in vitamins, antioxidants, fiber, & other nutrients) & grains (like organic sprouted quinoa & sprouted oats).   However, most of the "super-cleansing foods" (mentioned in chapter 6) have a low Glycemic load.[179]   Even a 60 gram serving of pitted prunes – which taste sweet – has a low GI (29) & a low GL (10).[179]

Thou shall include some amount of "super-cleansing proteins" & "super-cleansing fats" in most meals.   Examples of "super-cleansing proteins" & "super- cleansing fats" include raw ORGANIC:

- Nuts, seeds, sprouted lentils, sprouted beans, & others mentioned in chapter 6 (under "super-cleansing fats" & "super-cleansing proteins").

These "super-cleansing fat & protein" food sources contain very little "net carbs." Thus, they have a very low GL.   It should be recognized that none of the "Super-Cleansing foods/supplements" mentioned in Chapter 6 have or predispose you to a high GL meal.   **Including healthful fats & proteins in every meal can be a great way to prevent high GL meals.**

The most "God-made," _healthful_ (least harmful) "sugar substitutes" - for those who have the "weakness," craving, or addiction to add sweetness to their food - include the following 4 Raw Organic choices:

- **Apple(s)**. You can eat them whole, cut, chop, or even blend them with filtered water (remove stem & core, of course) & add to any food in the world (except melons –as discussed in "Commandment # 10"). They have a "God-given" sweetness, low GI (36),[177] & numerous health benefits. Be sure to consume them soon after cutting them to avoid their oxidation (turning brown).
- **Most fruit**. However, fruit can't be combined with "non-fruits" (as discussed in "Commandment # 10").
- **Honey**. As mentioned above, honey has a medium GI of approximately 61.[177] It also has numerous health benefits. However, you should use in moderation as honey (typically) contains no fiber &, therefore, consuming **over 2 Tablespoons** will create a harmful "**High GL meal!**"[74,177-179]
- **Cinnamon**. Daily intake of cinnamon has shown to reduce fasting blood sugar levels.[26,170]

Stevia (_Stevia rebaudiana_) is a "natural" plant/herb that is an extremely low (or no) GI/GL sugar substitute acceptable (in moderation) during the "Lifestyle Phase." However, stevia may have up to 300 times the sweetness of sucrose or glucose (with a longer after taste)![185] Two 2010 review studies found no health concerns with stevia or its' sweetening extracts.[186,187] In addition, a 2009 review study found that stevioside & related stevia compounds have the following actions:[188]

- Anti-hyperglycemic (reduced blood glucose levels ONLY when they were too high!); anti-hypertensive; anti-inflammatory; anti-tumor; antidiarrheal; diuretic; & immune-modulatory.

The U.S. FDA (as of 2012) has given a _no objection approval for GRAS_ (Generally Recognized as Safe) for the brands "_Truvia_" & "_PureVia_" (considered by the FDA as _highly purified products using rebaudioside A_ – a glycoside extract of Stevia).[189] However (despite being used by millions of Japanese for decades & billions in South Americans for centuries), the FDA will **not** give a GRAS rating to "**whole-leaf Stevia** or **crude Stevia extracts** _due to concerns on the reproductive, cardiovascular, & renal systems._"[189] The World Health Organization's joint experts Committee of food Additives has approved (based on long-term studies), an acceptable daily intake of **Steviol glycoside** of up to of up to 4mg/day per kg of body weight.[190] Therefore: a 100 pound human should not consume over 181 mg of steviol glycoside![190] Most stevia approved by the FDA as GRAS sold/added to foods is _not_ raw (or 100% "organic") &, therefore, unacceptable during the "Cleansing Phase." Non-raw stevia is permissible (in moderation) during the "Lifestyle Phase."

A **sugar substitute NOT 100% "God-made"** (that may be acceptable during the "Lifestyle Phase" – in moderation) is:

Xylitol (a sugar alcohol found in the fibers of certain fruits & vegetables) - & possibly some other sugar alcohols – is an extremely low-GI (7) & almost no GL sugar substitute.[191] Like stevia, xylitol doesn't contribute to high blood sugar levels or the resultant hyperglycemia caused by insufficient insulin response.[188,192] Like stevia, xylitol (& certain other sugar alcohols like erythritol) may, therefore, be helpful for those with Diabetes &/or "Metabolic Syndrome" (characterized by insulin resistance, hypertension, hypercholesterolemia, or an increased risk of blood clots).[188,192] Xylitol may also possess the following unique benefits: Dental health[193] Reduce the risk of Infections (especially ear & upper respiratory infections – as well as general sepsis);[194] & Reduce the risk of Candidiasis.[15,192] In contrast, "galactose," glucose, & sucrose may increase proliferation of the candida yeast (worsening candidiasis – due to their ability to raise blood sugar levels).[15,192]

However, most xylitol may be considered (like most, if not all sugar alcohols) "**_processed_**" by man (humans). Xylitol (like most sugar alcohols – but unlike stevia) has a **_laxative effect_** (lower than "mannitol" or "sorbitol" – but higher than "erythritol") because sugar alcohols are NOT fully digested or absorbed.[195] In humans (**unlike dogs**), no other side effects have currently been found from the ingestion of xylitol. Life-threatening hypoglycemia reactions & liver failure have been found **in dogs** after ingesting xylitol.[196] Since xylitol is not 100% "God-made," it is **_forbidden_** during "The Cleansing Phase" & should be limited (to only those with the "weak cravings of sweetness" – who for whatever absurd reason have not been satisfied by raw organic apples, most other fruits, honey, or cinnamon) during the "Lifestyle Phase."

There is a brand of chewing gum (called "*Peelu Chewing Gum with Xylitol: Cinnamon sass flavor*" found @ www.peelu .com) allowed after the "Cleansing Phase" that people may benefit from a piece or two after dinner (to possibly help with digestion, dental health, & other abovementioned benefits). This gum contains: *Xylitol, natural oil of cinnamon, peelu fiber, & rebiana (stevia extract)*. It is *dairy free, soy free, vegan, wheat free, sugar free, & aspartame free*. However, it is not raw or organic. Thus, I do not consider this acceptable during the "Cleansing Phase." Nor do I consider this a "super-food or supplement." Too much of this (like any xylitol product) may have a laxative effect. However, I must admit this "gum" may provide the abovementioned stevia & xylitol health benefits (such as dental health). If you have a "craving" or "weakness" to gum, I believe this is superior (less harmful) to most of the sugary or artificially sugared gum sold in most stores.

Keep in mind - the following truth about Stevia & Xylitol:
- You should always try to find them (as well as all "foods") as close to "**God-made**" (versus "man-made") as possible. They <u>should</u> be "**USDA Certified Organic**."
- **Future** research *may* show negatives – especially if the products become (or are) more "man-made" versus "God-made." Therefore, use them in moderation. There is already a lot of research that suggests almost all artificial sweeteners (usually 100% "Man-Made") have damaging effects on humans.
- **They don't come close to the other 4 in health benefits & may already possess harmful effects.**[189]
- Thus: <u>**try to use as 1st choice the natural sweetness of raw organic apples or other fruits (if not combining them with "non-fruits"); then the natural sweetness of raw organic honey; &/or cinnamon.**</u> These four choices mentioned have a lengthy list of wonderful health benefits & are considered 100% "God-made." The combination of raw organic honey with cinnamon (100% raw & organic) is probably one of the most powerful/healthful synergistic 100% God-made food combinations known currently to man! However, one should never consume more than 2 tablespoons of honey per "meal" as this will create a **harmful "High GL meal**!"[74,177-179]

We are "*FULL OF*" Diet Sodas!

Remember: most **diet sodas** (sold in the U.S.A.) do not contain honey or cinnamon (or even xylitol or stevia extract). Many diet sodas contain flame retardants – in addition to a slew of unhealthy ingredients – like genetically modified aspartame.[197] 4 major negative side effects of **drinking most diet sodas** may include:[197]

- **Kidney damage.** Harvard Medical School researchers studied over 3,000 women for 11 years & found that diet soda consumption (especially women who drank more than 2 diet sodas daily) had a positive correlation to kidney health decline (possibly due to the high sodium &/or artificially sweeteners).

- **Altered metabolism** – with a 34% increased risk of **belly fat**; & a 44% increased risk of **heart attack or stroke.**
- **Obesity** &, therefore, increased risk of **heart attacks & strokes**[183] – two or more cans of diet soda consumption was associated with a 500% increase in waistlines (possibly because the body receives/"ABSORBS" no calories or nutrients - & people then eat more food at meals to compensate. Again, the concept of ABSORPTION applies here!)!
- **Cell Damage** (due to diet sodas often containing mold inhibitors – not found in sugary sodas – often listed as sodium benzoate or potassium benzoate). These chemicals may cause **severe damage to the DNA** – as well as worsen hives, asthma, & other allergic reactions. Remember: aspartame is created using genetically modified bacteria (a "<u>GMO</u>" - which has been linked to cancer in rats).

Consuming one can/day of diet soda – usually containing aspartame – has shown to (based on a follow-up study on over 100,000 humans over 20 years):[198] Increase the risk of **leukemia** by 42% in men & women; Increase the risk of **multiple myeloma** by 102% in men; & increase the risk of **non-Hodgkin's lymphoma** by 31% in men.

In summary: Diet sodas are (for the most part) <u>usually</u> **diametrically opposed to being:**
- **100% "God-made" (They are usually 100% "man-made"); "Organic;" "Alive;" Or "healthful!"**

Therefore: my friends & family should avoid (in every phase) most –if not all current - diet sodas (as well as sugary sodas/drinks).

EXCEPTIONS: After the "Cleansing Phase," you may actually benefit from consuming a high-GL meal in the following situations:
- One: if you are suffering from a low blood sugar reaction.[179] However, a ***high-GI food* does NOT equal** a *high-GL meal*! Thus: this is truly not an exception of this "Commandment!" Ingesting a 1 gram cube of sugar (a 100 GI "food" – the highest GI food in the world)[177-180] *may* help quickly return *low* blood sugar levels to *normal*.[179] However, this 1 gram cube of sugar has a low GL of 1[177-179] - & will, hopefully, not raise your blood glucose levels above normal! Again: a teaspoon of watermelon (high GI food) or raw organic honey (medium GI food) would be a superior substitute to a cube of sugar.
- Two: if you are an athlete.[179] The more you exercise, the "higher" the GL you *may* be able to "afford" to eat (before & even after you exercise). Chromium (a trace mineral often in the form of chromium picolinate) 200mcg taken with this high GL food (before exercising) may help stimulate the sugar in the blood to transfer into the skeletal muscle cells to be burned for energy when exercising.[15] Chromium picolinate – along with carnitine are analyzed again in chapter 6 regarding their warnings & their ability to increase energy levels & help lose excess weight. This exception reiterates what "Commandment #1" states about avoiding gluttony. Consistent exercise helps you burn more calories – as well as reduce the burden of high GL meals.

Keep in mind, the other limitations of the GI & the GL include:[179]

205

- There is a scarcity & wide variation in GI measurements; Individual differences in glycemic response; & reliance on GI & GL may lead to <u>over</u>consumption of fat & total calories.

9. Thou shall Hydrate –but don't drink too much (just sip) when eating.

"YOU'RE NOT FAT. YOU'RE FULL OF:"

- <u>**Excess water (or other beverages) with your meals**</u> - preventing you from optimally absorbing/assimilating the nutrients in the food you are consuming!
- <u>**&/or Excess sodium chloride ("table salt"), sugar, &/or alcohol**</u> – that can predispose you to dehydration!

Preventing dehydration & keeping ourselves hydrated (with filtered water) is crucial to cleanse the entire body.   Keeping ourselves hydrated (with filtered water) seems crucial to cleanse the intestines - & keep the intestines clean – as colonic hydrotherapy often uses water to cleanse the intestines.[2,15,49]
Remember: ***if you are thirsty, you may already be dehydrated***!

During the "Cleansing Phase" or "Lifestyle Phase" the following <u>raw, organic</u> "foods" may be added to increase the overall ***cleansing*** effect of your filtered water: Lemon juice. Even the lemon peel (rinsed off with filtered water, of course) may be shredded and blended with the filtered water to increase the cleansing effect.

During the "<u>**Lifestyle Phase**</u>" (After the "Cleansing Phase") the following "foods" may be added to your filtered water to increase the overall cleansing effect of your filtered water:

- Organic Apple Cider Vinegar. Some people may have too much hydrochloric acid (HCL) – but most adults have a deficiency & may benefit from 1 teaspoon/week (or daily if needed).[15]
- Slippery Elm & Marshmallow powders. They may be very soothing to the throat –as well as the entire gastrointestinal system.[15]
- Organic Oregano oil. A few drops/day may be powerful enough to help people with candida, sinus problems, etc.[15]

Unlike beverages (like alcohol, "table salt" – sodium chloride, &/or sugar-added drinks) that may actually predispose you to dehydration, many of the "super-beverages" (like **kombucha** in the "Cleansing Phase" – or kefir in the "Lifestyle Phase") can rapidly hydrate the body.[1]   Fruits & vegetables (like the "super-food" broccoli = 91% water)[74] contain a high percentage of water & can also hydrate the body.   The effectiveness of each of your body's systems depends on proper hydration.   By using a high quality water filtration system: pesticides, toxic heavy metals, & other contaminates may be significantly reduced (&, hopefully, eliminated) from your everyday drinking supply.

You need to have a <u>**balance between your sodium and potassium intake**</u>. Most Americans are "***FULL OF***" excess sodium –due to our addiction to salty, processed foods. Excess sodium intake may lead to fluid retention, swelling/edema, bloating, etc. Due to the excess sodium in the S.A.D. (Standard American Diet), most of us would benefit from reducing our sodium intake. The "Cleansing Phase" automatically takes care of this.

   Don't drink too much – just sip – when eating to avoid interfering with your own body's digestive enzymes (as well as the digestive enzymes God already has put in the raw/living food you are eating)!   This includes kombucha (as well as perhaps other teas) & freshly juiced wheatgrass juice (or other fresh made raw vegetable juices) – which should be "swished" in your mouth to allow the amylase in your saliva help digest/absorb any carbs in the juice. Some nutritionists recommend drinking lots of water right before & during your meals in order to feel satiated (full) & avoid over-eating.   I believe this is bad advice. Drinking lots of water (or even fresh raw vegetable juices) right before eating - may actually put more stress on the gastrointestinal system (leading to mal-absorption & indigestion) as the water dilutes the digestive enzymes that God put in the healthful food you are consuming (as well as the digestive enzymes God gave you in your gastrointestinal system) necessary to digest/absorb the food!   Remember: you are not what you eat! *You are what you ABSORB*!

   If you do not absorb what you eat, you may deprive your body of necessary nutrients. Your brain will tell your body to keep eating more food. Unfortunately, you are consuming that food in an environment "***FULL OF***" intestinal waste matter due to the abovementioned bad advice.   This is like planting a seed in a deep puddle on top of the cement!   This waste matter can slow your metabolism & lead to obesity & a whole host of diseases.

If you want to "feel full" (satiated) to avoid over-eating:
- Eat low-starch vegetables (in the form of a salad) before & during the meal. This may be the most superior way to satiate you enough to avoid over-eating!
- Chew thoroughly & slowly (following Dietary Commandment # 1).

EXCEPTIONS: After the "Cleansing Phase," one may benefit from organic healthful soups, probiotic-enriched goat's milk, & kefir (from goat's milk) – which should still be chewed &/or "swished" in your mouth!   "Dead fruit juices" & "dead vegetable juices" (made over 1 hour ago – sold in stores - usually loaded with sugar & possessing NO enzymes or probiotics) should be avoided in either phase of this diet.   But if you do cheat, at least swish it in your mouth & avoid drinking too much of it near meal-time.

   Drinking **EXCESS Water** should be **avoided** due to the following reasons:
- Everyone should have an optimal BALANCE between the levels of potassium & sodium (as well as other important electrolytes) in their bodies.
- Drinking excess water may lower the level of sodium – as well as possibly other important electrolytes – in your body.

207

- Patients with kidney disorders - such as renal failure (usually requiring dialysis) -must limit the daily amount of water they drink. Of course these patients should ask their nephrologist about how much daily fluid/water to drink/consume.

10. Thou shall combine food correctly to ensure optimal ABSORPTION.

***"YOU'RE NOT FAT. YOU'RE FULL OF"* Incorrect FOOD COMBINATIONS -** preventing you from optimally absorbing & assimilating all the nutrients in the food you are consuming! Again: you are NOT what you eat. You are what you absorb (gastro-intestinally/physically – as well as intellectually & spiritually).

I intentionally saved this for last for the following reasons:
- The foundation & uniqueness of this "diet" is to achieve **optimal digestion/ABSORPTION** in order to help you maximally cleanse (achieve optimal health of) your body, mind, & soul! "Food-combining" diets focus on optimal digestion & absorption of the foods you eat. One may argue that this last commandment has very little scriptural basis. However, optimal ABSORPTION (I believe) is a fundamental aspect of the living word of God. As I have hopefully made clear throughout this book: if you eat the most healthful foods (or supplements) in the world –but do not digest/ABSORB them –it never really became part of you. It would be like *"planting a seed on the hard road."* We want to *"plant the seed on good soil."*
- This commandment is **somewhat controversial**.

One study showed that people on *a type of food combination diet* (in 6 weeks) had a significant decrease in:[199] Total body fat; waist-to-hip ratio; fasting blood glucose; total cholesterol; & blood pressure.

However, this same study showed *no superiority* (in reducing the above factors) to a "balanced diet." [199] Remember: **the optimal digestion/absorption aspect** of food-combining diets is NOT the characteristic that is controversial. In addition, this study did not use the below mentioned food combination rules in this "Commandment" or the other 9 "Dietary Commandments!" As one may have concluded by now: this "Diet" involves (in all "Phases"):
- "Optimal absorption/digestion" principles; "food-combining" principles; "balanced diet" principles, "raw/living (versus dead) foods;" Bible-based principles; avoiding high glycemic load meals; avoiding man-made chemicals; avoiding allergy-causing foods; avoiding toxic mucus-forming foods; & a whole lot more!
- This is the commandment that I see most ***people (including "so-called" health, nutrition, & diet-gurus) BREAK on a daily basis*** (if not multiple times per day)!
- This is probably the **most complicated** of all 10 commandments. Most food-combining diets include complicated pie charts/graphs, etc. However it really doesn't have to be so complicated. I have simplified it so you receive all the benefits without any of the negatives.

I have taken many food combination diets – such as the *"Fit for Life Diets"* (by the Diamonds – some of the pioneers in "food-combining" diets);[200] *"The Acid-Alkaline Diet"* (by C. Vasey);[201] & many food-combination articles – to create a simple & optimal way to food-combine.

Thus, after 19+ years researching these food-combining theories/diets, I have created the following 3 rules:

- **Rule # 1: Eat "fruits" with "fruits" & eat "non-fruits" with "non-fruits."** In other words: **Thou shall not combine fruits** (except for apples – see "Rule #2 below) **with non-fruits**.

I believe we should wait at least 30-60 minutes (depending on the quantity of the food & the metabolism of the person) before eating a "fruit" before or after eating a "non-fruit" (to ensure optimal digestion/absorption). For example: eating a couple of organic raw prunes may only require a 30 minute break before you start consuming your "non-fruits" (to avoid any interference with the digestion/absorption of these foods).

What is considered a "FRUIT" (enzymatically in your intestines)? I believe it is easier to understand this rule if everyone knows what is considered a "**FRUIT**" (enzymatically in your intestines). The only surprise to most is that: **TOMATO is considered a "FRUIT"** (enzymatically). Therefore, tomatoes should be eaten alone or with other "fruits" (to   ensure optimal digestion/absorption). Common food-combining *mistakes* with tomatoes include: Combining tomatoes with your vegetable salads or any other "non-fruits;" & drowning your "non-fruits" (like pasta & meats) with tomato sauce. These food combining mistakes may lead to digestive problems (including mal-absorption).

What is considered a "Non-Fruit" (enzymatically in your intestines)? This is also very simple. It includes seeds, nuts, legumes, vegetables, grains, & animal-based foods. The only surprise *to some* may be that the following are considered "**non-fruits**:"

- **Avocados, coconuts, olives, cucumbers, eggplant, peppers, & squash.**

- **Rule #2: is an exception to rule # 1. Apples are the ONLY fruit or food that can combine with fruits or non-fruits!**

Said otherwise, apples can be eaten with any food in the world – except melons (see below)! Considering apples' amazing unique food-combining property – as well the pectin, fiber, & hundreds of other healthful nutrients it contains – organic raw apples (not apple juice as it is predominantly sugar & lacking enzymes) are a "super-food!"

- **Rule #3: Eat melons alone or "leave them alone!"** Remember: melons include mangos, cantaloupes, Crenshaw melons, watermelon, honeydew, papaya, etc. Melons are considered enzymatic "snobs" of the food-combining world! After educating my friends & family, I would always ask them: "Now what is the only food in the world you can combine (eat with) watermelon?" The answer = only watermelon! The following humorous phrases may help you remember the above two rules: *Apples have a core & are a whore!* *Melons are snobs*! An apple "whore" will "combine" with anything! However, a melon snob (like the ones that live in Palm Beach, FL = "old money;" or Boca Raton, FL = "new money") will not associate (combine) with an "outside" whore! The mango snobs in Palm Beach, FL will only associate themselves with the mango Palm Beach snobs! I know this is low class & possibly insulting to those –but no harm intended! Just remember, the rules.

Sub-Rule: **When combining STARCHY "non-fruits"** (like carrots, potatoes, grains, lima beans & kidney beans) **with FAT or PROTEIN "non-fruits"** (like avocados, coconut, seeds, nuts, lentils, soybeans, & animal products): Adding NON-STARCHY vegetables will enhance the digestion/absorption of this combination.

The above is **NOT another rule**. However, the perfectionist (who strives to achieve optimal health & digestion) should be aware of this sub-rule (some may refer to this as "Rule #4").

EXCEPTIONS: Remember: quantity is important. Therefore, if you are going to break this commandment – do it very slightly. For example: if you are going to eat your organic vegetable salad (no tomatoes of course) with a home-made vinaigrette: the health benefits of having a couple drops of raw organic lemon as part of the vinaigrette probably outweigh the negatives. The negative would be a slight imperfection of absorption. However, if you added a whole lemon, tomato, or any fruit besides apple: the negatives (of mal-absorption) may outweigh the health positives! Again, "YOU ARE what you ABSORB!"

Final thoughts on these "10 Dietary Commandments"
Are you more or less confused? Remember: your brain's ability to learn is analogous to your digestive system's ability to digest/absorb the food you eat. If you try to learn too much, too quickly: you may get "intellectual indigestion." Go at your own pace. You have your life to achieve optimal health from your diet. We are ALL works in progress. We all fall short of the glory of God. However, now (at least) you are cognizant of (& hopefully understand) all the dietary rules (that I believe are the most superior dietary rules ever created). If you are still confused: don't worry. Worrying will not add a single second to your life (in fact: it is a SIN –as discussed in chapter 1– & can harm your health). Chapter 6 will list "super-cleansing foods/supplements" & chapter 7 will give you some examples of this diet in action from morning to night-time!

CHAPTER 6: "Super-*Cleansing* Foods/Supplements"

This chapter is written to bring everyone closer to God (& God's Love) & to help maximally cleanse (optimize the health of) our bodies, minds, & souls.

"What the peasant doesn't know - the peasant doesn't eat." (German proverb)   This is written here because many people do not consume many of the below-mentioned "super-cleansing foods & supplements" – because they are not cognizant of their powerful health benefits.

I. "Super-*Cleansing* Foods/Supplements"

Definition of a "Super-*Cleansing* Food/Supplement:" Any substance that may:
- Lower your "**_FULL OF IT_** Level of Disease, Obesity, &/or Chronic Pain!" &, therefore, directly or indirectly **CLEANSE** toxins from any part of your body. These "super-cleansing foods/supplements" may:
- **CLEANSE** your intestines of intestinal waste matter ("**IT**");
- **CLEANSE** your arteries of plaque &/or calcification ("**IT**");
- **CLEANSE** your brain, liver, kidneys, (or any other organ(s), body parts, or cells of your body) of bio-toxins – including, but not limited to, industrial pollutants & toxic heavy metals ("**IT**") – such as arsenic, mercury, aluminum, cadmium, & lead;
- **CLEANSE** your skin or any other part of your body of any & all physical toxins ("**IT**");
- **CLEANSE** your body of excess body fat ("**IT**");
- **CLEANSE** any &/or all your cells in your entire body of any &/or all free radicals ("**IT**");
- **CLEANSE** your body of inflammation to possibly **CLEANSE** your body of **chronic pain** – as well as **disease &/or obesity**;
- &/or Boost your immune system to help any &/or all cells in your body to **CLEANSE** anti-Godly free-radicals ("**IT**").

This definition applies in section II of this chapter when I refer to "**super cleansing: fats, proteins, carbs, fiber, teas, soy, milk, meats, shakes, & homeopathy.**"

Too often, society judges a food or supplement by the quantity of known *macronutrients* (vitamins, minerals, etc.) they contain.   However, it may be the powerfully healthful known (& currently unknown) **micro-nutrients** God put in His food to help us *cleanse our bodies* from harmful direct body toxins ("**IT**").

Are ALL Supplements SAFE?

If you believe ALL Supplements are 100% healthful & 0% harmful: "***YOU ARE FULL OF IT!***"

CAUTION: ALL of these foods & supplements have benefits.   However, they may also have negative side effects.   Remember: the term "natural" does NOT equal "Organic," beneficial, or SAFE!   The vitamin & herbal supplement industry generate tens of billions of dollars per year by selling products without warnings as to possible side effects &/or drug interactions. Researchers found that less than 6% of all over the counter herbal products contained an acceptable amount of safety information.[202]   Some of the **side effects from these foods &/or supplements** may only exist when they are:

- Consumed in excess;
- **COMBINED with other supplements or pharmaceuticals**;
- Consumed near surgery or trauma;
- Consumed by people who are allergic or sensitive to certain foods or supplements;
- &/or consumed when someone already has a disease that the supplement (or food) may worsen.

For example (as mentioned in "Dietary Commandment #6"): swallowing "natural" anticoagulant foods &/or supplements may increase the risk of bleeding when:

- Consumed in excess; Combined with other natural or pharmaceutical anticoagulants; Consumed near surgery or trauma; Consumed by people who are allergic or hypersensitive to them; &/or consumed by someone who already has a bleeding disorder.

Said differently, ***The Lamb of God shed His blood for ALL of us***. However, we currently shed our own blood (often hurting our own body = "*The Temple of the Holy Spirit*") by consuming an excess of natural anticoagulants!   This was analyzed thoroughly in "Dietary Commandment #6" (in Chapter 5).

Regarding excess: keep in mind your body needs a **dietary balance** between:

- **Acid versus alkaline forming** foods.   Eating an excess of foods (for a prolonged period of time that are "**Acid-Forming**" (such as alcohol, beans, cocoa, coffee, lentils, meat, cow's milk, oatmeal, organ meats, poultry, & prunes) can be harmful.[15]   In addition, consuming an excess of foods (for a prolonged period of time) that are "**Alkaline-Forming**" (such as avocados, fresh vegetables, raisins, & sprouts) can also be harmful.[15]   Here is that concept of balance again!
- Certain minerals like:
  - Sodium versus Potassium —especially important if one already has a kidney disorder;
  - Iron deficiency versus Excess Iron.   Iron deficiency may predispose you to iron-deficiency anemia (& possibly other bleeding disorders). Excess iron may predispose you to certain diseases of the liver, heart, pancreas, & the immune system![15]

- o & preventing bleeding versus preventing blood clots ("Dietary Commandment #6")!

This is why it is "vital" to see your physicians (or other health care professionals) & get certain **blood tests** - as well as having your **vital signs** measured on a regular basis – like:

- Percent oxygen saturation, heart rate, & blood pressure.
- Weight & Body Fat percentage.
- Feeling the strength of arterial pulses: behind knees (popliteal), inner aspect of ankles (posterior-tibial), & top of feet (dorsalis pedis). You may be able to do this on your own. Women are often better than men at this because women are trained at a young age to find things in their pocket books without seeing them!
- Capillary refill test of all ten toes. Again, your health care provider can show you how to do this.

You are paying your physician (as well as most health care professionals) to think. So ASK all the questions you should ask!

The U.S. FDA & "web MD" have recently developed a partnership in attempt to better inform the consumer of potential adverse effects of dietary supplements.[203] The law defines "dietary supplements" in part as:[203]

- Products taken by the mouth that contain a "dietary ingredient." "Dietary Ingredients" include:[203]
  - o *Vitamins, minerals, amino acids, & herbs or botanicals, as well as other supplements that can be used to supplement the diet. Dietary Supplements come in many forms including tablets, capsules, powders, energy bars, & liquids.*

"*YOU ARE FULL OF*" **Dietary Supplements – as well as Drugs (both OTC, prescribed, & illegal –shown in chapter 3)**! Not all dietary supplements "**ABSORB**" equally. If you believe that all dietary supplements are absorbed 100% - or equally in every person: "*YOU ARE FULL OF IT*!" Remember: if someone is "*FULL OF*" intestinal putrefaction, they will probably not absorb 100% of the dietary supplement – or the food they consume! Some dietary supplements (like those in powder or liquid form) may absorb better than others (like those in tablet form) for the general population. This may or may not – be remedied by emptying certain capsules into shakes (see part II of chapter 6 – as well as chapter 7).

As mentioned in the "10 Dietary Commandments," not all calories are created equally. This is why I do not believe in counting calories. As long as you are following all of the "10 Dietary Commandments," I do not believe you need to count any calories!

If you believe the **HEALTHFULNESS of all foods &/or supplements** are equal, then "*YOU ARE FULL OF IT*!" When you read or hear about research studies finding any food or supplement healthful or harmful, you should consider the following:

- How was it consumed: raw (alive) or cooked ("dead") with hydrogenated oils & trans-fats!?
- Was it 100% "USDA ORGANIC" or "**FULL OF**" pesticides, herbicides, artificial colors, flavors, sweeteners, & genetically modified organisms?
- Did the "subjects" consume it with healthful or harmful substances?
- In other words, did the "subjects" consume it following (or breaking) all of the "10 Dietary Commandments" shown in chapter 5?

For example: Raw organic pecans (washed with filtered water) – eaten alone or with other non-fruits – (in a peaceful state of mind & soul) are extremely healthful. Roasted non-organic pecans loaded with salt, sugar, & hydrogenated oils should be considered extremely harmful!

50% or more of American adults use dietary supplements on a regular basis, according to congressional testimony by the office of Dietary Supplements in the NIH (National Institute of Health).[203]   **My concern is that society has become so "Pro-supplements" that many patients are putting their health in harm's way by never asking their physician's opinion of combining these supplements (as well as OTC drugs) with their prescribed medications.** Your physician should be aware of ALL the supplements (& OTC drugs) you are taking!

If you see or hear of a dietary supplement that interests you (including one from my list of "Super-Cleansing Foods/Supplements") – write it down & do your research. "Buyer Beware" is the best practice. Go on the internet (such as www.webmd.com &/or www.wikipedia.org) for possible side effects & drug interactions.   The FDA suggests that you consult a Health Care Professional (such as your prescribing physician &/or pharmacist) before using any dietary supplement to determine if the supplement will be beneficial, ineffective, or worse dangerous![203]   Ultimately, the person most responsible for your health care = YOU!

As per the U.S. FDA:[203]
*It is not legal to market a dietary supplement product as a treatment or cure of a specific disease, or to alleviate the symptoms of a disease.   It is also illegal to advertise that they can **completely** prevent diseases.* However, it IS legal to advertise that some dietary supplements MAY be useful in *decreasing the risk* of certain diseases![203] Said differently: some "super-cleansing foods/dietary supplements" may reduce a person's "**FULL OF IT** Level of Disease(s), Obesity, &/or Chronic Pain!"   Taking a combination of supplements, using them with medications, &/or *substituting them in place of prescribed medications could lead to harmful – even life threatening results.*[203]

Federal law does not require dietary supplements to be proven safe to FDA's satisfaction _BEFORE_ they are marketed.[203]   In general, the FDA's role with dietary supplements begins _AFTER_ the product enters the marketplace.[203] Consumers & their Health Care Providers should contact the Dietary firm &/or the FDA (1-800-INFO-FDA or www.fda.gov/Safety/MedWatch/default.htm) with any serious or unexpected event associated with any dietary supplement!

Are "Natural" foods & dietary supplements SAFER than drugs?

Indubitably, YES!   Deaths in the U.S. from unintentional/accidental prescription drug poisoning (usually from accidental overdosing):[204]
- Has increased by 160% from 1999 to 2009.
- Has never been higher.
- & has become the number one cause of accidental deaths in the U.S. (over-coming motor vehicle accidents)!   On average 87 Americans die each day as a result of unintentional drug poisoning; another 2,277 are treated in emergency departments!   More than 60,000 young children are seen in emergency departments each year because they got into the medicines while their parents or caregivers were not looking!

According to the **2010** report of the American Association of Poison Control Centers (**AAPCC**), of the substances implicated in **fatal** poisonings in 2010: 84.6% were from pharmaceutical drugs, & only **0.8% came from (_ALL_) dietary supplements**.[205]

In the AAPCC's **2010** report, **zero deaths** were linked to _**vitamin & mineral supplements**_[205] - despite the fact that there were probably over 60 billion doses taken that year.[203]

Does the AAPCC's 2010 report prove that _ALL dietary supplements_ were 100% safe?   Indubitably, NO!
What the AAPCC's 2010 report failed to mention was whether (or not) these people with "_**drug-induced**_" _**fatalities**_ **also took dietary supplements**!?[205] Society – which includes our government departments - have a bias that all dietary supplements are healthful & safe.   This report simply used the phrase "_vitamin & mineral supplements_" _were linked to zero deaths in 2010_. It does **not** seem to include other forms of dietary supplements – such as "_**herbs/herbal medicines**_."

In addition, **the increased risk of death when certain dietary supplements are combined with pharmaceuticals is severely under-recognized**.   The increased risk of bleeding to death from combining "natural" & pharmaceutical anticoagulants is severely under-recognized (see "Dietary Commandment # 6" in chapter 5).   The AAPCC (in 2010) may blame bleeding fatalities on the pharmaceutical anticoagulants.   However, this bleeding fatality may have been due to the combination of the natural &

pharmaceutical anticoagulants (especially if one consumed an excess/"overdosed" on the natural &/or pharmaceutical anticoagulants).

Many supplements & foods can increase (& some can decrease) the effectiveness of the drug making it more dangerous.   Many supplements & foods can decrease the speed at which the liver breaks down the drug (keeping the drug in your "system" longer &, therefore, increasing the effectiveness & dangerous side effects of the drug).   Again: the AAPCC (in 2010) may blame the fatalities on the pharmaceuticals (without any recognition of any dangerous interactions that person may have received from the combination of the drug with the dietary supplement(s) or food(s)!

In addition, taking **dietary supplements near trauma or surgery may dangerously increase the risk of death**.   Some supplements (like Kava Kava & Valerian) may increase the sedative effects of pharmaceutical anesthetics &, therefore, increase the risk of coma – or even death – (when taken near the time of surgery).[120]   This death would probably be blamed on "the surgery" or the "anesthesia."   As mentioned in "Dietary Commandment #6:" The increased risk of bleeding (possibly to death) from consuming "natural" anticoagulants taken near the time of surgery or trauma is severely under-recognized!   These hemorrhagic deaths are not reported in the AAPCC's report because it is not considered a "poisoning."   These hemorrhagic deaths are usually blamed on (counted as) the surgery or trauma (without any recognition or knowledge of whether the deceased was taking natural anticoagulants or any other dietary supplements)!

Lastly: the absence of death (or even disease) – does not equal "optimal health!"   This same study found that "**vitamins**" were the substance category with **the 6th greatest rate of poison exposure <u>increase</u>** in the U.S.A.![205] In addition, "**Food/Food Products Poisoning**" & "**Food-Drug Interactions**" were reported in this report.[205]

I am always cautious to educate any friend or family about the existence of a "super-cleansing food/supplement."   *Most* of these "super-foods/supplements" should be eaten in moderation & cycled (perhaps every other day, etc.).   Like exercise: most people benefit from "rotating" different "super-cleansing foods/supplements" on a daily basis.   Cycling or rotating different super-cleansing foods/supplements on a daily basis may offer the following benefits:
-    May not create allergy reactions to these foods/supplements.
-    May benefit from the different nutrients in these foods/supplements.

Some people believe some of these foods would benefit them most when eaten every single day.   Any education as to frequency & duration (or which phase to consume) of any food or supplement is based on adults & is only educational (& not a recommendation).   Chapter 5 gave many examples of what foods are eaten in the "Cleansing Phase" versus "The Lifestyle Phase." Any health care advice (regarding putting or stopping to put things in your mouth) should be given by your qualified health care professional (such as your physician(s)).

In the end, you are the person most responsible for your health!

1.   **Probiotics** – live microorganisms that are beneficial –in fact, ESSENTIAL to LIVE & THRIVE!

I define the term "Probiotics" as:
- Live microorganisms that are benefit our intestinal microbial balance;
- & consumed as dietary supplements or as fermented foods (with specially added active LIVE cultures).

The amazing benefits of probiotics are severely under-recognized in society. The amazing benefits of probiotics (I believe) has a lot to do with its' relationship with **Menaquinone-7** (AKA "MK-7" = a type of **vitamin K2**).   All types of vitamin K have a coagulation effect.   Thus, all types of vitamin K may act to save your life from bleeding to death.   **However, vitamin K1 & K2 may be considered "God-made" & vitamins K3, 4, & 5 are "man-made" (synthetic).**   This will be discussed in "vitamin K2" ("super-cleansing food/supplement # 2").   **A type of Vitamin K2** ("MK-7") "produced" by probiotics in our intestines (the probiotics in our intestines *convert vitamin K1 to Menaquinone-7 – a type of vitamin K2*) & is found highest in natto – a probiotic food source.

The number one reason (I believe) God wants us to consume probiotics = **to stop, prevent, & save your life from bleeding (as well as anemia)**!   Said differently: Consuming Probiotics have shown to lower our "*FULL OF IT* **Level of**" bleeding &/or anemia!   The dietary intake of an umbrella of probiotics has shown to:
- Possibly **save your life from bleeding to death** in the ICU;[206]
- **Decrease rectal bleeding & ulcerative colitis**;[82,207,208]
- **Improve wound healing** – especially intestinal wound healing – decreasing GI bleeds;[209]
- **Decrease bleeding gums**;[210,211]
- **Suppress the helicobacter pylori** (the harmful bacteria believed to cause GI ulcers).[211]
- **Decrease intestinal mucosal injury** caused by hemorrhagic shock.[212]   Thus, probiotics may be helpful before & after surgery. Again, ask your surgeon's opinion about this.
- **Possibly prevent &/or treat anemia** as probiotic levels been found to be directly related to iron absorption.[213]   Probiotics also assist with the manufacture of vitamins B6, B12, & folic acid.[49,214]

217

Perhaps the best evidence that **preventing bleeding is the #1 purpose of probiotics in a human's life** is supported by the Committee on Nutrition of the American Academy of Pediatrics.[215]   As a result of the occurrences of vitamin K deficiency bleeding (which can be severe, leading to hospitalizations, blood transfusions, & death!), this Committee has recommended that 0.5 to 1.0 mg (500-1,000 mcg) of vitamin K1 be administered to all newborns shortly after birth.[215]   This vitamin K deficiency bleeding is mostly due to the sterility/*lack of probiotics in the guts of the newborns*.[215]   In addition, human milk appears to contain a low amount of vitamin K1 - & a **relatively much lower amount of vitamin K2**.[215]

The 2nd reason (I believe) God wants us to consume probiotics = to **help prevent atherosclerotic risk by decreasing the LDL/HDL & total cholesterol/HDL ratio levels** in patients with high & normal cholesterol levels.[89]   Lowering these ratios have shown to be extremely important in lowering our "***FULL OF IT* Level of" Atherosclerosis**![98,99]   Vitamin K2 ("produced" by probiotics in our intestines & found in natto- a probiotic food source) intake & levels are associated with **reduced risk of coronary heart disease, all-cause mortality, & severe aortic calcification**![85]   Thus, dietary intake of probiotics (or vitamin K2) can **reduce the risk of the aortic calcification side effect of certain pharmaceutical (vitamin K antagonist) anticoagulants**![85,86]   By preventing unstable/vulnerable atherosclerotic plaque (which can become an arterial blood clot),[216] probiotics (&/or vitamin K2) can ***indirectly*** prevent arterial blood clots!

This makes probiotics (& vitamin K2) so unique!   Probiotics (& vitamin K2) do NOT have anticoagulant properties (they do not directly interfere with the coagulation process).   In fact (as mentioned previously) their #1 purpose in our lives is to save us from bleeding!   Probiotics (& vitamin K2) reduce the risk of atherosclerosis and, therefore, *indirectly* reduce the risk of arterial blood clots (from unstable/vulnerable atherosclerotic plaque)!   This is why consuming probiotics (via supplements &/or food sources) is so important in creating an optimal balance between preventing bleeding & preventing blood clots (fulfilling "Dietary Commandment #6").

Sauerkraut (a probiotic food source) is high in the antioxidant enzyme S.O.D. – which may also help prevent atherosclerosis by **reducing the risk of LDL oxidation** (one of the most respected theories of atherosclerotic causes).[15,49,217]

Therefore, the 3rd reason why (I believe) God wants us to consume probiotics = **to help the gastrointestinal & immune systems - & prevent cancer**.   Probiotics (due to its' ability to "produce" vitamin K2 – convert K1 to K2) may decrease the risk of (& possibly help patients with):

218

- **Leukemia;**[218] **Liver cancer;**[219] **& Vitamin K-deficiency bleeding** that a startling 78% of patients with **advanced cancer** are prone to.[220]

Dietary intake of probiotics can help:
- **Bowel regularity;**[49,82,221]
- **Boost your immune system** by preventing pathogenic microorganisms from attacking the body;[49,82,221]
- **Prevent & treat bloating, gas, & diarrhea;**[49,82,222]
- & possibly **prevent inflammatory bowel disease.**[49,82,221,222]   Your gut & the probiotic organisms that live there may comprise over 80% of your immune system.[49]   Probiotics may possess anti-inflammatory & pathogen protection beyond the gastrointestinal tract.[49]   Dietary intake of probiotics (either via its' fermented/cultured food sources or supplementation) is also considered one of the best ways to **detox pesticides & other toxins from your body.**[8]   By ensuring your gut bacteria is in good health, your body is better able to combat invaders like the toxic pesticide chemicals (including the Bt-Toxin found in GMO crops)![23]

However, the European Food Safety Authority (EFSA) has so far rejected 260 claims on many of these potential benefits.[223]   This rejection by the EFSA supports my hypothesis that that reducing the risk of bleeding (&/or anemia) & atherosclerosis are the number one & two, respectively, reasons why God wants us to consume probiotics!

The 4th reason why (I believe) God wants us to consume probiotics = **to help reduce fracture risk, stop & reverse bone loss.**[224]   Dietary intake of natto (a probiotic food source) has shown to (via increasing circulating Menaquinone-7 or "MK7" – a type of vitamin K2) cause significant elevations of serum & -carboxylated **osteocalcin** concentration, a **biomarker of bone formation!**[224]   MK-7 (a type of Vitamin K2 found in natto & "produced" by the probiotics in our intestines) takes the calcium out of our arterial walls & puts in our bones! This is discussed further in "vitamin K2" ("super-cleansing food/supplement" # 2).

By seeing all of the abovementioned benefits of probiotics it is no wonder why the word "probiotic" comes from the Latin word: pro (**"for"**) & the Greek word bios (**"life"**)! If you want to live (& thrive): consume probiotics!

Quantity, Frequency, & Which Phase(s): The "daily value" of **probiotic supplements** has not been established. In my opinion, the best types of **probiotic supplements** should be ORGANIC:
- **Non-Cow's Milk** source.
- A probiotic **blend of over 1 billion active** (or live) **Lactobacilli** (the most prevalent beneficial bacteria in the small intestines) & **Bifidobacteria** (the most prevalent beneficial bacteria in the large intestines) cells per capsule or cup. It has been suggested that adults take 1-2 billion live cells/day of probiotics to treat or prevent uncomplicated diarrhea.[120, 222] However, it has been suggested that adults should consume 60-180 billion live probiotic cells/day to reduce the risk of atherosclerosis.[49]

- Most adults would benefit from **1 billion active** (or live) cells of **Saccharomyces *boulardii*** - a unique strain of probiotic derived from yeast that may survive stomach acid (possibly superior to other strains) to nourish the intestines.   This strain may possess "**prebiotic**" (see below) properties& may be the most beneficial probiotic strain to consume after finishing prescription antibiotics.[49]
- Some may benefit from a probiotic supplement that also contains **Inulin or FOS** (Fructooligosaccharides – which can be produced by degradation of inulin).[82] **Inulin & FOS are "prebiotics"** – meaning that they are scientifically proven to increase the activity of the beneficial bacteria as well as help prevent the growth of harmful bacteria in the digestive tract.[82]   **Inulin & FOS** – present in common fruits & vegetables (such as artichokes, asparagus, oat bran, oatmeal, & raisins) – are *good sources of natural soluble dietary fiber*, & fine for diabetics because they do not increase the glucose or insulin in the blood.[82]   However (as mentioned in "Dietary Commandment # 8"), consuming an excess of *instant oatmeal (not from rolled oats)* can create a **harmful** "**High Glycemic Load Meal**."[177-179]   This is mentioned to distinguish the dramatic difference between consuming a large bowl of instant oatmeal versus a probiotic supplement containing Inulin & FOS (that may have been derived from oatmeal or oat bran).

If the probiotic supplement is considered 100% alive (usually require storing in the fridge & does not include inulin or FOS or any "dead" ingredients): it ***can be consumed in both phases***.

Cautions of Probiotic supplements:
- ***Infants & children under 3 should NOT use*** over-the-counter commercial probiotic preparations unless directed by a physician.[120]
- Stupor with EEG-slowing has been reported with high oral doses in adult patients with the ***liver disease hepatic encephalopathy***.[120]
- & an ***excess of healthy bowel movements*** (sometimes ten times per day) & ***loss of their waist sizes/bellies*** (many consider this a huge positive – but it is still overwhelming for many)!   This is the most common complaint I have heard from my "friends & family" taking probiotic supplements.   This is probably because these people are "***FULL OF***" so much intestinal putrefaction ("***IT***") that gets "eliminated/pushed-out" by the probiotics. These people usually benefit from skipping days in between taking the probiotics.   The consumption of *large quantities of Inulin or FOS* (or even 1 gram of FOS – in particular by sensitive or unaccustomed individuals) can lead to *gaseous discomfort*![82]   However, these people may not get this side effect when ingesting the FOS (1 gram or less per day) in a probiotic food supplement (which may help eliminate the gaseous discomfort)![82]
- If ***you are taking warfarin*** (or other vitamin K antagonists), you should discuss consuming natto (a probiotic food source high in **vitamin K2**) &/or green leafy vegetables (high in vitamin K1) with your physician as **all forms of vitamin K can decrease the effect of warfarin** (& other vitamin K antagonist anticoagulants) – lowering the INR.[225]   Experts[226,227] now advise that **patients on warfarin should consume a *CONSISTENT* amount of vitamin K1 &/or K2** so they can better monitor the effectiveness of the warfarin.

Based on the abovementioned "Cautions," the natural Probiotic food sources *may* be considered the best. The **most healthful probiotic (cultured/fermented) food sources** include ORGANIC:

- *"Cultured Coconut milk"* –best to wait until the *"Lifestyle Phase."*
- *Kombucha* – can be consumed in *any phase*.
- *Low Sodium vegetables* such as: sauerkraut, pickled beets, carrots, & cucumbers (AKA "pickles") – may be consumed any phase.
- *Soybeans* such as natto (the best in my opinion), doenjang, & tempeh – best to wait until the *"Lifestyle Phase."*
- *Goat's milk sources* such as: probiotic goat's milk; buttermilk; kefir; & yogurt (no fruit added - except apple of course). Probably best for most people to wait until the "Lifestyle Phase" (& avoid in the "Cleansing Phase"). These probiotic goat's milk sources are considered "super-cleansing milk" & are discussed in section II of this chapter.

All of the abovementioned probiotic food sources may be considered the #1 "super-foods" in the world! They are all much easier to digest than their non-fermented/uncultured food sources.[1,78] However, most of these food sources *never disclose to the consumer the QUANTITY of probiotics contained (per serving) in them*! This is a huge negative to most probiotics' food sources. Imagine your boss tells you that you will get paid every 2 weeks & your pay-check will "contain money" – without specifying the exact dollar amount!

Additional growth of probiotics is encouraged by:[82]
- Vitamin C; Pectin; & roughage/fiber – especially Inulin & FOS sources (mentioned earlier).

This is important since friendly bacteria can die within five days unless they are continuously supplied.[82]

Conversely, the numbers of healthy bacteria **(probiotics) in the digestive tract can be diminished by factors such as**:[49,82]
- Poor diet; Travel; Illness; *Stress***;* & the use of antibiotics. Many nutritionists (& even physicians) recommend their patients consume probiotics (often via yogurt) one hour before or after the antibiotics to help "replenish" the probiotics killed in the intestines by the antibiotics. Remember (from Chapter 3): Americans unintentionally consume **pharmaceutical antibiotics (found in our drinking water, non-organic animal products,** etc.)!

***The above justifies why this book – learning how to maximally *cleanse your body, mind, & soul* - is so important in achieving optimal health! ☺

2. Vitamin K2 (Menaquinones) = the supplement of 2023!

Society is very aware of the ability of vitamin K1 (phylloquinones – found in mostly green leafy vegetables) to prevent &/or stop bleeding.[225-227] However, vitamin K2 (like all types of vitamin K) also prevents &/or stops bleeding. In addition, vitamin K2 has a whole host of other benefits making it superior to vitamin K1 (& making it a "super-cleansing food & supplement").

As mentioned previously (in "probiotics"), the amazing benefits of vitamin K2 are severely under-recognized.   Vitamin K2 (like probiotics - due to probiotics' ability to convert K1 to K2 in the intestines) has been found to lower the "*FULL OF IT* Levels of:"
- *Arterial calcification, atherosclerosis, all-cause mortality;*[85,86]
- **Leukemia,**[218] **Liver Cancer,**[219] **Bleeding**[220] (&/or **anemia**), & **Osteoporosis/bone loss,** & even **aging** (see below)!

One may say that vitamin K2 takes the calcium out of:[85,86,228-230]
- The arteries' the inner lining – or "intima" –where atherosclerotic plaque accrues;
- The arteries' middle smooth muscle layer;
- & the heart valves (especially the aortic valve – which can cause aortic stenosis).

Vitamin K2 appears to "put" this calcium into the bones (& teeth) where it belongs![224]   "*Vitamin K2* appears to be the most important factor in *steering calcium into the bone & away from heart valves & the arterial system*."[228]   By preventing pathological tissue calcification, vitamin K2 may confer *anti-aging effects throughout the body*.[228]

Remember: the level of vitamin K2 (Menaquinones) in your body *may* be increased by consuming probiotic food sources.[15,215,224]   Probiotics in your intestines convert vitamin K1 to menaquinone-7 (a type of vitamin K2).[15,215,224] Consuming probiotics may, therefore, increase your body's level of menaquinones.[15,215,224]   This is why "probiotics" are considered the #1 "super-cleansing food/supplement."

Vitamin K2 (AKA "*The Elusive X-Factor*") is superior & more healthful than vitamin K1 (phylloquinone –found in mostly green vegetables) due to the following 3 facts:[231]
- Fact # one: **Superior absorption**. Humans appear to have a finite ability to absorb vitamin K1 from plant foods. Humans may NOT possess the ability to absorb much more than 200 micrograms of vitamin K1 per day from vegetables.   Whereas the absorption of vitamin K2 from natto is nearly 100%, the absorption of vitamin K1 from servings of green vegetables may only be about 10-15%. Our absorption of vitamin K1 declines as the amount we consume & supports the interpretation that we might only be able to absorb about 200 micrograms of vitamin K1 per day.
- Fact # two: **Intake of vitamin K2 is inversely associated with atherosclerosis in humans, while intake of vitamin K1 is NOT!**[85]
- Fact # three: **Vitamin K2 (Menaquinone-7) may be at least 3 times more effective than vitamin K1 at activating proteins related to skeletal metabolism.**   In fact, one large multicenter randomized placebo-controlled trial showed that heavy doses of supplemental vitamin K1 had no effect on bone density of post-menopausal women with osteopenia![232]   Daily intake of **Menaquinone-4 (**AKA "MK4" – the other major type of vitamin K2) has been

approved by the Ministry of Health in Japan since 1995 for the treatment & prevention of osteoporosis. Other studies have shown that daily intake of Menaquinone-7 (AKA "MK7" – a type of vitamin K2 found especially high in Natto) has: reduced fracture risk, prevent, & reversed bone loss.[224,233]

Keep in mind: the vital benefits of **saving our lives from bleeding have been found by dietary intake of either vitamin K1 or K2 (&/or their food sources)**![120,215,220] In addition, there is no known toxicity (&, therefore no "tolerable upper intake level = "UL" has been set) associated with high doses of phylloquinone (vitamin K1) or menaquinone (vitamin K2) forms of vitamin K.[234] Very high doses of vitamin K2 (or probiotics) have never shown to increase the risk of blood clots.[235] In summary: probiotics, vitamin K2, & K1 protect you from bleeding – but do NOT increase your risk of blood clots! In fact, probiotics & vitamin K2 (unlike vitamin K1) actually decrease the risk of atherosclerosis &, therefore, indirectly decrease the risk of arterial blood clots!

As mentioned previously: Experts[226,227] now advise that **patients on warfarin _SHOULD_ eat a consistent amount of vitamin K1 or K2** so they can better monitor the effectiveness of the warfarin (measured via the PT/INR blood tests). Considering the abovementioned superiority of MK-7 (over vitamin K1), it seems obvious *these patients would be better off consuming a consistent amount of MK-7 (such as 100mcg/day - via a supplement)*!

Remember: Vitamins K3, 4, & 5 are not recommended for my "friends or family" as they are synthetic ("man-made") & have all shown toxicity.[15]

Quantity, Frequency, & Which Phase(s): The RDA for vitamin K1 & K2 combined is 65 micrograms per day for adult females & 80 micrograms per day for adult males.[228] Consuming **100 micrograms per day of the MK-7** form of vitamin K2 can provide greater benefits than higher potencies of other forms of vitamin K1 & K2.[228] The **MK-7 form** of vitamin K2 *remains in bloodstream longer* than other forms of vitamin K - & **reaches levels 7-8 times higher**.[228] **100 Micrograms of MK-7** can be taken as a **supplement every day after the "Cleansing Phase" (during the "Lifestyle Phase").**

Sources: MK4 is found in meat (especially goose livers), eggs, & dairy products.[231,236] MK7 is converted from Vitamin K1 by probiotics in the intestines[15,215,224] & is found in probiotic food sources (extremely high in natto).[215,224] However, probiotic-derived menaquinones (MK7) appear to contribute minimally to overall vitamin K status in ADULTS (especially the elderly)![114] This probably has to do with the S.A.D. (Standard American Diet) of adults not consuming enough healthful greens & probiotic food sources (or probiotic supplements)! Vitamin K2 is found in the following foods (from highest to lowest) – which should be ORGANIC:[231,236]

- **Natto**: 100 grams contain <u>1,103 micrograms</u> of vitamin K2 (**100% as MK-7**)! May eat 3-4 days per week (if you can find it) <u>during</u> the "Lifestyle Phase."
- **Goose Liver paste** (pate): 100 grams contains <u>369 micrograms</u> of vitamin K2 (**100% as MK4**).   May be eaten during the "Lifestyle Phase" a gram per day amount ***ONLY if you have a diagnosis of anemia & are low in iron*** (confirmed & approved by your physician)! ☺   Goose liver extract (Organically raised) contains all the elements needed for red blood cell production.[15]   This is discussed in "super-cleansing meats" later on in this chapter.   The debate as to whether or not one's personal serum cholesterol will be raised by consuming foods high in cholesterol is discussed later in this chapter (under "super-cleansing fats" in section II of this chapter).
- **Goat Cheese**: 100 grams contains <u>56.5 micrograms</u> of vitamin K2 (6.5% as MK4 & **93.5% as MK7**).   May be eaten during the "Lifestyle Phase" in moderation – possibly 2 tablespoons per week or less.
- **Goose Leg**: 100 grams contains the highest animal "meat" (flesh) source of <u>31 micrograms</u> of vitamin K2 (**100% as MK4**). This "super-cleansing meat" may be eaten in moderation (2 meals per month – if you can find free-range goose) during the "Lifestyle Phase."   "Super-Cleansing Meats" are discussed further in section II of this chapter.
- **Goat's milk butter or egg yolk** (in the U.S.A.): 100 grams contain approximately <u>15 micrograms</u> of vitamin K2 (**100% as MK4**).   May be eaten during the "Lifestyle Phase" in moderation (possibly 3 eggs/week or less). Eggs should be eaten soft boiled so that the yolk is liquid & orange. However, those more concerned about neurological diseases may benefit from more than 3 eggs per week (possibly due to the phosphatidyl choline, lecithin, B vitamins, or other nutrients eggs possess).
- **Chicken or beef**: 100 grams contain slightly more than <u>8 micrograms</u> of vitamin K2 (**100% as MK4**).   Adults may benefit from consuming free-range chicken 3 meals per week & beef 2 meals per month during the "Cleansing Phase."   However, if diagnosed with iron-deficiency anemia – adults may benefit from consuming these "super-cleansing meats" on a daily basis to replenish the iron lost.[15]   These "super-cleansing meats" are discussed further in section II of this chapter.

In summary (of frequency, duration, & phase): most American adults (due to the difficulty finding natto & society's fears –either rational or irrational over the consumption of high cholesterol foods) would benefit from a **menaquinone-7 supplement of 100 micrograms per day (usually derived from natto)**. **MK-7 *may* be considered the superior form** of vitamin K as the MK-7 form remains in the bloodstream longer & reaches levels **7-8 times higher**![228]

Cautions for vitamin K2 (as well as vitamin K1):
- *If you are taking warfarin*, you should always discuss consuming any type/source of vitamin K with your physician as all forms of vitamin K (K1, K2, etc.) can decrease the effective of warfarin (& any other vitamin K antagonistic anticoagulants) – lowering the INR.[225] As mentioned in "probiotics," **experts now advise that patients on warfarin SHOULD consume a *CONSISTENT***

<u>amount of vitamin K2 &/or K1</u> (from their food sources &/or supplements) so they can better monitor the effectiveness of the warfarin (measured via the PT/INR blood tests).[226,227]

- *If you are taking pharmaceutical Antibiotics*: this can produce vitamin K deficiency bleeding either because:
    - Pharmaceutical Antibiotics (a "vitamin K antagonist"[113,114] mentioned in "Dietary Commandment #6" in Chapter 5) can reduce the "production" of MK7 by intestinal probiotics (by nearly 74%).[237]
    - Or pharmaceutical antibiotics may also inhibit the enzyme within the human body that recycles vitamin K.[231]

Remember: Americans unintentionally consume pharmaceutical antibiotics (found in our unfiltered drinking & bathing water, non-organic animal products, etc.) which *may* increase the risk of this vitamin K deficiency (which can cause bleeding & harm our health in other ways - as discussed above).

3. Vitamin C

The 1st reason (I believe) God wants adults to consume vitamin C (either from food sources or via a supplement discussed later) = **to help PREVENT bleeding (&/or anemia)**.[15,82,120]   Vitamin C (unlike probiotics or vitamin K) will <u>NOT STOP</u> the bleeding if you are **currently** bleeding.   Dietary intake of **vitamin C** may:[15,02,120]

- **Help wound healing** (especially important after surgery);
- **& strengthen the walls of the blood vessels & capillaries to PREVENT blood from leaking out of them.**   Remember: bruising is usually a warning sign that your blood may be too thin or your blood vessel walls may be too weak. Thus, vitamin C works to prevent future bleeds.[15,82,120]
- Help **prevent &/or treat anemia** (like probiotics) because vitamin C **increases iron absorption**.[82,120]

As mentioned in super-cleansing food #1, vitamin C encourages the growth of healthy intestinal flora (probiotics)![82]

The 2nd reason (I believe) God wants adults to consume vitamin C = **to help reduce the risk of atherosclerosis** (&, therefore, indirectly help prevent arterial blood clots).[120]   Dietary intake of Vitamin C:

- **May decrease arterial stiffness in patients with diabetes.**[238]
- Acts as an **antioxidant** in vessels & **inhibit the inflammatory process –** **reducing LDL oxidation**.[120]   It prevents certain white blood cells from absorbing LDL & is, therefore, a *first-line defense against atherosclerosis*.[7]
- Is correlated with a **decreased risk of cardiovascular disease, ischemic heart disease, & increased life expectancy**.[239]
- Helps to **synthesize carnitine**[240] – needed to transport fatty acids into mitochondria during the break down of lipids (fats) for the generation of metabolic energy.[105-107]   Vitamin C's synthesis of carnitine may, therefore, be helpful for patients with **congestive heart failure, high triglycerides, & recovery from a heart attack**![1,105-107]
- May protect against atherosclerosis when **one has high cholesterol** levels.[82]

225

- Is believed by some nutritionists[82] to lower the incidence of blood clots in the veins!
- Prevent atherosclerosis via its' natural **chelation effect**.[45] This **chelation effect** (as mentioned in "Dietary Commandment #5") **may remove toxic heavy metals from the body**[43] – lowering your *"FULL OF IT* Level of Diseases" – especially cardiovascular, neurological, & immune-related diseases**.[15,45-47]
- **Cleanse the liver** – as <u>lemons & limes</u> (good vitamin C sources) are considered some of the best liver-cleansing foods (which may indirectly help decrease your risk of atherosclerosis – as well as help your overall body detoxify).[90]
- **Helps with allergies & <u>chronic pain</u>** as it *decreases the amount of histamine released with allergies & chronic pain (high histamine = more pain; less histamine = less pain)!*[7]

The 3rd reason (I believe) God wants adults to consume vitamin C (as mentioned above & earlier in chapter 5) = to **cleanse your entire body from toxins**! Vitamin C has been found to lower lead blood levels & reverse some of the oxidative damage caused by lead.[241] **When combined with vitamin E**, vitamin C has been found to reduce neonatal brain tissue damage from **arsenic** in one study of rats.[242] Vitamin C's natural chelation effect can help the immune, neurological, & cardiovascular systems – as well as the rest of the body.[15,45-47] Lemons & limes (good vitamin C sources) can help cleanse the liver – to help your overall body detoxify.[90]

Quantity, Frequency, & Which Phase(s): **Buffered or Acid-Free Vitamin C 500 mg supplement two to times daily with food** (**during the "Lifestyle Phase**") may be the optimal dosage for most adults. An acid-free or buffered form is considered the best so as to not create any acid reflux, heartburn, or other gastrointestinal problems.[15] As humans & primates do not produce our own vitamin C, other nutritional experts suggest 500 mg (of buffered or acid free form) 4 times daily with food.[7]
For adults with the rare (in the U.S.A.) bleeding disease scurvy (due to a vitamin C deficiency), the AMA recommends:[120]
- 100mg 3x/day for 1 week – then 100mg/day for several weeks until tissue saturation is normal.

The recommended dosage (for adults) for wound healing is 1,000mg to 1,500mg/day![120]
The recommended dosage of vitamin C for adults to prevent atherosclerosis is 45mg to 1,000 mg/day.[120]

As mentioned in "Dietary Commandment # 7," vitamin C should be combined with vitamin E for increased synergistic antioxidant benefits:[7,15,242]
- ***Vitamin C is water soluble***, *working both in the intracellular & extracellular water-soluble places.*[7]
- ***Vitamin E is a fat soluble antioxidant***, *acting in the fatty or lipid places of your body.*[7] *Estimates are that 69-93% of adults do not even get the recommended daily intake of vitamin E, let alone the antioxidant level that may be desired.*[7] *Vitamin E allows us to exercise as it neutralizes the increase in free radicals when we breathe heavier.*[7] *D-alpha-tocopherol is considered*

226

the best/most natural source (dl-alpha-tocopherol is synthetic – man made).[7,15] However, the combined antioxidant activity from a variety of fruits & vegetables might still provide the best antioxidant required to prevent disease. In addition (as mentioned in "Dietary Commandment # 6"), vitamin E has anticoagulant properties.[15,82,110,120]   60 to 200 I.U. of supplemental vitamin E daily may be safe (may prevent blood clots & not increase the risk of bleeding) for most individuals.[15,82,110,120]   However, 200 I.U. (or more) of vitamin E may increase the risk of bleeding[15,82,110,120] for people:

- o   Taking other natural or pharmaceutical anticoagulants;
- o   Undergoing surgery or near trauma;
- o   &/or who already have a bleeding disorder/disease.

As mentioned in "Dietary Commandment #6," vitamin C should be taken with vitamin E to also greatly reduce this bleeding risk of vitamin E!

Some of the highest *common* healthy **food sources of vitamin C** (from highest to lowest all containing 50mg or more of vitamin C per 100grams) include ORGANIC, raw (if edible):[243]

- **Acerola cherries; Green Chili pepper+++; Guava; Red pepper; Red Chili pepper+++; Parsley; Kiwifruit; Broccoli; Brussels sprouts; Wolfberry (Gogi); Lychee; Papaya+++; Strawberry; & Orange.**   If these foods are 100% alive/raw & organic: they can be eaten in both phases.   Many of these **foods +++** are also good natural sources of **vitamin E.**   Other foods high in vitamin E that may be combined (with foods high in vitamin C) for optimal synergistic antioxidant effect include sunflower seeds, almonds, asparagus, spinach, Swiss chard & leafy greens (Like turnip greens, mustard greens, & collard greens).[74]

The negatives to some of these natural food sources (of vitamin C) is that some people may have gastrointestinal difficulty with the acidity or "spiciness" of *some* of these food sources.   This is why many adults may prefer 500mg of the buffered or acid-free supplement version of vitamin C twice daily with food (after the "Cleansing Phase").   However, 60mg of vitamin C in food (1/2 cup of broccoli) quenches about as many free radicals as 900 mg in supplement, because of the additive effect of all the other healthful macro & micronutrients! [7]

You may need extra vitamin C if you:[82] Live in a city (as carbon monoxide destroys vitamin C); Are on "the pill;" Take aspirin (which triples the excretion rate of vitamin C – predisposing you to an even greater risk of bleeding); Consume lots of sugar &/or have high blood sugar levels; [244] &/or want to reduce *the duration* of the common cold.[245]

4.   "Super-Green Vegetables"

"And to everything that moves on the earth which __has LIFE__, I have given every __GREEN plant__ for food." (Gen 1:29-30)

Most dark green leafy vegetables contain one of God's most powerful antioxidant enzymes: **Superoxide Dismutase (S.O.D.).**   **S.O.D.** (found highest in **_wheatgrass & barley grass_** – as well as *sauerkraut & most dark green leafy vegetables*) may:[15]

- Reduce inflammation; Decrease oxidative stress; &, therefore, decrease the risk of atherosclerosis (as well as boost the immune system & decrease the risk of all diseases)!

Wheatgrass, barley grass, chlorella, & spirulina are all dietary sources of **Chlorophyll**.[15] In experiments with anemic animals, blood counts returned to normal after 4-5 days of receiving **chlorophyll** (whose molecular structure resembles that of hemoglobin)![15]

Greens (especially when freshly juiced) **help neutralize acid buildup in the blood** from a typical Western diet (high in acidic-forming foods such as meats, dairy, & grains).[1,15,82]

Cautions to most, if not all green vegetables: When taking *pharmaceutical vitamin-K antagonist anticoagulants* (like warfarin), you should definitely consult your physician as these green vegetables high in vitamin K1 may interfere with warfarin's effectiveness.[225] However (as mentioned earlier in "Vitamin K2"), **experts now advise that people on warfarin should consume a CONSISTENT amount of vitamin K1 &/or K2 (from the food sources &/or supplements**) so they can better monitor the effectiveness of the warfarin (measured via the PT/INR blood tests).[225-227]

4a. **Wheatgrass** (Organic & raw) **Juice = *"God's chemotherapy"*** (drink within 30 minutes after juicing with a wheatgrass juicer)
Organic wheatgrass juice is a rich nutritional food that was popularized by the late Ann Wigmore, an educator & founder of "Hippocrates Institute" in Boston (as well as West Palm Beach, FL & other places).[15] It is a good source of vitamin K1, iron, S.O.D., & chlorophyll.[15]
Quantity, Frequency, & Which Phase(s): An ounce of prevention is worth a pound of cure! Therefore, I drink an **ounce or more (EVERY DAY in BOTH PHASEs**) of raw organic wheatgrass juice – within 30 minutes after juicing it with a wheatgrass juicer.

4b. **Cilantro** – Organic & raw (AKA "**Coriander leaves**," or "**Chinese Parsley**")
100 grams (3.5 ounces) of cilantro contains:[246]
- 388% of the U.S. RDA for vitamin K1; 3 grams of dietary fiber; 45% of the U.S. RDA for vitamin C; & 16% of the U.S. RDA for iron.

Cilantro is also considered to possess the following properties:[246]
- Moderately high "anti-inflammatory;"
- Extremely healthful (very high in antioxidants) – given a "5 out of 5 stars" for "optimum health;"
- & an extremely high "fullness factor (satiating effect)" – given a "5 out of 5 stars" for their capacity to produce "weight loss!"

Cilantro is also considered to possess the **most powerful "chelation" properties** (of all the foods) in the world to effectively bind & *remove mercury, lead, aluminum, & other toxic heavy metals* from our nervous system (& perhaps other parts of our body).[49,84] Cilantro is also considered to possess the most powerful chelation properties (of all the foods in the world) to *remove bacterial infections* – as the infectious organisms use the metal toxins to protect themselves from antibiotics![84]   Cilantro's powerful chelation properties (as well as its' antioxidant, anti-inflammatory, & weight loss capabilities) may make it the most important food in the world to decrease the risk of atherosclerosis,[217] neurological diseases, & cancer (as well as boosting the immune system)![15,45,49,84]

Quantity, Frequency, & Which Phase(s): Adults may benefit from **juicing at least an ounce a week** (may be juiced with the wheatgrass juice) **during BOTH "Phases."**   After that, it is the preference, needs, & desires of the person.   My own opinion is that those with – or at risk for - neurological, cardiovascular, or immune diseases: may benefit from this food at least 3 days per week!   Some find it delicious on salads or lettuce wraps (with avocado & other goodies inside).

Caution for Coriander spice: The coriander in a spice grinder (NOT the coriander leaves) has been found to cause an allergic reaction (although very rare & the allergy was not via consumption but possibly via inhalation or touch - & was probably not organic or raw).[247]

4c. **Iceberg Lettuce** (raw, Organic) – the *"Rodney Dangerfield"* of Green Vegetables!

The myth/misunderstanding (which probably began in the mid 1980's about iceberg lettuce having *"no nutritional value"* is a falsehood!   One would have to consume half a medium head (6" diameter) of iceberg lettuce to receive:[74] 3 grams of fiber; 1 gram of iron; 60 micrograms of vitamin K1, & over 77 micrograms of folic acid.

It is true that Romaine lettuce contains a greater amount of all these (as well as almost all other "macro-nutritional value").[74]

However (as mentioned in "Dietary Commandment # 4"), iceberg lettuce is the only food (that I am aware of) that has all 5 of the properties listed in "Dietary Commandment # 4!"   Therefore, **Iceberg lettuce** may help prevent:

- **Bleeding & anemia** (if one eats a considerable amount –such as half a head as stated above).[15,225]
- **Atherosclerosis & therefore, arterial blood clots** (**indirectly** by decreasing the "stress" on the gastrointestinal, immune, & cardiovascular systems).[78]
- **Constipation.**[78]   Many patients of mine complain of being constipated for days. They often suffer with a dangerous drop in blood pressure after finally having a bowel movement (removing that "pressure/stress"). Remember, the "King of Rock & Roll" (Elvis Presley) was believed to have passed away from this (ironically, the "King" died on the throne)!   Cleansing the colon may **decrease the stress** on the **gastrointestinal, lymphatic, immune, & cardiovascular systems!**[49,78]
- **Venous blood clots** (**indirectly** by purifying the lymph which decreases the risk of edema (& possibly lymphedema)! [78]

229

Quantity, Frequency, & Which Phase(s): Most adults would benefit from consuming iceberg lettuce at least 1 day per week during BOTH phases. Those who suffer with more "congestion" (in their respiratory - sinuses, gastrointestinal, &/or lymphatic systems) may benefit from greater amounts &/or frequencies.

4d. **Green Powders/Drinks** – Organic

Most green powders are good sources of vitamin K1, C – as well as minerals, enzymes, & other important nutrients.[15]   A good green powder should contain (per serving –usually 3 teaspoons):[15]

- **Over 1 billion live probiotics.**
- Good **detoxifiers** – like the **chelation agent pectin** (found in apples, beets, carrots, cabbage, dried peas, okra, etc.). **Pectin** (a natural chelation agent) **helps remove harmful metal toxins, helps lower cholesterol, & reduces the risk of heart disease & gallstones.**
- **Blood cleansers & chlorophyll** sources (such as wheatgrass, barley, chlorella, &/or spirulina).   Spirulina contains tyrosine which may naturally boost your dopamine levels (to possibly help you lose weight, lift your moods, & increase energy levels).
- **Wheatgrass & barley juice powder** – possibly 2 of God's highest sources of the **powerful antioxidant enzyme S.O.D.**

Quantity, Frequency, & Which Phase(s): **During the "Lifestyle Phase**:" these green powders can be added to one's water & sipped throughout the day. My preference is to make a smoothie in the morning with filtered water, 1 teaspoon of a greens powder product, 1 organic apple, & raw Brazil nuts (or raw creamy almond butter).   There are thousands of other smoothies one can make & some are mentioned in Chapter 7.

4e. **Other "Super Green Vegetables"** – Organic

Most people would probably benefit from a variety of different types of vegetables of different colors (possessing a variety of beneficial macro- & micronutrients).   There are too many healthful vegetables to discuss or even list. Almost all vegetables have wonderful health benefits. Some of the other healthful "Super Green Vegetables" include Organic:

- **Parsley** is a good source of vitamin K1, C, copper, fiber, & glutamine (the amino acid that may help heal ulcers &, therefore, help anemia)![15]
- **Broccoli & Brussels sprouts** are also good sources of vitamin K1, C, copper, & fiber. **Broccoli sprouts** contain 20 times more cancer-fighting sulfurophane than broccoli.[7,173]
- **Mustard greens & turnip greens** are good sources of vitamin K1, C, folic acid, copper, & fiber.[74]
- **Asparagus** is a good source of:[74] iron, folic acid, & the fiber *Inulin* (a prebiotic – mentioned earlier – that stimulates the growth of intestinal probiotics)![82]
- **Jerusalem Artichokes** are also a good source of the fiber *Inulin* - & may be considered one of the highest antioxidant-rich foods.[166]

- **Celery** may be considered one of the top foods in the world for weight loss as it:[248]
  - o   May actually take more calories to chew & digest than you gain from it.
  - o   May also quickly satiate your hunger.
  - o   & is also a good source of vitamin C, calcium, & apigenin – a compound that reduces the risk of ovarian cancer.

Quantity, Frequency, & Which Phase(s): **If raw – during BOTH phases**. Most would benefit eaten once per week. For example, one may benefit from parsley juice one day & broccoli the next day (& asparagus the next day; etc.) **If cooked – during the "Lifestyle Phase**." Again, rotate them daily.

5.   **Superoxide Dismutase (S.O.D.) – as a supplement (must be combined with glutathione)**

As mentioned previously, S.O.D. is an antioxidant enzyme found in most dark green leafy vegetables (as well as sauerkraut).   As per Phyllis Balch (in her book *Prescription for Nutritional Healing*) this enzyme may:[15]

- Decrease inflammation. When people smoke cigarettes: the level of their free radical activity has been found to raise dramatically – as do the SOD levels![7]
- Decrease oxidative stress &, therefore, decrease the risk of cancer,[7] atherosclerosis (as well as boost the immune system &, therefore, decrease the risk of all diseases)!
- Help with wound healing – especially after a burn.[7]
- Revitalize cells & reduce the rate of cell destruction.
- Neutralize the most common, & possibly the most dangerous, free radicals – superoxide.[7] S.O.D.'s levels tend to decline with age, while free radical production increases.   Thus, it may possess anti-aging benefits! **A good supplement source should contain "Catalase" & "Glutathione peroxidase" to inactivate/break down the free-radical hydrogen peroxide**.[7]

Quantity, Frequency, & Which Phase(s): During the "Lifestyle Phase," one may benefit from 2,000 "McCord" units every other day. **If one consumes enough "greens" (daily)** such as: 2 ounces of raw wheatgrass juice; some raw broccoli; & a greens powder drink loaded with barley grass: **you may not need to take this supplement**!

Cautions: SOD produces hydrogen peroxide (another powerful free-radical) in its wake, & **must be combined with glutathione** (which inactivates this free radical)![7]   This is why some may prefer to consume (during any phase) this powerful antioxidant enzyme via its' raw natural organic sources (such as fresh wheatgrass juice, barley grass juice, & most dark green leafy vegetables – as well as sauerkraut)!

6.   **Glutathione supplement**

Glutathione is an amino acid that may be considered the most powerful antioxidant, liver/blood cleanser, & chelation supplement in the world to **cleanse inflammatory toxins (such as toxic heavy metals, industrial**

chemicals, drugs, etc.) from your body.[7,15,45]   Since this **inflammatory load** is believed to be the #1 cause of chronic diseases (mentioned in chapters 3 & 4), glutathione may be the most important supplement to help **reduce the risk of chronic diseases**.   Glutathione is a powerful antioxidant that inhibits the formation of, & protects against cellular damage from, free radicals.[15]   Thus, glutathione may help you *"CLEANSE"* toxins out of your cells - especially your brain (as a chelation agent) – as glutathione is the major free radical scavenger in the brain![249,250]   Therefore, supplementation of oral glutathione may satisfy ALL "10 Dietary Commandments"- except # 3 – which is why it should only be consumed in the "Lifestyle Phase."

  Research suggests that glutathione supplementation may be effective in the treatment &/or prevention (reducing our *"FULL OF IT Level"*) of:
- Psychological diseases – such as Schizophrenia & bipolar disorder![250]
- Neurological diseases – such as Parkinson's disease & cerebral-reperfusion injury diseases.[7,241,242]
- Cancer,[15] AIDS, Sepsis, Trauma, Burns, & even athletic over-training.[251] Where selenium (needed to make glutathione) soil levels are the highest (e.g. South Dakota), cancer rates are the lowest.[7]
- & **aging**. *"The rate at which we age is directly correlated with reduced concentrations of glutathione in cellular fluids; as we grow older, glutathione levels drop, resulting in a decreased ability to deactivate free radicals."*[7]

  Glutathione, as mentioned previously, protects the cells of your body by *"inhibiting the formation of, & protecting against cellular damage from, free radicals."*[15]   Therefore, Glutathione helps the body defend against damage from:[15]
- Cigarette smoking; Radiation exposure; Cancer chemotherapy; Alcohol; Toxic heavy metals (like mercury, arsenic, & lead)[7,241,242] & Drugs (such as acetaminophen).[7]   Therefore, it aids in the treatment of blood & liver disorders.
- **& STRESS** – both psychological & physiological stress from all the mind, body & soul toxins we become *"**FULL OF**."*   In stress, the level of glutamine (which is necessary for our bodies to make glutathione) decreases.[7]   In healthy people, glutathione is in every cell at very high concentrations.[7]

"Glutathione protects not only individual cells but also the tissues of the arteries, brain, heart, immune cells, kidney, eye, liver, lungs, & skin against oxidant damage."[15]

Quantity, Frequency, & Which Phase(s): During the "Lifestyle Phase," adults may benefit from **500mg/day of glutathione (powdered form)** combined/mixed with the following:
- **Organic wheatgrass juice** (high in SOD) freshly made or filtered water
- **500mg of powdered glycine** (as glycine is one of the major amino acids the liver uses to produce glutathione).[15]
- **500mg of glutamine powder** (another major amino acid the liver uses to produce glutathione).[7,15]   The abovementioned combination seems to have synergistic properties creating one of the **most powerful mixtures in the**

world to help cleanse your liver & the rest of your body from inflammatory body toxins!

We also have to have sufficient **selenium** to make glutathione.[7]   Selenium 200mcg/day may be taken with the abovementioned combination or taken with lunch as part of a multivitamin (or simply by eating raw Brazil nuts – mentioned later on this list).   Some nutritionists suggest that taking **N-Acetyl Cysteine** (500mg/day with water – never exceed 1,000mg/day) may raise glutathione levels better than taking glutathione itself.[15]   However, **N-Acetyl Cysteine** may have side effects (especially in Diabetics).   Therefore, I prefer the abovementioned "Super-*CLEANSING* Combination" as I believe this may be the more "natural" way to ingest it. Of course the most natural way to consume glutathione may be to eat its' natural, organic food sources (like **avocados**)![88]

Cautions: Like everything in this book, people should first consult their health care providers before taking this or any supplement.

7.   **Avocado** – (*Persea Americana*) Organic* & raw (of course!)
*As mentioned in "Dietary Commandment #2," non-organic avocados can be consumed during the "Lifestyle Phase" as they're part of the "Clean 14" (least sprayed with pesticides).[54]

If you believe eating avocados will make you fat, then "*YOU ARE FULL OF IT*!"   I know many people who followed this book's diet as "vegans" & consumed multiple avocados per day & actually lost too much weight! Avocados are a good source of:[74] Folic acid, fiber, & extremely healthful fats – like mono-unsaturated fats ("MUFAs" – discussed in section II of this chapter).

Avocados are considered by many to be **one of the best foods in the world to reduce** one's "*FULL OF IT Level*" of **obesity**.[248]

As mentioned in "Dietary Commandment # 6," avocados are considered one of the top 4 best liver-cleansing foods[90] – probably because they are high in glutathione (a powerful antioxidant/chelation agent mentioned earlier)![88]   Avocados have an extremely low glycemic index/load (like almost all "super-cleansing foods/supplements").[74,177-179]

Most importantly: avocados contain substances that may help stabilize blood sugar levels –preventing high blood sugar spikes (hyperglycemia) – as well as preventing low blood sugar levels (hypoglycemia)![15,252]   As mentioned in "Dietary Commandment #8," this amazingly unique ability of avocados may significantly lower the "*FULL OF IT Level*" of:[174,175] Type II Diabetes, atherosclerosis, & age-related macular degeneration.

Quantity, Frequency, & Which Phase(s): My opinion/quote for the past 17 years regarding avocados = "*An avocado & apple* (mentioned next) – *per day* (during BOTH phases) *can keep the doctor away*!"   They both satisfy all 10 "Dietary Commandments!"   As mentioned in "Dietary Commandment # 10," they are enzymatically considered a "non-fruit" &, therefore, should be combined with other non-fruits.

8. Apples (Organic & raw)

Apples are high in flavonoids, antioxidants, minerals, dietary fiber, beta-carotene, & phytosterol (which may inhibit various cancers & help lower cholesterol).[9]   Red Delicious, Granny Smith, & Gala apples may possess some of the highest amounts of *antioxidant capabilities* of all the foods in the world.[166]   Numerous research studies have shown apples to lower the "***FULL OF IT* Level**" of cancer/ tumors![169]   Thus, apples help fulfill "Dietary Commandment # 7."   Apples are high in pectin - an amazing type of soluble fiber that helps *chelate metal toxins* from the body.[15,248]

Apples are considered **one of the best foods in the world for**:[253]

- **Increasing Dopamine levels naturally.** Apples contain quercetin – which may prevent neuro-degeneration & boost dopamine. Dopamine is the "feel-good" substance in your body that helps control weight, energy levels, & supports brain & heart health.   Thus, a deficiency may contribute to obesity, depression, & fatigue.
- **Weight loss.**[248] This may be due to the pectin – a soluble fiber – which can satiate your appetite longer (as well as help prevent colon cancer).[248]

Apples are also considered one of the top 4 healing foods in the world to **detox your body** naturally due to the following reasons:[9]

- Apples are a great source of the fiber pectin (which as mentioned above can help **chelate metal toxins**).[15,248] Thus apples help fulfill "Dietary Commandment # 5."
- Apples contain a variety of powerful phytochemicals such as D-Glucarate, flavonoids (like Phlorizidin which helps regulate the production of bile in your liver – to help remove toxins from the body), phytosterols, & terpenoids – all of which play a role in the natural detoxification process.

However, the most amazing quality of apples may be their unique ability to "**combine**" with all non-fruits (as well all fruits –except for melons)!   This was mentioned in "Commandment #10."

Quantity, Frequency, & Which Phase(s): Same as avocados – mentioned previously.

Caution: Avoid consuming apple seeds as they contain a small amount of cyanide. I prefer to cut apples four ways & throw out the core, stem, & seeds.

9. Sprouted Beans & Lentils (Organic & Raw)

Sprouted lentils & beans are a good source of iron, copper, folic acid, & fiber.[74] Despite the fact that sprouted lentils & beans contain less than half of these nutrients (& calories - when compared to un-sprouted lentils & beans),[74] they are still a great source of these nutrients.   Thus, they may help reduce the "***FULL OF IT* Level**" of atherosclerosis (due to their high fiber content)[15,82,103] & anemia (due to their high iron, copper, & folic acid content).[15,49]

In addition, raw sprouted beans & lentils are considered an enzyme-rich vegetable & are, therefore, easier to digest (& possess "No toxic mucus-forming activity" - fulfilling "Dietary Commandment # 4") –than un-sprouted beans & lentils.[49,78]

Beans & Lentils produce L-methione – a chelation agent – in good quantities[45] &, therefore, help fulfill "Dietary Commandment # 5." This ability of sprouted beans & lentils to possibly help remove metal toxins from the body may help neurological diseases & atherosclerosis (as these metal toxins may damage the walls of arteries).[45,49,217] Maybe this is why Esau sold his "birthright" to Jacob in exchange for Lentil stew (Genesis 25:33)! ☺

Small Red Beans, Red Kidney Beans, Pinto Beans, & Black Beans may also possess some of the highest antioxidant capabilities in the world.[166] Therefore, these sprouted beans may fulfill "Dietary Commandment # 7."

Quantity, Frequency, & Which Phase(s): Both phases every other day may benefit most adults.

10. Cocoa (Raw, Unprocessed, & Organic)

Discussing beans above creates a perfect Segway to mention Cocoa (as cocoa or cacao is a bean also). *"Raw, unprocessed cocoa bean"* may possess one of the highest antioxidant capabilities in the world.[26,166] Therefore, it may also fulfill "Dietary Commandment # 7." Since it is a bean, it may also fulfill "Dietary Commandment # 5."

The healthiest cocoa (rare to find) should be:
- Raw. Most cocoa found in the stores is not raw.
- Unprocessed. Most of the cocoa found in stores is "**processed**." In fact, if you read the ingredients of most brands of chocolate sold –it will state the words: *"Processed with* (often alkali or something else)." Having the cocoa **processed** *may* decrease or eliminate its antioxidant abilities.[26,166]
- Organic. Most chocolate/cocoa/cacao found in stores does not state "USDA Certified Organic."
- Sugar-free. Most cocoa found in the stores contain sugar. This breaks "Dietary Commandment # 8!"
- Cow's milk-free. Most cocoa found in the stores contain cow's milk. This violates/breaks "Dietary Commandments # 4 & 5" – as the high toxic-mucus capability of cow's milk may interfere with the absorption of the healthful macro & micro-nutrients (including the antioxidant capabilities) of the cocoa![78]

However, even raw, unprocessed organic cocoa can be acidic & act as a gastrointestinal irritant to some when taken in high amounts. Goat's milk yogurt &/or cultured unsweetened coconut milk yogurt may neutralize this acidity &, therefore, may be added (in the "Lifestyle Phase") to chocolate "super-shakes." Raw organic almond butter may neutralize this acidity &, therefore, may be added (in any phase) to create chocolate shakes &/or "brownie balls."

My *"Super-Chocolate Brownie Balls"* are vegan & mostly raw (&, therefore, should wait until the "Lifestyle Phase") & are homemade via the following recipe: Mix filtered water with raw, organic, un-processed 100% cocoa &the following 100% organic ingredients:

- Extra-virgin coconut oil; Raw almond butter; A dash of cinnamon, vanilla, & stevia (or raw honey). Stir them all together until smooth, roll into balls, & then put in the fridge for 1 day. Then eat! They are nutritious & delicious!

Quantity, Frequency, & Which Phase(s): Both phases in minimal amounts once a week or as tolerated gastro-intestinally.

11. "Super-Nuts" = Almonds, Brazil Nuts, & Pecans (Organic & Raw)
Most nuts are a good source of iron, fiber, & copper.[74] Thus, they may help reduce the "***FULL OF IT* Level**" of atherosclerosis (due to their high fiber content)[15,82,103] & anemia (due to their high iron & copper content).[15,49] As will be shown later in this chapter under ("super-cleansing fats"), the consumption of nuts has shown to lower the "***FULL OF IT* Level**" of atherosclerosis (due to their high "healthful fat" content – see section II of this chapter).[100] Pecans (as well as almonds) are rich with antioxidants.[26,166] Brazil Nuts are a good source of selenium – a known antioxidant trace mineral – which may protect your body from fluoride exposure & oxidative stress.[254] Therefore, pecans & Brazil nuts may fulfill "Dietary Commandment # 7."

"Smooth Raw Almond Butter" may make the almonds easier to absorb for many people (as it requires less chewing).[49,78] Walnuts contain the amino acid arginine & the omega 3 fatty acid Alpha Linolenic Acid – which helps liver function.[255] However, people at risk for bleeding need to be cautious of walnuts as omega 3 fatty acids possess anticoagulant properties.

Unlike most nuts that are "**Low-Level Acid Forming**," **Almonds & Brazil Nuts** are considered "**Low-Level Alkaline Forming**."[15] This concept of "balance" was discussed earlier in this section.

Quantity, Frequency, & Which Phase(s): Both phases –alternating these 3 different nuts each day would probably benefit most adults. All raw nuts possess health benefits. I simply chose the above 3 as they *best* satisfy all "10 Dietary Commandments."

12. Garlic (Organic & Raw)
Garlic may fulfill "Dietary Commandments # 5 & 6" as it is considered one of the world's best chelation agents[45] & liver cleansers.[88,90] Aged garlic extract has actually been shown to suppress LDL oxidation to help prevent atherosclerosis (&, therefore, prevent arterial blood clots).[256] Garlic's anticoagulant properties may help prevent the formation of all types of blood clots (see below under cautions).[110,117,132,133] Aged Garlic Extract may

boost its' antioxidant potential &, therefore, may fulfill "Dietary Commandment # 7."[15]   Garlic contains a natural antibiotic (also found in onions, radishes, & leeks) that can destroy disease-causing germs without harming the good bacteria (probiotics) in your body![82]   Garlic has been claimed to:[257]

- Boost immunity, decrease blood pressure, eliminate toxins, combat cancer & harmful bacteria.
- & be one of the 4 best ways to *cleanse* toxins from your gut[9] – as well as the rest of your body.

Caution: Garlic (as mentioned in "Dietary Commandment #6") also has anticoagulant properties & may, therefore, decrease the risk of a blood clot.[110,117,132,13?] Therefore, garlic may also increase the risk of bleeding when taken:[110,117,132,133]

- In excess; with other natural anticoagulants; with pharmaceutical anticoagulants; near the time of surgery or trauma; &/or when one already has a bleeding disorder.

In addition, garlic may be irritating to the gastrointestinal systems of some people - especially when taken in excess.

Quantity, Frequency, & Which Phase(s): Raw, Organic Garlic may be consumed in both phases - 1-3x/week. Aged Garlic Extract may be consumed in the "Lifestyle Phase" as tolerated.

13. Turmeric & Ginger (Organic & Raw) = "super-*cleansing* spices"

These two "super-cleansing spices" are grouped together due to their similar benefits to the human body.   If Turmeric is *"King of the spices,"* then Ginger root is a *"close cousin"* to the King![170]   Turmeric & ginger root may both possess health benefits greater than pharmaceuticals (without the toxic side effects).[258]   The health benefits these spices both share may include the following:

- Have **anti-inflammatory** properties (due to the curcumin found in Turmeric - & the gingerols found in ginger).[15,170,258,259]   These anti-inflammatory benefits can help:[15,259]
  - Decrease "**joint pains**" & increase mobility for those with osteoarthritis & rheumatoid arthritis
  - Decrease "**muscle pains/strains/soreness**."   The compounds gingerol, shogaol, & zingerone found in ginger may be more effective than NSAIDs – in reducing "muscle soreness."
- Decrease the risk of (& help to treat those who already have) **diabetes, Alzheimer's, Cardiovascular diseases, & numerous cancer types.**
- Possess **antioxidant & anti-cancer** properties (as mentioned above).[7,15,26,170-172,258,259] Ginger root may kill ovarian & prostate cancer cells **better than chemotherapy**![171,172]
- *Cleanse* the **colon & the liver**.[15,90]
- Possess **anti-bacterial properties** – helping **fight colds** to reduce coughing, sore throats, nasal congestion, & nausea.[15,259]

237

-   & possess **anticoagulant properties** & may, therefore, **reduce the risk of a blood clot**.[110,112,117,122,123,159]

Despite their great similarities regarding their health benefits, differences do exist.

Turmeric extract (similar to the spice cinnamon in this regard) may be more effective than ginger root at fulfilling "Dietary Commandment #9" as it considered a "miracle solution" in **preventing and treating diabetes**.[260]   In a study in which 240 participants received either a placebo or 250mg of turmeric extract (curcumin) every day for 9 months, the results revealed:[260] *16.4% of the placebo group were diagnosed with type 2 diabetes mellitus, whereas **none were diagnosed with type 2 diabetes mellitus in the curcumin-treated group**!*   Turmeric has been found to be **superior to mouthwash** for oral health to help prevent & treat **gingivitis, mouth cancer, plaque, toothaches (& other inflammatory diseases), & microbial dental infections**.[261]   Turmeric has also shown to prevent breast cancer, promote fat loss,[248] detoxify the liver,[90] & help **fight depression** –as well as *positively impact over 581 different diseases & conditions*![170,172]

Ginger root may be useful (possibly more effective than drugs) for **combating vertigo, motion sickness, dizziness, & nausea**.[15,259]   As a physical therapist specializing in Vestibular Rehabilitation: hundreds of my "friends & family" have praised **ginger root** for these benefits.   Some other health benefits that may be unique to **ginger root** (that may also be considered more effective than pharmaceuticals) include:[259]

-   **Relieves heartburn/acid-reflux** (without the osteoporosis, cancer, & mal-absorption side effects/risks common with pharmaceutical proton pump inhibitors – PPIs)
-   **Relieves upset stomach/helps digestion** (*ginger tea may be mixed with a few sprigs of mint leaves & a teaspoon of raw honey to subdue an upset stomach*)
-   **Relieves headaches/migraines** (*the tea may be mixed with peppermint & cayenne pepper to help relieve headaches &/or migraines*).
-   **& relieves toothaches** (raw ginger root can be rubbed on the painful tooth for relief).

Ginger & turmeric are both spices (non-fruits) & should, therefore, be consumed with other non-fruits for superior absorption (as mentioned in "Dietary Commandment # 10").   Turmeric is fat-soluble & should, therefore, be **consumed with healthful fats** to optimize the absorption of this amazing spice.[172]

Caution: Turmeric & ginger have anticoagulant properties (as mentioned above & in "Commandment # 6") & may, therefore, decrease the risk of a blood clot. Therefore, turmeric & ginger may also increase the risk of bleeding when taken:[110,112,117,122,123,159]

238

- In excess; with natural or pharmaceutical anticoagulants; near the time of surgery or trauma; &/or when one already has a bleeding disorder.

In addition, an excess of these spices may be irritating to the gastrointestinal systems of some people – especially when taken in excess.

Quantity, Frequency, & Which Phase(s): Raw, Organic Turmeric & Ginger Root may be consumed in both phases – as tolerated (regarding their anticoagulant & gastrointestinal "spicy-ness"). Turmeric & ginger root capsules may be consumed in the "Lifestyle Phase" as tolerated.

14. **Carnitine:** in its L-Carnitine form or N-Acetyl Carnitine forms
Carnitine is an amino acid that chemically attracts long chain fatty acids to be burned within the mitochondria of skeletal muscle cells to provide energy. Therefore, Carnitine may:
- Improve energy levels by increasing the use of fat as an energy source.[107]
- Protect against atherosclerosis via helping to prevent fatty buildup in the heart & arterial vessels – as well as helping to prevent lipid peroxidation;[105,106]
- Improve exercise ability of those with angina;[105,106]
- Help prevent fatty buildup in the heart, liver, & skeletal muscles.[15,107]
- Help ease the pain of intermittent arterial claudication, a condition in which a blocked artery in the leg decreases the supply of blood & oxygen to leg muscles, causing pain –especially with physical activity.[105,106]
- & **decrease body fat mass** & aid in weight loss.[15,107] Therefore, carnitine helps "*CLEANSE*" fat out of your organs, arteries, waist, hips, & the rest of your body! I am not familiar with any other substance in the world that "burns fat." The levels of carnitine in the body decline with age.[15] This may be one contributing factor to why many people have trouble losing excess body fat as they age. This may also be one contributing factor to why heart disease becomes more prevalent as we age.

I have educated thousands of adults (usually desiring to lose excess body fat) about L-carnitine since the mid-1990s. The other supplement I have educated adults desiring to lose excess body fat about (since the mid-1990s) is:

Chromium picolinate (AKA "Glucose Tolerance Factor") – is a trace mineral involved in the metabolism of glucose that may help with blood glucose levels. However, chromium (unlike carnitine) should not be considered a "*fat burner*." As carnitine stimulates fat to enter skeletal muscle cells to be burned for energy, chromium stimulates sugar to enter skeletal muscle cells to be burned for energy.[15] This is why these two supplements/ingredients are often recommended for weight loss – as well as found in "sports/energy drinks." It has been estimated that only 10% of Americans have an adequate amount of chromium (150-400mcg/day) in their diet due to the following reasons:[15]
- o Much of the chromium found in foods is lost during processing
- o High quantities of sugar, refined flour, & junk foods in the diet cause a loss of chromium from the body

239

o   & a lack of chromium in our water & soil.

***Cautions* for Chromium picolinate:** Most adults will benefit from a multivitamin containing approximately 200mcg of chromium during their lunch (diabetics & those who consume more fruit juices/sugars may benefit from taking this separate from their multivitamin during a meal).   However, excessive intake of chromium may lead to:[15]

- Dermatitis (some people develop a slight skin rash)
- Gastrointestinal ulcers
- Kidney & liver impairment
- Low blood sugar reactions – especially in diabetics taking insulin simultaneously.   As with everything you put in your mouth, diabetics (& everyone else) should consult their health care providers to determine the correct amount of this trace mineral for you.

Caution: My personal warning **about carnitine** is that I have seen many people lose a lot of body fat %age with this supplement.   As mentioned & referenced in chapter 4, it has been suggested, that men should have approximately 12% & women 18% body fat for optimal health.   Once one goes below these levels, I would not take L-carnitine.   Remember, there isn't a perfect 100% correlation between health & fitness.   For example, marathon runners with 2% body fat who get heart attacks at age 45 are extremely fit – but, unfortunately, not very healthy.

Quantity, Frequency, & Which Phase(s): Men over 12% body fat - & women over 18% – may benefit from taking 500-1,000 mg/day with water (only in the "Lifestyle Phase").

15. Coenzyme Q10 (AKA CoQ10 or ubiquinone or ubidecarenone)

CoQ10 is a component of the electron transport chain & participates in aerobic cellular respiration, generating energy in the form of ATP (95% of the human body's energy is generated this way!).[262]   It also possesses antioxidant (& anti-atherosclerosis) properties due to its ability to suppress LDL oxidation[108,109] &, therefore, fulfills "Dietary Commandments # 6 & 7."

It is believed[15,120] that as many as 75% of people over 50 may be deficient in CoQ10, which may be one reason why cardiovascular disease increases in incidence as we age!   Studies have shown that supplementation of CoQ10 may benefit patients having cardiovascular surgery such as:[120]

- Coronary Artery Bypass Graft (CABG), cardiac valve replacement, & repair of abdominal aortic aneurysms.

Unlike other antioxidants, CoQ10 inhibits **both the initiation & propagation** of lipid oxidation of LDL,[109] therefore lowering the risk of heart attacks, ischemic strokes, & overall atherosclerosis.

CoQ10 may also reduce the "***FULL OF IT* Level**" of the following:

- Migraine headaches (when taken 150-300mg/day).[263]
- & Hypertension – may have the potential in hypertensive patients to lower systolic 17 mm Hg & diastolic 10 mm Hg without significant side-effects.[264]

- Side effects of Statins (drugs) because these pharmaceuticals can reduce serum levels of Coenzyme Q10 by up to 40%.[265,266] Golomb & Evans[266] have extensively reviewed & documented the role of statin side effects & very strongly associated them with the CoQ10 depletion!   This statin-induced depletion of CoQ10 leads to depleted **anti-oxidant activity** as well as (CoQ10's important role in) electron transfer phosphorylation in **cellular respiration!**[266]
- Low Percent Oxygen Saturation as CoQ10 may increase oxygenation of all tissues.[87] This is common in anemia/blood loss. Thus, CoQ10 may indirectly protect against arterial blood clots - as well as help people with anemia/blood loss to increase their oxygen saturation![87] Thus, <u>**CoQ10 is truly an amazing "Super-Cleansing Supplement" as it may protect against atherosclerosis (&, therefore, arterial blood clots) & may help people with anemia/blood loss improve their oxygen saturation**</u>!

My personal opinion (based on experience & the research of CoQ10's strong involvement in aerobic cellular respiration) is that Co Q10 is extremely important for individuals with low percent oxygen saturation (93% or lower = a "D" or lower).

Caution: In the author's opinion, this supplement is not needed in people who always have excellent SpO2 (percent oxygen saturation measured by a pulse oximeter) of 98% or higher (grade "A" or higher).   Keep in mind, many older adults have excellent oxygen saturation sitting &/or standing – but poor when lying down (possibly predisposing themselves for sleep apnea)! Of the thousands of patients I have measured (with an *accurate* pulse oximeter –possessing an accuracy light sensor, wire, & finger probe), I would estimate over 50% of all adults over the age of 70 have their percent oxygen saturation levels significantly drop (over 4 percentage points - or "grades") when they lie down.

Drug Interactions: CoQ10 may decrease the anticoagulant effect of warfarin.[120]

Quantity, Frequency, & Which Phase(s): In the "Lifestyle Phase," 1 mg per pound of body weight per day in an oil based capsule (if % oxygen saturation is not always excellent –see above cautions).   For example: If an adult weighs 200 pounds with an oxygen saturation below 94%, 200 mg/day of coenzyme Q10 may improve their oxygen saturation (& possibly prove to be a "life saver")![87]   This 200mg/day of coenzyme Q10 is way below the 1,200 mg/day "Observed Safe Level."[267]

16. Vitamin D3 (cholecalciferol)

As mentioned previously in chapter 5, the body can synthesize vitamin D3 (from cholesterol) when **exposed to sunlight**.[1,30,31] The most conclusive evidence of benefit for vitamin D3 supplementation is for:[268]

- Bone health; A boost of the immune system; & a prevention of the influenza. This mostly comes from research suggesting that a deficiency of vitamin D (in which most Americans are)[30,31] leads to an increased risk of contracting a cold or flu, & even depression.[30,32,33,37,39]

Some research results have suggested that adding vitamin D to a reduced-calorie diet will lead to increased weight loss in individuals with low vitamin D levels.[39]

Caution: The Institute of Medicine (IOM) as of 11/30/10 has set the Tolerable Upper intake Level (TUL) to 4,000 IU/day for ages 9-71 years.[268] The TUL is defined as the highest average daily intake of a nutrient that is likely to pose no risk of adverse health effects for nearly all persons in that generation.   Vitamin D overdose (published cases of toxicity usually involve vitamin D doses of 40,000 IU/day) can cause hypercalcemia – which may lead to nausea, vomiting, weakness, insomnia, nervousness, & ultimately renal failure.[268]

Quantity, Frequency, & Which Phase(s): In the "Lifestyle Phase," 1,000 – 2,500 IU/day of supplemental vitamin D3 may benefit most adults. In both phases, some exposure to sunlight may benefit all adults.   Twenty minutes/day of ultraviolet exposure in light-skinned individuals (3-6 times longer for pigmented skin) has caused the concentration of vitamin D precursors produced in the skin to reach an equilibrium (in which further vitamin D that is produced is actually degraded).[31]

17. Magnesium (in the form of orotate, gluconate, amino acid chelate, oxide, or citrate)

This has to be considered a "super-cleansing" mineral as it has so many vital health functions –including helping to move your bowels!   Magnesium is a vital catalyst in enzyme activity, especially the activity of those enzymes involved in **energy production**.[15]

Magnesium (a beneficial metallic mineral) has been shown to "***CLEANSE***"/chelate harmful toxic heavy metals – such as:[7]
- Lead. Magnesium has been shown to decrease the absorption of lead.
- Cadmium. Magnesium has been shown in animal studies to prevent cadmium-induced testicular tumors.
- & other metal carcinogens.

Magnesium carries out over 300 functions in the body including, but not limited to, the following additional possible benefits:[269]
- Assists in the uptake of other beneficial minerals – like calcium & potassium[15] - as well as vitamin B6; Helps with detoxification;
- Boost energy; Make healthy teeth & bones; Improve symptoms of PMS & menopause for women; Reduce Migraines; Lowers High Blood Pressure; Helps eliminate constipation; Helps reduce an abnormal heart rate; Helps Diabetes Mellitus Type II; Helps insomnia & depression.   This may be because magnesium has a natural muscle relaxant effect to help sleep – as well as possibly help **reduce muscle strains**.   Thus: The "old wives tale" of taking an Epsom salt (magnesium sulfate) bath to "relax your muscles" is not a fallacy.

Therefore: Consuming magnesium (as a supplement or from its' food sources) may lower your "***FULL OF IT*** Level of <u>Chronic Pain</u> – as well as **Diseases &/or Obesity!**" Some "super-cleansing foods" that are rich in this vital mineral include Organic:[269] Brown Rice bran; Dark chocolate; Dark leafy greens; Sprouted beans & lentils; & Avocados.

Caution: Taking **excess** magnesium may have too strong a laxative effect. **Excess** intake of magnesium hydroxide (AKA "Milk of Magnesia" = "MOM") may decrease the absorption of iron & folic acid.[270]   This may be why magnesium (when taken in **excess**) is claimed to have a side effect of increased bleeding times.[120]   When combined with ibuprofen for a prolonged period of time, magnesium may increase the activity – and GI bleeding risk – of ibuprofen (possibly by increasing the gastric pH & creating an environment conducive to absorption)![15]

Many people are aware of magnesium sulfate ("Epsom salt") & "Milk of Magnesia" (MOM) & their laxative effects. They used to add MOM to certain dietary ice creams to "keep you thin!"   However, the consumer was still eating the toxic cow's milk & sugar!   Some of my patients have reported a dangerously strong laxative effect (over 10 bowel movements per day) by simply applying Epsom salt (used as a muscle relaxant) <u>to the skin</u> over their strained muscles for only 15 minutes per day!

Quantity, Frequency, & Which Phase(s): In the "Lifestyle Phase," 350mg – 800mg/day (in the supplement form of orotate, gluconate, or amino-chelate) may provide a daily protective level of magnesium.   Supplementation may not even be necessary if you consume enough magnesium via your "God-created foods" (like the magnesium-rich foods mentioned above).   Over 40% of Americans get less than 75% of the USRDA of magnesium (400mg per day).[7]
Sugar & alcohol consumption both will increase urinary excretion of magnesium, leading to a magnesium deficiency.[7,15]

II.   Super-*Cleansing*: Fats, Proteins, Carbs, Fiber, Teas, Soy, Milk, Meats, Shakes, & Homeopathy

The reader should take note that there is a lot of categorical sharing of foods as many super-cleansing fats, proteins, etc. are found in the previous section as "super-cleansing foods." In addition, many "super-cleansing fats" may also be found in the "super-cleansing proteins" section.   These dietary categories are all considered "super-cleansing" as they are all capable of lowering one's "***FULL OF IT*** Level of **Disease(s), Obesity, &/or Chronic Pain!**"   Said differently, all of these dietary

243

categories are all capable of *"__cleansing__"* your body (in some manner already discussed in the 1st section of this chapter) to help optimize your physical health.

II.A. 4 "Super-*Cleansing* Fats"
"Go, Eat of the FAT!" – Nehemia 8:10

Despite being numbered from most to least beneficial for the cardiovascular system, all 4 fat sources can be considered healthful (& probably vital)! However (like even the "super-cleansing foods/supplements" mentioned in the first section of this chapter), moderation is still the key! However, the **type of fat** is much more important than the quantity! These 4 "Super-Cleansing Fats" have cardiovascular benefits – as well as other health benefits. Not all categories of fats are equal. In fact (as shown below), not all Saturated Fatty Acids (SFAs) are equal. All 4 "Super-Cleansing Fats" must be "organic" or "organically raised." If their food sources are 100% alive, they may be eaten in any phase. If they are not 100% alive, they may be eaten after the "Cleansing Phase."

If you believe these 4 "Super-Fats" will harm your heart – or make you fat, you may be *"**FULL OF IT!**"*
If you believe all fats (as well as carbs, proteins, &/or calories) are equally healthful or harmful, *"**YOU ARE FULL OF IT!**"*

These "super-cleansing fats" (like the other "super-cleansing foods") are known to have wonderful God-given benefits to our health - & our waistlines. This is especially true when eaten in obedience with all of the "10 Dietary Commandments!"

1. **Lauric Acids (a type of SFA) found in <u>PROBIOTIC</u> food sources such as <u>fermented/cultured</u>: "coconut milk"** (best source as lauric acid makes up the greatest percentage of coconut's fat content) available in a yogurt-like consistency (assuming no sugar added; usually high in fiber; -& no reduction of the natural coconut fat has occurred) **& goat's milk (such as plain goat's milk yogurt & kefir).** Replacement of carbs with <u>lauric acid</u> (found in coconut fat/oil, palm oils, & dairy fat –to a lesser degree) has resulted in significantly lower total cholesterol/HDL & lower LDL/HDL ratios,[100] two of the strongest predictors to decrease atherosclerosis risk![98,99] Since the abovementioned lauric acid fat sources are also **probiotic** food sources, we may also get the amazing benefits of preventing atherosclerosis – as well as bleeding, anemia, & osteoporosis (as well as boosting the immune & gastrointestinal systems)!

2. **EPA/DHA (Eicosapentaenoic acid & docosahexaenoic acid) – the type of omega 3 fatty acids found mostly in fatty fish.**

Regular dietary intake of EPA/DHA may decrease the risk of:
- Blood clots, CHD (Coronary Heart Disease),[68] ischemic & thrombotic strokes,[64] & secondary & primary heart attacks.[65,66]

Despite possibly NOT having the same benefit on LDL/HDL ratio as the other 3 "super-cleansing fats,"[100] EPA/DHA probably has the strongest anticoagulant ability to prevent a blood clot![146,147]

Caution: As mentioned in "Dietary Commandment # 6," its' strong anticoagulant properties make it a bleeding risk (especially if over 3 grams of the EPA/DHA are taken).[64,69] As EPA/DHA is being added to so many foods – as well as the feed of chickens & other animals, the anticoagulant properties (as well as the bleeding risks) of these foods (including the eggs of chickens) is being increased.

3.   3a. Non-Trans, Non-Hydrogenated **Omega 6 fatty acids** & 3b. **Alpha-Linolenic Acid (the type of Omega 3 fatty acid** found mostly in <u>non-marine</u> food sources).

The most favorable effect on total cholesterol/HDL ratio has been found when carbohydrates intake has been replaced by foods:[100]

-    High in non-trans, non-hydrogenated Omega 6 fatty acids found in **NATTO*** - as well as **safflower oil (not high-oleic) & sunflower oil (or edible safflower & sunflower seeds);**
-    &/or high in Alpha Linolenic Acid (ALA) – the omega 3 fatty acid found in the whole food – or highest in the oil of: **flaxseed, chia seed, kiwifruit seed, hemp seed**, etc.

These fats also lowered total cholesterol, LDL, & triglycerides; & increased HDL levels when they replaced carbohydrate intake.[100]   These fats are also considered to be extremely helpful in detoxing the liver.[255]

*I strongly doubt any of these studies used NATTO to replace the carbs. However, Natto is high in Omega 6 fatty acids. Natto also contains a very high amount of fiber, probiotics, & the highest vitamin K2 (in the form of MK7) in the world!   Therefore, Natto is not only a "super-cleansing fat" source – it is a "super-cleansing food."   This is why it was mentioned earlier in this chapter. Some may consider natto the #1 food in the world! It is a food commonly eaten in Japan & has an "acquired" taste, texture ("gooey") & aroma (foul)!

Caution: As mentioned in "Dietary Commandment # 6," the Omega 3 fatty acid ALA has anticoagulant properties. ALA's anti-platelet properties (& bleeding risks) have not shown to be ***as strong*** as that of EPA/DHA.[146,147] However, ALA (&, therefore, its' food sources) has antiplatelet properties[76,143] & can increase bleeding time.[120] Typically/usually, the higher the percentage of ALA found in the food source, the higher/*stronger* its' antiplatelet properties[76,143] (&, therefore, its' bleeding risk).[120] In addition, ALA is converted to the stronger anticoagulants EPA/DHA in the human body – albeit with an efficiency below 5% in men,[148] and at a greater percentage in women.[149] Therefore, women get a greater anticoagulant benefit – as well as a greater bleeding risk – from consumption of these ALA food sources. ALA is considered an omega 3 "ESSENTIAL" fatty acid because (unlike EPA/DHA) the body can't produce it - &, therefore, needs to be consumed.

As the omega 3 fatty acid ALA is being added to many foods – as well as the feed of many animals – the anticoagulant properties (as well as the bleeding risks) of these foods (including the eggs of the chickens) is being increased!

Nattukinase is an enzyme derived from Natto that possesses thrombolytic properties.[15] Therefore, Nattukinase may increase the risk of bleeding – especially cerebral hemorrhage.[142] However, Natto (as a whole food) does not have any known anticoagulant properties or bleeding risks. As already mentioned, this is probably because of the extremely high amount of probiotics & vitamin K2 it possesses!

As mentioned in "Dietary Commandment #6," if you believe we should be so paranoid of blood clots & negligent of bleeding risks that we should consume an excess of natural &/or pharmaceutical anticoagulants, then:

"***YOU ARE FULL OF IT!***" Again, the principle of a healthy balance is the goal.

245

4. Non-trans, non-hydrogenated **Mono-Unsaturated Fatty Acids ("MUFAs")**.

Replacing carbohydrate intake with foods high in MUFAs – such as **extra-virgin olive oil, high-oleic safflower oil** (an acceptable cooking oil mentioned in "Dietary Commandment #3), **rapeseed oil, AVOCADO** (a "super-cleansing food"), & raw **NUTS** (Brazil, Pecans, & Almonds are all "super-cleansing foods") – has resulted in:[100] Increased HDL levels; Decreased LDL levels; & decreased triglyceride levels.

While PUFAs (Poly-Unsaturated Fatty Acids) –like the previously mentioned Omega 3 & 6 fatty acids ("super-cleansing fats" # 2 & 3) have a stronger effect on reducing cholesterol levels, in vitro assays suggest the effects of MUFAs on reducing **LDL oxidation** are the most beneficial.[100] This ability of MUFAs to reduce LDL oxidation may make MUFAs the most important fats to consume to reduce the risk of atherosclerosis!

An important observation to make is that the **abovementioned 4 fats** have shown to reduce the risk of heart disease when they replaced carbohydrate intake. One may conclude the following:

- Obviously the **calories** from these "super-cleansing fats" are **heart healthful** – as well as **reducing our waist lines** – when compared to the **harm from carbohydrates** (especially refined carbohydrates/sugars).
- The original (1970s) & even most revised (2011) "**Food Guide Pyramid**" may be "**FULL OF IT**!" As mentioned earlier in this book, the original "Food Guide Pyramid" (1970s) recommended we eat more carbohydrates than any other food category. The newly revised USDA approved (2011) Food Guide Pyramid (called "My Plate") recommends 30% of our diets be from grains. "My Plate" also recommends breaking &/or neglecting most – if not all 10 – of the "10 Dietary Commandments!"

Controversy over the relationship between the level of cholesterol in the blood & the incidence/risk of atherosclerosis

The vast majority of doctors & medical scientists consider there is a link between the level of cholesterol in the blood and the incidence/risk of atherosclerosis.[99,271] A small (but growing) group of scientists question this link[272] – possibly due to the results of the *Framingham Heart Study*![273] The *Framingham Heart Study* found:[273]

- For men **47 or younger**, there **WAS** an association between high levels of blood "total cholesterol" & increased likelihood of **future heart attacks**.
- However, this study found **NO** relationship – for men **over 47** – between high levels of cholesterol & **dying** of a heart attack.

Keep in mind, there are other atherosclerotic events (like ischemic strokes & TIAs) besides heart attacks – which the "Framingham General Cardiovascular Risk Profile" *currently* takes into account.[273]

High ratios of LDL/HDL & total cholesterol/HDL are considered 2 of the strongest predictors of atherosclerotic disease.[98,99] Remember, you can't calculate the first ratio without measuring the "total cholesterol!" Ultimately, the decision is between you & your physicians.

Obesity, triglyceride levels, insulin sensitivity, endothelial function, & thrombogenicity (tendency to get a blood clot &/or embolus), among others, that play a role in atherosclerosis, although it seems, in the absence of the abovementioned 2 adverse blood lipid ratios, the other known risk factors may only have a weak atherogenic effect.[98]

The most harmful fats (a fact that is NOT controversial) are the trans-fats &/or hydrogenated oils! Trans-fats increase the risk of CHD (Coronary Heart Disease) more than any other macronutrient, conferring a substantially increased risk at even low levels of consumption (1-3% total energy intake)![93] **Replacing healthful fats** (like the "super-cleansing fats" mentioned above) in our diets (in the past 40 years) **with refined carbohydrates & hydrogenated oils &/or trans-fats** (all strongly correlated to an increased risk of atherosclerosis) is definitely a factor in why society has developed a severe case of "*Blood Clot Paranoia*"(as mentioned in "Dietary Commandment #6")!

No FAT Lives on an Island!

The American Heart Association[274] (as well as most medical, heart-health, & government authorities) advises that dietary intake of <u>saturated fat</u> is a risk factor for atherosclerosis. However, there are many major flaws with this general advice (In my humble opinion):

- Replacement of carbs by lauric acid (a type of SFA found abundantly in coconut oil, palm oil, & somewhat in goat milk fat) has actually resulted in a significantly lower total cholesterol/HDL & lower LDL/HDL ratios![100] In fact (as mentioned previously), if these fats are cultured as a PROBIOTIC food source – as well, then they will possess the amazing heart healthful benefits (as well as overall benefits) as other probiotic food sources. Thus, "cultured coconut milk" & "cultured goat's milk yogurt" are "super-cleansing fats" & "super-cleansing foods!"
- Despite often decades of efforts & thousands of people randomized, there is still only *limited & inconclusive evidence* of the effects of consuming foods high in SFAs on cardiovascular morbidity &/or mortality![275] Despite the fact that consumption of ALL types of SFAs raise the 3 types of blood cholesterol measurements (total cholesterol, HDL, & LDL), none of the SFAs have shown to raise the most important[98,99] blood cholesterol ratios (total cholesterol/HDL & LDL/HDL).[100] In fact (as already mentioned), one type of SFA called lauric acid (found high in coconut oil & less in dairy fat) actually improves (lowers) these important ratios![100]
- Dietary fats & oils always consist of a mixture of fatty acids, & each fat & oil has its own characteristic fatty acid composition. No fat lives on an island! Sesame seed oil is healthful as it has almost a 1:1 ratio of MUFAs & PUFAs (omega 6 fatty acids) – as well as other types of fatty acids.
- Breaking versus Following all "10 Dietary Commandments" when consuming fat sources are diametrically opposed to each other (regarding the health/harm effect to your body).   See the example/study below.

One study[276] showed that substituting carbohydrates for nuts (same calories) was associated with a 30% reduction in CHD (Coronary Heart Disease) risk; &

substituting SFAs for nut fat (same calories) was associated with a 45% reduction in CHD risk! However, we must keep in mind that many nuts (like Brazil nuts & cashews) possess slightly over 20% of their total fat composition as SFAs (Saturated Fatty Acids)![74]   Studies[277] that have shown a heart health benefit from replacing the intake of most SFAs with non-trans, non-hydrogenated PUFAs (Polyunsaturated Fatty Acids) were (most likely) **NOT** done with 100% "unsaturated" "PUFA" food sources!   No fat lives on an island!!

Therefore, any study that claims the healthfulness or harmfulness of any of the fats (or carbs) should make us wonder:

- How do the studies **define what a SFA, PUFA, or MUFA food source** is? In the abovementioned study[276] raw nuts were considered a MUFA & PUFA food source.   What were the SFA food sources in this - & all the other studies?
- How do they **define what a carbohydrate food source** is? No carbohydrate lives on an island either! Consuming the carbs of raw organic prunes & apples is a world more healthful than the refined carbs found in soft drinks!
- What was the **quality of the food sources**? Was it organic/organically raised? Were the goats or cows fed organic grass?   Were the animal food sources fed sugars -including grains & donuts?! Were the animal food sources injected with hormones or antibiotics?
- How were the **food-sources prepared**? Were they fried with hydrogenated or trans-fat oils?
- A soft boiled "free range" egg (from a chicken raised on organic feed & without injections of antibiotics or hormones) should NOT be lumped together with non-organic eggs fried with hydrogenated &/or trans-fat oils!   Both are high in SFAs. However, one may heal you & the latter may harm you!
- Raw, unprocessed unsweetened organic cocoa should NOT be lumped together with roasted, processed, non-organic cocoa with dairy & sugar added to it! One may heal you & the latter may harm you!
- Raw organic nuts should NOT be considered in the same "category" of food source as non-organic nuts with salt, sugar, & roasted with hydrogenated oils. The first may heal you & the latter may harm you!
- "Super-cleansing meats" (mentioned later on) cooked with water or extra-virgin coconut oil (baked or broiled) should not be put in the same category as non-organically raised meats (with added hormones & antibiotics) fried with hydrogenated oils!   Again, the first may heal you & the latter may harm you!

II.B. "Super-*Cleansing* Proteins"

All below mentioned "super-cleansing protein" food sources should be "Organic" or "Organically Raised."   "Super-Cleansing Protein" food sources during the "**Cleansing Phase**" would include:

- Raw Nuts – especially almonds, pecans, & Brazil nuts; Raw Sunflower & Pumpkin Seeds; Raw Sprouted Lentils & Beans - including sprouted soybeans; &raw Cocoa Powder.

Super-Cleansing Protein" food sources during the "**Lifestyle Phase**" would include:

- Probiotic Goat's Milk Yogurt (no fruit added) & Kefir; Probiotic Soybeans – Doenjang, Tempeh, & Natto; & Eggs (preferably soft boiled with yolk liquid & orange), Goose Meat, Chicken, Turkey, Lamb, & Beef!

Remember: **amino acids** are the building blocks of protein.   When amino acids are "free-form" (meaning they are in their purest form – needing no digestion & are absorbed directly into the bloodstream)[15] & taken with water (without food): they can have powerful effects on the body.   The effects of **Glycine, Glutamine, Glutathione** (working synergistically with Glycine & Glutamine), & **Carnitine** were already shown earlier.   Other examples of amino acids affecting the body include:[15]

- **Arginine** may be helpful in treating sterility in men – as well as helping in maintaining a proper nitrogen balance. Similar to the way nitric oxide works, arginine may lower blood pressure – as well as help with impotence. *Cautions*: As per Phyllis Balch (Author of *Prescription for Nutritional Healing*, 5th Edition), *Supplemental arginine should be avoided by:[15] People with viral infections such as herpes; Pregnant & lactating women; & People with schizophrenia should avoid amounts over 30mg/day. Long-term use, especially of high doses, is not recommended as several weeks of large doses may result in thickening & coarsening of the skin.*
- **L-lysine** may possess anti-viral benefits – making it useful in fighting cold sores & the herpes viruses. This amino acid *works synergistically with vitamin C & bioflavonoids to effectively fight &/or prevent herpes outbreaks (especially if arginine is avoided).*

II.C. "Super-*Cleansing* Carbohydrates"

Like fat, protein, & calories - no carbohydrate lives on an island either! **Healthful fruits** would include all raw, organic fruits. Some "**super-fruits**" (already mentioned & referenced earlier in this chapter) would include raw organic:

- Apples (do not eat the seeds), prunes, raisins, & the following berries:
    - Acai; Himalayan Gogi; Blueberries; Cranberries; Black berries; Raspberries; & Strawberries.

Harmful fruit may include **fruit juices, non-organic bananas**, & "**sulphured**" fruits.[78] Non-organic bananas & dried sulphured fruits are man-made & moderate in "toxic-mucus" Most, if not all, **fruit juices** bought in the store are dead (have been made over 24 hours) & are, therefore, lacking in living enzymes. Most fruit juices have no fiber, are high in simple sugar (even if none is added), & are, therefore, high in glycemic load.

      Healthful "super-grains" would include organic sprouted: quinoa, millet, oats, & brown rice.   If these grains are raw they can be consumed during the "Cleansing Phase."   Remember (as mentioned/referenced previously in this chapter), sprouting these grains converts them into vegetables with an almost complete elimination of toxic mucus capacity!

      Harmful grains would include non-organic corn, wheat, gluten, French fries, potato chips, mashed potatoes (in excess), etc. As will be mentioned later in "super-cleansing meats," animals fed a diet high in grains (like these harmful grains) become fatter. Therefore, if you are looking to gain body fat = eat more grains.

Remember, some adults need to gain body fat to achieve optimal health. However, the majority of adults need to lose (because they ***ARE FULL OF*** excess body fat!)!

    <u>Healthful Vegetables</u> would include almost all organic vegetables. If they are edible/digestible raw, they should be eaten raw! Sprouting the beans, peas, lentils, & grains converts them into vegetables & (for the most part) eliminates the toxic mucus. Thus, "**super-cleansing vegetables**" would be considered any organic, raw, sprouted: vegetable, beans, peas, lentils, & even grains! The "**super-cleansing vegetables**" pickled beets & pickled carrots are a probiotic food source & are, therefore (if low in sodium), also a "super-cleansing food!"

    <u>Harmful Vegetables</u> would include non-organic fried vegetables (especially if fried with hydrogenated oils &/or trans-fats).

    "**Super-Carbohydrate Drinks**" would include raw organic:
-    Kombucha; & Vegetable juices like wheatgrass, cilantro, & barley grass juice. Other green vegetable juices would be included here as well. They should all be consumed fresh within 30 minutes of juicing.

<u>Harmful High Carbohydrate Drinks</u> would include:
-    Diet sodas; Sugary Sodas & off the shelf energy drinks (dead & full of caffeine, sugar, corn syrup, & sometimes even turpentine!); & Fruit juices off the shelves (dead & full of sugar).

Just look at the contents & see how many grams of sugar they contain per serving (& be careful as to serving size). Many fruit juices – or other store-brand juices & "energy" drinks contain close to 100 grams of sugar in one 16 ounce bottle! The caffeine may give you an un-natural nervous energy rush temporarily. However, it may interfere with your sleep, memory, & overall health long-term (especially those loaded with sugar & who knows what else).

    Caffeine gives you energy (often a nervous energy that acts as a vasoconstrictor & heart rate accelerator as it stimulates the sympathetic – "flight or fight response" – nervous system). Panax Ginseng Root Extract (on the other hand) is an adaptogen that may give you energy when you *need it*! So if I feel run down (during the "Lifestyle Phase") – or believe I am going to have a "high stress" day: I take natural, God-created adaptogens like organic Ginseng Root Extract (also needs to be raw – if during the "Cleansing Phase")!

II.D. "Super-*Cleansing* Fiber"

"**Super-Cleansing Fiber**" food sources (already mentioned & referenced previously in this chapter) would include raw, organic: Vegetables; Fruits; Sprouted peas, lentils, & beans – including sprouted soybeans & cocoa beans; Wheat-free grains like sprouted quinoa & sprouted oats. Sprouted grains (such as sprouted: oats, millet, & brown rice) are also "super-cleansing fiber" food sources that – when cooked - may be consumed in the: "Lifestyle Phase." If they are 100% raw, they can be consumed in the "Cleansing Phase."

Remember: sprouting the beans, peas, lentils, vegetables, & grains usually reduces their fiber content.[74] However, the sprouting process also eliminates (for the most part) any "toxic mucus!"[78] The more fiber you consume from these "super-cleansing fiber" food sources, the more toxins you cleanse from your intestines – as well as your entire body.[8,23] Increasing your fiber content from these "super-cleansing fiber" food sources is considered one of the top 7 ways to detoxify pesticides from your body.[8]

If you are trying to find fiber on the labels of raw food containers, consider the following:

- "**Soluble Fiber**" can be found in the above. This type of fiber "absorbs" the toxins from inside the body & moves it "out of the body" & **into the intestines**.
- "**Insoluble Fiber**" can be found in the above also. This type of fiber simply acts as an "intestinal broom" to push the toxins **out of the large intestines** (& into the toilet bowl).

As one can see, both types of fiber have value.

Harmful Fiber food sources would include dead, non-organic:[80]
- Whole Wheat, wheat bran, etc.;[78,80] High fiber breads & cereals containing wheat, gluten, &/or genetically modified corn; Fiber supplements (dead) containing chemicals similar to those used in anti-freeze!

The truth about why the abovementioned fiber food sources should be considered harmful was illustrated in the "10 Dietary Commandments." The lies about these harmful fiber food sources being healthful are just another example of how we have become more "*FULL OF IT*" than ever before!

II.E. "3 Super-*Cleansing* Teas"

Realize there are many other varieties of tea in the world that have specific health benefits. In fact, there are many other varieties of tea that may be able to "detox" you as well – or greater – than these three. However, I am choosing these simply as my own preference for the purpose of detoxification ("cleansing"). Remember: all adults (& probably most adolescents) need to "cleanse their bodies of toxins" as they are "*FULL OF IT*"

These 3 teas may be rotated on a daily or weekly basis – as they all have amazing health benefits.

1. **Organic Green Tea**. Believed to have antioxidant properties – as well as possibly weight loss & blood sugar control benefits. Green tea may also be considered one of the best natural liver-detox foods.[88]

2. "***Organic Mulling Spices by R.W. Knudsen.***" This tea contains all organic ingredients – including: cinnamon, cloves, ginger, orange peel, & lemon peel. These spices (especially clove & cinnamon) may have the most antioxidants (by weight) of any "food."[26] Besides being loaded with these "super-cleansing herbs/spices," it tastes great! In addition, I don't believe this violates "Dietary Commandment #10" as they use the peel/skin of the orange & lemon – versus the fruit/pulp. However, if you do believe this violates "Dietary Commandment #10," then consider **Kombucha** tea (or the above or below) as a healthful replacement. **Kombucha** tea is a fermented probiotic-rich food/tea that (as mentioned previously) is a super-cleansing food/tea & tastes great!

3. "***Essiac Powder Formula from Rene M. Caisse, RN***." This tea contains all organically grown herbs – including burdock root, sheep sorrel leaves, slippery elm bark, & Indian rhubarb root.[278] Consuming burdock root (in this tea form) is considered one of the best 7 ways to detox pesticides from your body.[9] "*Burdock root helps flush toxins through urination & perspiration*."[8] This amazing combination of "cleansing" herbs tastes great & has been used for decades to help reduce the "*FULL OF IT* Level*" of cancer![278]

II.F. "Super-*Cleansing* Soy" versus "Harmful Soy:" The Great versus the Ugly
"**Super-Cleansing Soy**" food sources would include organic:
- **Raw Sprouted Soybeans** = an enzyme-rich healthful food that is easily absorbed.[78,279]

251

- **Natto, doenjang, & tempeh**.[78,279] These cultured/fermented "super-cleansing foods" are also a great source of probiotics. Miso is also a soy-based "super-cleansing food" – but is usually very high in sodium.

As the world has become more integrated, Americans (in the past 20 years) have been including soybean-based foods (as well as other foods) to their diets. The problem is that most Americans don't consume the abovementioned extremely healthful soybean based foods. We have been lied to - once again (making us *__FULL OF IT__*)! I have come to disclose the truth. Hopefully the below shows you *the truth - & sets you free!*

Americans have been adding to their diets **non-fermented &/or un-sprouted, processed "Ugly" soybean-based foods** (with high toxic mucus capability)[78] such as:[279]

- **Soy-milk; soy-cheese; soy-burgers; soy-ice cream**; etc.

Some major problems with these non-fermented, un-sprouted processed "**ugly**" soybean-based foods have been listed by Fallon S & Enig M (in an article in *Newlife* entitled *"How Safe is SOY?"*):[279]

- As mentioned in "Dietary Commandment #4:" They are almost as "**toxic mucus-forming**" (**& constipating**) as non-fermented (non-cultured) cow's milk products (the most "toxic mucus-forming" & constipating of all foods)![78] Thus, these processed non-fermented, un-sprouted soybean-based foods create almost as much intestinal putrefaction as non-fermented cow's milk.[78,279] Fermented soybean-based foods & sprouted soybeans (on the other hand) are easy to digest for most people.[78]
- *Vegetarians who consume them as a substitute for meat risk severe mineral deficiencies.*[279]
- *Oriental children who do not get enough meat to counteract the effects of a high phytate diet (found in processed soy-based foods), frequently suffer rickets & stunting of their growth. "Parents would do well to ask their six-year old boys whether they would prefer to be six-foot-one or five-foot-seven when they grow up, before substituting eggs & meat products for soymilk & tofu."*[279]
- They have no anti-carcinogenic effects. Isoflavone a-glycosides are anti-carcinogenic substances found in fermented soybean products. *However, in non-fermented soybean-based foods (such as tofu & soymilk), the isoflavones are present in an altered form as beta-glycoside conjugates, which have no anti-carcinogenic effects!*[279]

II.G. "Super-*Cleansing* Milk"

"**Super-Cleansing Milk**" Food sources would include organic &/or organically-raised (fed organic feed –mostly grasses & not injected with any hormones or antibiotics) – if applicable:

- **Cultured coconut milk** – unsweetened & full of healthful probiotics.
- **Cultured Goat's Milk** containing at least 1 billion viable probiotic cells per cup. This includes **goat's milk yogurt; acidophilus goat's milk; & kefir from goat's milk**.
- **& cultured plain, unsweetened, Cow's milk yogurt** - with at least **50 billion viable probiotic cells (organisms)** per cup – to reduce the toxic-mucus capability of the cow's milk to less than 1%.[78] However, very few brands ever disclose to the consumer how much they contain. The reader may argue that the abovementioned "super-cleansing milk" food sources seem to all have the consistency of yogurt or a "milk-shake" (pertaining to the kefir) due to them containing the "super-cleansing probiotics." The above may be "liquefied" in a blender with filtered water added – if a thinner consistency is desired.

Jordan Rubin, N.D., C.N.C. (in his book *The Maker's Diet*) outlines below some of the superior (when compared to cow's milk) health benefits attributed to goat's milk consumption:[1]

- *Goat's milk is less allergenic, does not suppress the immune system, & is easier to digest than cow's milk.* As mentioned in "Dietary Commandment #4:" Goat's milk has an estimated 20% toxic mucus capability & cultured goat's milk (with at least 1 billion viable probiotic cells per cup) has an estimated 5% (or less) toxic mucus capability.[78] This is dramatically lower than the estimated 100% toxic mucus capability of cow's milk (or the 50% toxic mucus capability of a cultured cow's milk yogurt containing 1 billion viable probiotic cells/organisms per cup).[78] *Goat's milk may digest in a baby's stomach in 20 minutes, whereas pasteurized cow's milk may take 8 hours.*
- Goat's milk has more **buffering capacity than over-the-counter antacids.** The USDA & Prairie View A & M University in Texas have confirmed that goat's milk has more acid-buffering capacity than cow's milk, soy infant formula, & non-prescription antacid drugs![280]
- Goat's milk **alkalinizes the digestive system & the blood stream** *because it is the dairy product highest in glutamine!*
- Goat's milk contains **twice the healthful medium chain fatty acids**, such as capric and caprylic acids – which may help prevent/treat candida albicans (a disease caused by a yeast fungus).
- Goat's milk is a **rich source of the trace mineral selenium** – a necessary nutrient noted for its' immune modulation & antioxidant properties.[7,15,49,82]
- There may be an **iron deficiency (& bleeding for infants) risk with cow's milk.**[165] The American Academy of Pediatrics (AAP) recommends that children under 1 year old not drink cow's milk (unfortified = without iron added to it) because the consumption of unfortified cow's milk by infants & toddlers has been found to interfere with iron absorption & cause internal bleeding in about 40% of otherwise healthy infants![165] The loss of iron in the form of GI bleeding from cow's milk apparently stops after the age of 1.[165] The combination of the high amount of casein & calcium in unfortified cow's milk products (includes ice cream, cheeses, etc.) interferes with iron.[165] In addition, most "non-organic" dairy products contain additives that interfere with iron absorption[15] &, therefore, may worsen (or increase the risk of) iron deficiency anemia. Again (as demonstrated in "Commandment #6), you need a balance between preventing an excess – versus a deficiency - in iron.

Remember, the abovementioned "super-cleansing milk" food sources are also probiotic food sources – which (as mentioned earlier in this chapter) may actually help lower the "_**FULL OF IT**_ Level" of bleeding, anemia, atherosclerosis, gastrointestinal disorders, immune disorders, & possibly osteoporosis!

II.H. "Super-*Cleansing* Meats"

"Super-Cleansing Meats" would include the following animal meats organically fed/raised – without injections of hormones or antibiotics:
- Turkey; Chicken; Goose; Goat; Lamb; Veal; & Beef.

These "super-cleansing meats" (because they are not "alive") must be eaten in the "Lifestyle Phase." As mentioned in "Dietary Commandment # 3," adults may benefit from a digestive enzyme supplement to break down/absorb these meats better.[1,15,49] A good digestive enzyme supplement should contain Pancreatin (supplying **protease** to break down the protein, **amylase** to help break down the amylase, & **lipase** to help break down/absorb the fat in the food).[1,15,49] Some people may benefit from a digestive enzyme that also contains HCL.[1,15,49] This was analyzed thoroughly in "Dietary Commandment #3."

These "super-cleansing meats" possess the following benefits:
- They contain the heme form of iron – believed to be the **easiest form of iron for humans to absorb**.[15] The heme form of iron is also considered **the fastest**

way to __restore__ iron in the blood to normal.[15]   Thus, may help **prevent anemia**. Remember, we always need a balance between preventing an excess - versus a deficiency - of iron.

- They contain *cysteine, glutathione, coenzyme Q10, MSM, & carnitine*![1] Lamb & goat meat represent two of nature's best sources of **carnitine**[1] – to possibly cleanse (help burn) the excess fat off your body.   Thus, these red meats may actually help **prevent atherosclerosis & obesity**!
- Goose meat - & to a lesser extent beef & chicken – is a good source of *Menaquinone-4 (a type of vitamin K2* mentioned earlier in this chapter). Thus, they may help **prevent bleeding, atherosclerosis, & osteoporosis**! In addition, this vitamin K2 (as mentioned previously in this chapter) is absorbed far greater than vitamin K1 (found abundantly in green leafy vegetables!
  - The protein from these "super-cleansing meats" may represent nature's best![1]

Keep in mind: light/"white" meat turkey & chicken (without the skin) tends to contain much lower amounts of iron, cholesterol, & saturated fat than the other "super-cleansing meats."[74] Therefore, most adults *may* benefit from consuming them (during the "Lifestyle Phase") a few times per week. The other "super-cleansing meats" *may* benefit many adults on a less frequent basis.

Grass-fed versus Grain-Fed

When the abovementioned animals are grass-fed (as compared to grain-fed), their meats usually contain more of the omega 3 fatty acids.[281]   However, the 0.03 grams of omega 3 fatty acids in a 3 ounce serving of grass-fed lean meats & turkey is truly insignificant.[282]

However, grain-fed beef & lamb (when compared to grass-fed beef & lamb) have been found to be fatter – higher in total fat & saturated fat.[283,284]   In most countries, lamb is grass-fed.   In the U.S., lamb is often "finished" (i.e. fattened before slaughter – to make extra money as they sell the lamb per pound) with grain![284]   We can learn a lot from the animals!   If grains make the animals fatter, is there really any doubt that a high-grain diet will make humans fatter!?

Keep in mind, these "super-cleansing meats" become harmful when they are cooked with trans-fats &/or hydrogenated oils!   As mentioned earlier, it is best to bake or broil them with **extra-virgin COCONUT oil**[1] -or boil them with filtered water.

II.I. "Super-*Cleansing* Shakes"

Slowly chewing (& "swishing" in your mouth to assure some sublingual absorption) of these "Super-Cleansing Shakes" may be the best way to **optimally absorb the healthful micronutrients** (as well as the healthful macronutrients) in our healthful/super-cleansing foods & supplements!

Super-Cleansing Shakes – during the "**Cleansing Phase**" may include any combination of the following raw, vegan, organic ingredients (mixed thoroughly in a powerful blender):

- Filtered water; Apple(s) (cut out the core to assure no seeds are consumed as apple seeds contain a small amount of cyanide); "Super-Nuts" mentioned earlier in this chapter (let the nuts soak in the filtered water in the blender for at least a few minutes. Some nutritionists believe the nuts become even easier to assimilate if soaked overnight); Seeds (Pumpkin &/or Sunflower); Sprouted beans; Pea, sunflower, &/or broccoli sprouts; Unprocessed, raw cocoa (may be found in powdered form); &/or freshly juiced wheatgrass juice.

254

Super-Cleansing Shakes – during the "**Lifestyle Phase**" may add the following organic ingredients:
- Greens powders (which should contain wheatgrass & barley grass juice powder; pectin; spirulina &/or chlorella; & 1 billion live cells of probiotics per serving); Soft Boiled egg(s) – most adults would probably benefit from at least 1 per week; Any of the "super-cleansing teas" (can even substitute the filtered water); Any of the "super-cleansing milk" food sources***; Protein Powder free of gluten, dairy, sugar, cane juice, & soy; Dash of cinnamon – may have glucose control benefits & may, therefore, help prevent type II diabetes & weight gain; Fenugreek & thyme powder (great nasal decongestants –can empty the contents of the capsules). Fenugreek may also have glucose control benefits & may, therefore, help prevent type II diabetes & weight gain; Maitake mushroom (antioxidant properties); Marshmallow &/or slippery elm bark (soothing for the gastrointestinal system); Milk Thistle; Turmeric powder; Ginger root powder; Resveratrol powder; &/or any other herbs &/or foods deemed beneficial to you.

Realize in any phase, raw & organic vegetables (including herbs like ginger) may be added to these "super-cleansing shakes." The herbs in capsule-form can be emptied during the "Lifestyle Phase." Remember: these *shakes must be CHEWED & consumed slowly* to assure optimal absorption. The blender pitcher (container) should be clear & colorless glass (not plastic – as mentioned in chapter 3).

***Adding these "super-cleansing milk" food sources to the shakes creates somewhat of a "milk-shake" consistency. Freezing them (& then allowing them to thaw out for an hour or so) can create a delicious "super-cleansing dessert" similar to an "Italian Ice" or "ice cream" consistency. The more "super-cleansing milk" food sources added to the "super-cleansing shake" will create more of an "ice cream" consistency. The more filtered water used will create more of an "Italian ice" consistency. These are truly delicious desserts you should never feel guilty about eating!

II.J. "Super-*Cleansing* Homeopathy"

Many nutritionists & homeopathic physicians believe that homeopathic "medicines" can be extremely powerful healing/cleansing agents. However, they are also believed to be among the safest preparations to medical science.[15] The majority of these homeopathic preparations are derived from plants – with the intention of seeking to stimulate the body's own natural healing processes.[15]

Homeopathic physicians may recommend "Super-Cleansing Homeopathic" preparations to help:
- Lower one's "*FULL OF IT* Level"
- & cleanse your liver, bowels, sinuses, &/or any other cell/organ/organ system in the body from allergens, free-radicals, toxic heavy metals, etc.

Almost all herbs & other supplements can be taken in a homeopathic form. This may be the safest way to consume herbs & other supplements –like glandular extracts such as:[285]
- Thymus gland extract to boost the immune system. The thymus gland shrinks from adolescence on & becomes a "*shadow of its former self by middle age.*" This may be one reason many immune disorders begin at middle age.

- Thyroid gland extract to help control our metabolism if diagnosed with hypothyroidism. This should only be taken (like anything that goes in your mouth) if approved by your physician (preferably one that is familiar with homeopathy).

Two of the most respected companies that prepare & sell "super-cleansing homeopathic" preparations include "Des-Bio" (www.desbio.com) & "Bio-Active Nutritional" (www.bioactivenutritional.com).

CHAPTER 7: Dietary Examples of the
"YOU'RE FULL OF IT - DIET"

Remember: these are simply **examples** of the diet friends, family, & I have been successful with over the past 17 years or so. There are so many variations of these foods – as well as when & how much to consume. These have already been addressed in Chapters 5 & 6. You have to create your own taste. Don't focus on what you should not eat. That is like trying not to think of a purple cow. See- now you are thinking of a purple cow! Focus on the thousands (if not hundreds of thousands) of variations of healthful foods (with their allowed combinations) that you find delicious!

I.   The "Cleansing Phase"

Remember you must follow all ten of the "10 Dietary Commandments" during the "Cleansing Phase." **No EXCEPTIONS**!!   Therefore, all food must be 100% alive, vegan, organic (preferably USDA certified), combined correctly, eaten in a God-pleasing manner, etc.

Wake up & immediately drink freshly juiced organic wheatgrass juice (1 ounce or so for prevention/2-4 ounces for curative purposes).   May juice organic raw cilantro, raw barley grass, &/or raw organic broccoli sprouts with the wheatgrass juice.   These can all be juiced together with most wheatgrass juicers.   You should consume these juices within 30 minutes of juicing them.   Some people may prefer to drink these juices later in the day – or after meal #1 (for example).   In fact, some may prefer to add these live juices to their "super-cleansing shakes" as part of that meal!   That's why they have menus at restaurants (to each their own).

If you drink the 1-4 ounces of the abovementioned live juices separate from your "super-cleansing shake," wait 5 minutes before (or after) consuming meal #1.

Remember to drink "**CLEANSING WATER**" throughout the day (1 hour before & after meals of course).   Cleansing Water in the "Cleansing Phase" is filtered water with the following added raw, vegan, organic, cleansing ingredients:

- Lemon. Of course wash off the lemon with filtered water, cut it open, & squeeze out the fresh lemon juice into your clear glass container throughout the day.   Remember, lemon is a "fruit" enzymatically & can't be sipped with your "non-fruit" meals!
- Oregano. Should use a blender to liquefy the raw, organic oregano. Oregano drops can suffice in the "Lifestyle Phase."
- Ginger. Again, a blender should be used for optimal absorption.
- &/or Honey.

I prefer most "meals" (many would consider them "snacks" – my Jewish family members consider it "noshing") to have a fair amount of "super-cleansing fat & protein" food sources (mentioned in section II of chapter 6) to avoid breaking "Dietary Commandment #8."

Meal #1: A raw, organic "super-cleansing shake" (mentioned in last chapter).   My favorite = the raw *cocoa shake*!

Meal #2 (2-3 hours after the 1st meal): An organic lettuce "super-wrap." Best lettuces for these wraps would include organic: iceberg (a "super-cleansing food" mentioned in the last chapter & "Dietary Commandment #4"), romaine, green leaf, etc.   Put organic avocados, raw sprouted beans, raw almond butter, raw organic cilantro, slices of red, yellow, &/or orange pepper (&/or whatever other raw vegetables/foods you enjoy).

Meal #3 (1 hour after the 2nd meal): An organic "super-salad" with organic scallions, avocados, & whatever other vegetables you enjoy (no tomatoes).

Meal #4 (1-3 hours after the 3rd meal): A handful of washed raw "super-cleansing nuts" (such as Brazil, Almonds, or pecans (mentioned in last chapter) – or edible seeds (such as raw sunflower or pumpkin seeds).   Remember to was off with filtered water before consuming.

Two hours after finishing last meal, drink 16 ounces of "cleansing water" in a clear colorless <u>glass</u> mug/bottle/container.

Meal #5 (1 hour + after finishing water): Raw sprouted quinoa with raw edible organic "super-seeds" (sunflower, pumpkin, etc.), raw sprouted beans, raw organic chopped celery, &/or whatever other raw, organic vegetable (non-starchy) you desire.

Meal #6 = Dessert! A glass of filtered water is recommended for most adults –as it is recommended that most adults avoid dessert –especially during the "Cleansing Phase." However (for those who are not as disciplined as some), dessert is permissible during the "Cleansing Phase." An example of an acceptable dessert during this phase includes:

- Raw *Chocolate Brownies*! Mix in a clear glass bowl 3 tablespoons of raw organic cocoa powder; 3 tablespoons of raw organic almond butter; 1 teaspoon of raw organic honey; & add enough filtered water to stir until powder not seen. Put in the fridge for 1 night or more & then shape into rectangular pieces (brownies) or balls (I call them "*Uncle David's cocoa balls*"). Delicious, nutritious, & should satiate your hunger due to the high fiber content.
- Another dessert allowed during the "cleansing phase" are my <u>raw vegan</u> "**super-cleansing shakes**" <u>**frozen**</u> (& let thaw out before consuming). See "super-cleansing shakes" in section II of chapter 6.

Notes: Meal #2, 3, or 4 may simply be a raw "super-cleansing fruit" bowl. This may include raw organic prunes, raisins, berries, apples, etc. This may also simply be a raw melon. This "fruit substitution" should **NEVER** be your last meal of the day/night. Fruit should be limited for most adults choosing to lose weight. However, substituting a protein/fat meal with this fruit meal may benefit someone before exercising. Remember meal #1 ("super-cleansing shake") may include an apple. Therefore (even if you avoid fruit the rest of the day), you will still be getting the revitalizing/rejuvenating property of fruit via meal #1.

Remember: these are only examples! There are such a great number of "permissible" foods &, therefore, permissible combinations of foods. These are simply examples. Think of these diet examples as furniture/decorations in a house (or biblically, a "*temple of the Holy Spirit*"). You don't have to decorate the house/temple the same as others!

II.   The "Lifestyle Phase"

This phase also obeys the "10 Dietary Commandments" –but allows their exceptions. Again, these are simply examples.

Remember the "Cleansing Water" in the Lifestyle Phase can use the same ingredients in the "Cleansing Phase" – as well as (or replaced by) the following cleansing organic ingredients to your clear, colorless glass container:

- Oregano oil. Two to three drops/day may be potent enough to help cleanse fungus & yeast (such as Candida Albicans) from your body.
- Apple Cider Vinegar. One teaspoon/day may be enough to help cleanse your body from harmful microorganisms – to help prevent colds, the flu, etc. Adults (including adults that actually suffer with acid reflux) may be deficient in HCL! Those adults actually report better digestion/absorption of their food when they consume a teaspoon of this vinegar with their meals. However, not every adult is deficient in HCL (Hydrochloric acid). Those adults who have too much HCL should probably avoid apple cider vinegar as this may exacerbate acid-reflux problems in those people. Again, *ask your physician & buyer beware & that's why they have menus in restaurants*!
- Slippery Elm Bark & Marshmallow capsules emptied into the bottle to create a gastrointestinal soothing effect from mouth to anus.

Meal #1: Any "super-cleansing shake" (mentioned in last chapter). Remember, one can add the 1-4 ounces of freshly juiced wheatgrass – with or without cilantro, barley grass, &/or broccoli sprouts into these "super-cleansing shakes."

Meals #1-6 can be very similar to the meals in the "Cleansing Phase." However, consider the following benefits of the "Lifestyle Phase:"

- Now you can add healthful, <u>non-raw</u> foods such as: the "super-cleansing: foods, supplements, fats/oils, proteins, carbs, fiber, teas, soy, milk, meats, & shakes" mentioned in chapter 6. Gradually adding ("re-introducing") these non-raw foods one day at a time may help you determine if you are allergic to them.
- You still want to try to have the majority of your "plate" to be raw (& organic).
- Remember, most adults benefit from a digestive enzyme taken during a cooked "super-cleansing meat" (mentioned in chapter 6).
- Most adults also benefit from a multivitamin swallowed during meal #2, 3, or 4.
- Many adults benefit from swallowing a **food-based** calcium citrate & magnesium oxide with (or immediately after their dinner) to facilitate a restful sleep. Remember: green leafy vegetables (eaten @ Dinner time) provide your body with natural calcium & magnesium. I would consider these God-made greens superior to any man-made supplements.

Consider the following examples of "Lifestyle Phase" meals:

"**Jewish Penicillin:**" Rub extra-virgin coconut oil on the bottom of the pot. Sautee cut up onions & garlic. Then, add free-range chicken (organically raised without the injections of hormones or antibiotics) to pot. Add spices such as turmeric & oregano. Flip chicken over after is brown. Add spices to this bronzed side. Then flip over again, add water, & close lid. Let boil for 20 minutes & then flip over & cook for 20 more minutes with lid on top. Add cut up washed vegetables. Cook for 20 more minutes until chicken is edible. Delicious & nutritious.

- **Mulligatawny Soup**: Same as above – but I use - already cooked cut up chicken & potatoes - & add celery, apples, & a pinch of thyme.
- "**Uncle David's Cocoa Balls:**" Can add extra-virgin coconut oil, "super-cleansing milk" food sources, & a dash of cinnamon & vanilla to these to make them tastier (& a smoother, creamier texture).
- "**Uncle David's Lettuce Salad:**" Prepare the vinaigrette with: healthful organic oils (such as extra-virgin olive, sesame seed, sunflower seed, safflower seed, etc.) add goat cheese, avocado, oregano, & black pepper. Stir & then add raw pecans, lettuce, &/or any other vegetables (after washing them with filtered water of course) to this vinaigrette. Mix all together & make it into the shape of a heart for the people you love (including yourself)! If you don't want the vinaigrette to be so thick – then add sliced avocado & sprinkled goat cheese on top afterwards.
- "**Uncle David's Dip:**" Use the same thick vinaigrette as a dip for veggies, nuts, or any other non-fruit you desire.

259

- *"**Heavenly Pizza**:"* Use a gluten-free, wheat-free (& preferably yeast-free) bread/toast/dough as your base.   Add goat's cheese, extra-virgin coconut oil, & sliced red peppers. If desired, add other veggies (no tomatoes of course as tomatoes are enzymatically considered fruit).   After broiling a couple minutes (or until done – with the consistency of your choosing), remove from broiler & let sit until no longer dangerously hot.   Once cooled down a bit, feel free to apply healthy liquid oils (such as extra-virgin olive oil, sesame seed oil, safflower seed oil, or sunflower seed oil).   Rice cheese (mozzarella flavor/texture) may be substituted for the goat's cheese.   Delicious & nutritious!
- *"**Brooklyn's Delight Lettuce Wrap**:"* This is named after my beautiful cat Brooklyn (who converted me into a huge cat –as well as all-animal lover) & her favorite foods.   Use Iceberg lettuce as the wrap. Add free range turkey slices & a soft boiled egg (egg yolk should be liquid orange – not yellow or clumpy).   This will be messy (not for cats as they eat with their mouth) so you may want to use a spoon to consume!
- **Reuben Sandwich**: Can use organic tempeh or turkey – grilled with rice-based mozzarella cheese on gluten-free, wheat-free (& preferably yeast-free) toast. Add raw almond butter & healthful oils (such as extra-virgin olive, sesame seed, sunflower, or safflower oil).   Enjoy!

ENDNOTES

Acknowledgements

[i] Rubin J (2005). *The Maker's Diet*. Lake Mary, FL: Siloam – a Strang Co.

[ii] Balch PA (2010). *Prescription for Nutritional Healing*, 5th Edition. New York, NY: Avery – a Penguin Group Inc.

[iii] Pronsati MP (1991 January 14). "Aide Channels Frustration to Help People with Disabilities." *ADVANCE for Physical Therapists* **2**(2): 5.

[iv] Charla L (1990 Fall Issue). "SUNY Student Invents Robotic Arm." *PT Bulletin* volume S4: 13.

[v] Alpine WE (1991 February). "Ten Who Make a Difference - Highlighting student leaders: A Robot that Brushes Teeth." University @ Stony Brook – *Currents* **9**(1): 9.

CHAPTER 1: *"YOU'RE FULL OF"* SIN – causing More Diseases, Obesity, & Chronic Pain than ever before

All biblical references taken from
The Zondervan Corporation (2000). *New American Standard Bible.* Grand Rapids, Michigan: Zondervan Publishing House.

[1] Kohl HW 3rd, Craig CL, et al. (2012 July 21). "The pandemic of physical inactivity: global action for public health." *Lancet* **380**(9838): 294-305.
[2] Garber L (2012 July 19). "Physical Inactivity Killing 5 Million a Year." (http://naturalsociety.com/physical-inactivity-killing-5-million-a-year/)
[3] Andreyeva T, Sturm R, Ringel JS (2004). "Moderate and Severe Obesity Have Large Differences in Health Care Costs." *Obesity Research* **12** (12): 1936-1943.
[4] Barrett M (2012 July 7). (http://naturalsociety.com/portion-sizes-restaurants-quadruple/)

CHAPTER 2: Why *"YOU'RE FULL OF"* more *Mind & Soul* Toxins than ever before

[1] Rothman RH (1984). "A Study of Computer-Assisted Tomography." *Spine* **9**(6): 548.
[2] Webber H (1983). "Lumbar Disc Herniations: A Controlled Prospective Study with Ten Years of Observation." *Spine* **8**: 131-140.
[3] USDA (2011 June). (http://fnic.nal.usda.gov/dietary-guidance/myplatefood-pyramid-resources)
[4] CBNNews.com (2012 August 16). (http://www.cnb.com/cbnnews/us/2012/August/More-Americans-Identifying-asAtheists/)
[5] Barrett M, Natural Society (2013 February 17). (http://naturalsociety.com/leading-geneticist-human-intelligence-slowly-declining/)
[6] Aronson D (2009 November). "Cortisol – Its Role in Stress, Inflammation, & Indications for Diet Therapy." *Today's Dietitian* **11** (11): 38.
[7] *The Week* staff (2011 October 28). (http://theweek.com/article/index/220754/taxing-the-rich-a-guide-to-the-controversy)
[8] Joffe-Wal C (2013). "Unfit for work: The startling rise of disability in America." *Planet Money* (http://apps.npr.org/unfit-for-work/)
[9] Merline J (2013 April 25). "Record 8.9 Million People Now on Disability." (http://news.investors.com/042513-653555-disability-rolls-continue-to-explode.htm)
[10] Strauss S (2012 May 20). "America: Slouching Towards Third World Status." (http://www.huffingtonpost.com/steven-strauss/america-third-world-b_1531492.html).
[11] Stewart H (2010 September). (http://fivethirtyeight.blogs.nytimes.com/2010/09/19/consumer-spending-and-the-economy/)

CHAPTER 3: *"YOU'RE FULL OF"* more Direct *Body* Toxins than ever before

[1] Greenfield L (2012 March – last revision). "Over the Edge: Biological Stress & Chronic Conditions – A Self Instructional Program" - Continuing Educational for Healthcare Professionals. (http://www.consultantsforthefuture.com).
[2] Rubin JS (2005). *The Maker's Diet.* Lake Mary, FL: Siloam – a Strang Co.
[3] Beck L (2012 Copyright). "Finally: An Affordable, Valid & Reliable EMF Pollution Solution!" Grounding: skin to soil (http://www.becknaturalmedicine.com/).
[4] Evans A (2012 June 1st). (http://naturalsociety.com/living-a-disease-free-life-solutions-todaily-health-risks-that-lead-to-disease/)

[5] Barrett M (2012 May 17). (http://naturalsociety.com/average-american-diet-infographic/)
[6] Rogers SA (2002). *Detoxify or Die*. Prestige Publishing (www.Kospublishing.com/html/detox.html).
[7] Garber L (2012 September 19). (http://naturalsociety.com/bpa-making-you-fat-fueling-obesity/)
[8] Renter E (2013 June 27). (http://naturalsociety.com/6foods-ingredients-sold-u-s-banned-other-countries/)
[9] Marty D (2002 Jan – Feb). "Getting on Our Nerves." *The Environmental Magazine*.
[10] Bassil KL, et al. (2007 Oct). "Non-cancer health effects of pesticides: Systemic review & implications for family doctors." *Can. Fam. Physicians* **53** (10): 1712-20.
[11] http://www.epa.gov/pesticides/health/human.htm
[12] Sparrow CP & Olszewski J (1993 July). "Cellular oxidation of low density lipoprotein is caused by thiol production in media containing transition metal ions." *J. of lipid research* **34** (7): 1219-28.
[13] Marquez T (2004 Oct/Nov). "Organic Choices Clarified." *New Life Journal*.
[14] Steinman D & Epstein SS (1995). *The Safe Shopper's Bible: A Consumer's Guide to Nontoxic Household Products, Cosmetics, & Food*. New York: Hungry Minds, Inc.
[15] Centers for Disease Control and Prevention (2013 July 2). "Policy Impact: Prescription Painkiller Overdoses" (http://www.cdc.gov/homeandrecreationalsafety/rxbrief/).
[16] CDC Vital signs (2013 July). (http://www.cdc.gov/vitalsigns/PrescriptionPainkillerOverdoses/index.html)
[17] Joffe-Walt C (2013). "Unfit for Work: The startling rise of disability in America." *Planet Money* (http://apps.npr.org/unfit-for-work/)
[18] Garber L (2012 July 19). (http://naturalsociety.com/5-air-purifying-plants-your-home/)
[19] U.S. Environmental Protection Agency (2010 Oct. 12). "A Citizen's Guide to Radon." (http://www.epa.gov/radon/pubs/citguide.html)
[20] Environmental Working Group (2005, July). "Body Burden: The Pollution of Newborns." (http://www.ewg.org/reports/bodyburden2)
[21] Rauch M ((2004, Sept.-Oct.). "Pesticides Pollute Children." *Mothering*.
[22] Centers for Disease Control and Prevention (2009). "Chronic Diseases: The Power to Prevent, the Call to Control: At a Glance 2009." (http://www.cdc.gov/chronicdisease/resources/publications/aag/chronic.htm#)
[23] Fassa P (2013 July 17). (http://naturalsociety.com/12-tips-extinguishing-disease-causing-inflammation/)
[24] Kohl HW 3rd, Craig CL, et al. (2012 July 21). "The pandemic of physical inactivity: global action for public health." *Lancet* **380** (9838): 294-305.
[25] Garber L (2012 July 19). (http://naturalsociety.com/physical-inactivity-killing-5-million-a-year/)
[26] Aronson D (2009 November). "Cortisol: It's Role in Stress, Inflammation, & Indications for Diet Therapy." *Today's Dietitian* **11** (11): 38.
[27] Williams KJ, Tabas I (1995 May). "The Response-to-Retention Hypothesis of Early Atherogenesis." *Arteriosclerosis, thrombosis, & vascular biology* **15** (5): 551-61.
[28] Sparrow CP & Olszewski J (1993 July). "Cellular oxidation of low density lipoprotein is caused by thiol production in media containing transition metal ions." *J. of Lipid research* **34** (7): 1219-28.
[29] Brownstein D (2006). *Iodine: Why You Need It – Why You Can't Live Without It*, 2nd Edition. West Bloomfield, Michigan: Medical Alternatives Press.
[30] Wilson L (2012, August). "Detecting Toxic Metals." (http://drlwilson.com/Articles/DETECTING%20METALS.htm)
[31] Balch PA (2010). *Prescription for Nutritional Healing*, 5th Ed. New York, NY: Avery- a Penguin Group Inc.
[32] Sears ME, Kerr KJ & Bray RI (2012). "Arsenic, cadmium, lead & mercury in sweat: a systematic review." *J. Enviro.n Public Health* **1155** (2012): 184745.

[33] Genuis SJ, et al. (2011 August). "Blood, urine, and sweat (BUS) study: monitoring and elimination of bio-accumulated toxic elements." *Arch. Environ. Contam. Toxicol.* **61** (2): 344-57.

[34] Paris S, Nyberg R, Irwin M (1993). *S2 Course Notes: Advanced Thoracic, Lumbar & Pelvic Spines – Evaluation & Treatment.* St. Augustine, FL: Institute of Physical Therapy.

[35] Rothman RH (1984). "A Study of Computer-Assisted Tomography: Introduction." *Spine* **9** (6): 548.

[36] Webber H (1983). "Lumbar Disc Herniations: A Controlled Prospective Study with ten years of Observation." *Spine* 8:131-140.

[37] Paris S & Loubert P (1990). "Foundations of Clinical Orthopaedics." St. Augustine, FL: Institute of Physical Therapy.

[38] Turpie AGG (Author); Porter RS, Kaplan JL, et al. (editors) (2011). "Peripheral Venous & Lymphatic Disorders." *The MERCK MANUAL of Diagnosis & Therapy*, 19th Edition. Whitehouse Station, NJ: Merck Sharp & Dohme Corp. PP. 2224-36.

[39] Zuther J (2003 July 7). "Lymphedema- Taking Flight: How airline travel can affect patients with lymphedema." *Advance For Physical Therapists & Assistants*: 41-43.

[40] Zuther J, etal (2003). "Lymphedema Management Seminar Course Manual." Academy of Lymphatic Studies.

[41] McNamara D (2006 June). "Strong Link Seen Between Depression & Inflammation." *Clinical Psychiatry News*.

[42] Renter E (2012 September 15). (http://naturalsociety.com/cleaner-purer-air-try-air-cleaning-plants-nasa/)

[43] Libby P (Author); Longo DL, et al. (editors) (2012). "The Pathogenesis, Prevention, & Treatment of Atherosclerosis." *Harrison's Principles of Internal Medicine*, 18th Edition. New York, NY: McGraw-Hill Co., Inc. Pp. 1983 92.

[44] Garber L (2012 October 2). (http://naturalsociety.com/flouride-treatment-5-ways-to-detox-flouride/)

[45] Gucciardi A (2011 February 7). (http://naturalsociety.com/common-food-items-could-contain-180-times-more-flouride-than-tap-water/)

[46] Fassa P (2013 June 29). (http://naturalsociety.com/ditch-toxic-sunscreen-use-cocnut-oil-instead/)

CHAPTER 4: *"YOU'RE FULL OF"* Myths about OBESITY – as well as Nutrition

[1] USDA (2011 June). (http://fnic.nal.usda.gov/dietary-guidance/myplatefood-pyramid-resources)

[2] CDC NCHS (2010). "National Obesity Trends." (http://www.cdc.gov/obesity/data/trends.html)

[3] Mayo Clinic (2008 March 27). "Normal Weight Obesity: An Emerging Risk Factor for Heart & Metabolic Problems." *Science Daily* (http://www.sciencedaily.com/releases/2008/03/080327172025.htm)

[4] Muth ND (2009 December 2). (http://www.acefitness.org/blog/112/what-are-the-guidelines-for-percentage-of-body-fat/)

[5] OECD (2010). "Health at a Glance: Europe 2010." OECD Publishing.

[6] http://evolution.berkeley.edu/evolibrary/article/evo_2

[7] Blackburn GL, Walker WA (2005 July 1). "Science-based solutions to obesity: What are the roles of academia, government, industry, & health care?" *The American J. of Clin. Nutr.* **82** (1): 207-210.

[8] Weight Information Network (2006). "Statistics related to overweight & obesity: Economic costs related to overweight & obesity." (http://win.niddk.nih.gov/statistics)

[9] Kohl HW 3rd, Craig CL, et al. (2012 July 21). "The Pandemic of Physical Inactivity: global action for public health." *Lancet* **380** (9838): 294-305.

[10] Garber L (2012 July 19). (http://naturalsociety.com/physical-inactivity-killing-5-million-a-year/)

[11] Weiss J (2006). "Why we eat … and why we keep eating."

(http://insulitelabs.com/articles/Why-We-Eat.html)

[12] Barrett M (2012 July 7). (http://naturalsociety.com/portion-sizes-restaurants-quadruple/)

[13] Aronson D (2009 November). "Cortisol – It's Role in Stress, Inflammation, & Indications for Diet Therapy." *Today's Dietitian* **11** (11): 38.

[14] Greenfield LS (2012 March – last revision). "Over the Edge: Biological Stress & Chronic Conditions – a Self-Instructional Program" – Continuing Education for Healthcare Professionals. (www.consultantsforthefuture.com)

[15] Brownstein D (2006). *Iodine: Why You Need It, Why You Can't Live Without It*, 2nd Edition. West Bloomfield, Michigan: Medical Alternatives Press.

[16] Patterson S (2012 December 6). (http://naturalsociety.com/worried-about-flouride-exposure-protect-yoyrself-selenium/)

[17] Barrett M (2012 May 17). (http://www.naturalsociety.com/average-american-diet-infographic/)

[18] Balch PA (2010). *Prescription for Nutritional Healing*, 5th Edition. New York, NY: Avery – a Penguin Group Inc.

[19] Garber L (2012 September 19). (http://naturalsociety.com/bpa-making-you-fat-fueling-obesity/)

[20] McNamara D (2006 June). "Strong Link Seen Between Depression & Inflammation." *Clinical Psychiatry News*.

[21] American Heart Association (2007). "Inflammation, heart disease, & stroke: The role of C-Reactive Protein." (http://www.americanheart.org/presenter.jhtml?identifier=4648)

CHAPTER 5: "Natural" & "Super-Natural" Cleansing Methods; & CHAPTER 6: "Super-*Cleansing* Foods/Supplements"

The references for Chapter 6 are combined with Chapter 5's references. This is because Chapter 6 shares so many references with chapter 5 &, maybe, thought of as an extension or continuation of chapter 5.

[1] Rubin JS (2005). *The Maker's Diet*. Lake Mary, FL: Siloam – a Strang Co.

[2] Edwards J (2012 December 26). (http://www.naturalsociety.com/7-methods-holistic-detox-cleansing-body-toxic-exposure/)

[3] Barrett M (2012 March 9). (http://www.naturalsociety.com/infographic-why-you-need-more-sleep/)

[4] Gallagher P (2012 April 23). (http://www.naturalsociety.com/how-lack-of-sleep-affects-your-metabolism/)

[5] Avela J & Komi PV (1998 October). "Reduced stretch reflex sensitivity & muscle stiffness after long-lasting stretch – shortening cycle exercise in humans." *Eur. J. Appl. Physiol. Occup. Physiol.* **78** (5): 403-10.

[6] Paris SV & Loubert PV (1990). *FCO: Foundations of Clinical Orthopaedics*. St. Augustine, FL: Institute Press.

[7] Greenfield LS (2012 March). "Over the Edge: Biological Stress & Chronic Conditions. A Self-instructional Program." Continuing Education for Health Care Professionals. (http://www.consultantsforthefuture.com)

[8] Renter E (2012 November 18). (http://naturalsociety.com/how-to-detox-pesticides-body-7-ways/)

[9] Renter E (2013 January 1). (http://naturalsociety.com/4-simple-steps-detoxifying-gut/)

[10] Gans RE (2013). The American Institute of Balance: Continuing Education Courses for Health Care Professionals. (http://dizzy.com/education_without_boundaries.htm)

[11] Beck L (2012). "Finally: An Affordable, Valid, & Reliable EMF Pollution Solution!" (http://www.becknaturalmedicine.com/)

[12] Garber L (2012 July 19). (http://naturalsociety.com/physical-inactivity-killing-5-million-a-year/)

[13] Kohl HW 3rd, Craig CL, et al. (2012 July 21). "The pandemic of physical inactivity: Global action

for public health." *Lancet* **380** (9838): 294-305.

[14] Haas E & Levine B (2006). *Staying Healthy With Nutrition*. Berkley, California: Celestial Arts Publishing.

[15] Balch PA (2010). *Prescription for Nutritional Healing*, 5th Ed. New York, NY: Avery – a Penguin Group, Inc.

[16] Nichols JS, et al. (1997 March). "Magnetic Resonance Imaging: Utilization in the management of central nervous system trauma." *J. Trauma* **42** (3): 520-3; discussion 523-4.

[17] McGaffin PA (1996 May). "Hazards of hypoxemia: How to protect your patient from low oxygen levels." *Nursing* **26**(5): 41-6; quiz 47.

[18] Elsevier Saunders (2012). "Cyanosis; Hypoxemia." *Dorland's Illustrated Medical Dictionary*, 32nd Ed. Philadelphia, PA: Elsevier Saunders. Pp. 452, 908.

[19] O'Brien JM, Lam JYT, & Hallett JW (Authors); Porter RS, Kaplan JL, et al. (editors) (2011). "Pulse Oximetry, Atherosclerosis, & Peripheral Artery Disease." *The MERCK MANUAL of Diagnosis and Therapy*, 19th Ed. Whitehouse Station, NJ: Merck Sharp & Dohme Corp. Pp. 1856, 2081-86, 2218-21.

[20] Nonin Medical, Inc. (2003 November 6). "Nonin Medical, Inc. Announces U.S. Military Approval for Onyx® & Palmsat® Pulse Oximeters." (http://www.nonin.com/documents/onyx-palmsat%20Military%20approval.pdf)

[21] Undersea & Hyperbaric Medical Society. "Exceptional Blood Loss = Anemia." (http://www.uhms.org/ResourceLibrary/Indications/ExceptionalBloodLossAnemia/tabid/277/Default.aspx.)

[22] Garber L (2012 October 2). (http://naturalsociety.com/flouride-treatment-5-ways-to-detox-flouride/)

[23] Renter E (2013 January 7). (http://naturalsociety.com/5-steps-avoiding-detoxing-bt-toxin-found-gmo-crops/)

[24] Sears ME, Kerr KJ, Bray RI (2012). "Arsenic, cadmium, lead, & mercury in sweat: a systematic review." *J Environ Public Health* 2012: 184745.

[25] Genuis SJ, Birkholz D, Rodushkin I, Beesoon S (2011 August). "Blood, urine, & sweat (BUS) study: monitoring & elimination of bio-accumulated toxic elements." *Arch. Environ. Contam. Toxicol.* **61**(2): 344-57.

[26] Garber L (2012 August 31). (http://naturalsociety.com/top-5-antioxidant-rich-foods-aging-cancer/)

[27] Renter E (2012 October 6). (http://naturalsociety.com/what-is-detox-bath-how-take-one/)

[28] Barrett M (2013 February 19). (http://naturalsociety.com/home-remedies-for-hemorrhoids-6-natural-treatments/)

[29] Russell R (1996). *What the Bible Says about Healthy Living*. Ventura, CA: Regal Books. Page 241.

[30] Office of Dietary Supplements, NIH (2011, June 24). Dietary Supplement Fact Sheet: Vitamin D. (http://ods.od.nih.gov/factsheets/VitaminD-HealthProfessional)

[31] Holick MF (2007 July). "Vitamin D Deficiency." *The New England J. of Medicine* **357**(3): 266-81.

[32] American Society of Clinical Oncology (ASCO) (2012). "Seasonal Mortality in terminally-ill cancer patients." (http://meetinglibrary.asco.org/subcategories/2009+ASCO+Annual+Meeting)

[33] Falagas ME, et al. (2009 October 19). "Seasonality of mortality: the September phenomenon in Mediterranean countries." *CMAJ* **181**(8): 484-6.

[34] Pella JP, et al. (1999 July 30). "Seasonal variation in out of hospital cardiopulmonary arrest." *Heart* **82**(6):680.

[35] Murphy NF, et al. (2004). "Seasonal variation in morbidity & mortality related to atrial fibrillation." *International J. of Cardiology* **97**(2): 283-8.

[36] Medical News Today (2009 January 17). "Seasonal variation in Blood pressure." (http://www.medicalnewstoday.com/releases/135805.php)

[37] CNN (1999 July 12). "Summer sun for winter blues." (http://www.cnn.com/HEALTH/alternative/9907/12/sun.depression/)

[38] CDC (1995 December 22). Hypothermia-related deaths – New Mexico, October 1993 – March 1994." *MMWR MORB Mortal Weekly Rep.* **44**(50): 933-5.

[39] Gucciardi A (2012 May 1). (http://naturalsociety.com/vitamin-d-tied-toweight-loss/)

[40] Spiegel K, et al. (1999 October 23). "Impact of sleep debt on metabolic & endocrine function." *Lancet* **354**(9188): 1435-1439.

[41] Mehta KC (2013 Copyright). "Neil-Med Sinus Rinse." (http://www.neilmed.com)

[42] Goldhaber N & Raja S (2003). "Nasal Saline Irrigation" instructional hand-out from *Ear, Nose, & Throat Associates of South Florida.* (http://www.entsf.com)

[43] American Cancer Society (2008 November 1). (www.cancer.org/treatment/treatmentsandsideeffects/complementaryandalternativemedicine/pharmacologicalandbiologicaltreatment/chelation-therapy)

[44] American College for Advancement in Medicine (2002 August 14). Press release: "Physician Group Backs New NIH Chelation Therapy Study for Heart Disease." (http://www.acam.org/press_releases/20020814.htm)

[45] All4NaturalHealth.com (2011 Copyright). "Natural Chelation – Nature's Own Chelation Therapy." (http://www.all4naturalhealth.com/natural-chelation.html)

[46] Natural Standard Professional Monograph (2013 Copyright). (http://www.naturalstandard.com/monographs/monoframesmonograph=/monographs/alternativemodalities/chelation)

[47] Masters SB, Trevor AJ, & Katzung BG (2008). *Katzung & Trevor's Pharmacology: examination & board review.* McGraw Hill Medical. Pp: 481-483.

[48] Bridges S (2006). "The promise of chelation." *Mothering.* Pp: 54-61.

[49] Watson B (2010). *The Road to Perfect Health: Balance Your Gut, Heal Your Body.* Palm Harbor, FL: Renew Life Press & Information Services.

[50] Brownstein D (2006). *Iodine: Why You Need It, Why You Can't Live Without It,* 2nd Ed. W. Bloomfield, Michigan: Medical Alternatives Press.

[51] Garber L (2012 December 9). (http://www.naturalsociety.com/nutritional-value-of-food-risk-vegetables-less-nutritious/)

[52] Garber L (2012 September 10). (http://www.naturalsociety.com/simple-ways-avoid-pesticides-in-food-exposure/)

[53] Garber L (2012 October 13). (http://www.naturalsociety.com/7-nasty-effects-of-pesticides-in-food-exposure/)

[54] Coy K (2012 July 24). (http://naturalsociety.com/dirty-dozen-fruit-vegetables-clean-15/)

[55] Gucciardi A (2011 July 7). (http://naturalsociety.com/common-food-items-could-contain-180-times-more-flouride-than-tap-water/)

[56] Renter E (2012 July 28). (http://naturalsociety.com/top-10-worst-GMO-foods-list/)

[57] Gucciardi A (2012 September 19). (http://naturalsociety.com/france-launches-investigation-gmos-following-tumor-study/)

[58] Gucciardi A (2013 January 10). (http://naturalsociety.com/india-signs-mandatory-gmo-labeling-into-law/)

[59] Renter E (2013 July 7). (http://naturalsociety.com/5-steps-avoiding-detoxing-bt-toxin-found-gmo-crops/)

[60] Gucciardi A (2013 January 21). (http://naturalsociety.com/global-treaty-signed-mercrury-fda-allows-in-your-food/)

[61] Sarich C (2013 September 9) (http://naturalsociety.com/3-gmo-foods-likely-in-your-multi-vitamins/)

[62] Renter E (2013 June 27) (http://naturalsociety.com/6-foods-ingredients-sold-u-s-banned-other-countries/)

[63] Renter E (2012 September 27) (http://naturalsociety.com/5-foods-not-eat-sick-battling-cold/)

[64] Iso H, Rexrode KM, et al. (2001). "Intake of fish & omega-3 fatty acids and risk of stroke in women." *JAMA* **285** (3): 303-312.

[65] Bucher HC, et al. (2002). "N-3 polyunsaturated fatty acids in coronary heart disease: a meta-analysis of randomized controlled trial." *Am. J. Med.* **112** (4): 298-304.

[66] Burr ML, et al. (1994 August). "Diet & re-infarction." *European Heart Journal* **15**(8):1152-1153.

[67] Brown M. (1999 August 7). "Do vitamin E & fish oil protect against ischemic heart disease?" *Lancet* **354** (9177): 441-2.

[68] U.S. FDA (2004 September 4). "FDA announces qualified health claim for omega-3 fatty acids" (Press release). (http://www.fda.gov/SiteIndex/ucm108351.htm)

[69] Lewis CJ; U.S. FDA (2000 October 31). "Letter regarding Dietary Supplement Health Claim for Omega-3 Fatty acids & coronary heart disease." (http://www.fda.gov/ohrms/dockets/dockets/95s0316-Rpt0272-38-Appendix-D-Reference-F-FDA-vol205.pdf)

[70] Consumer Lab.com (2005 March 15). (http://www.consumerlab.com/results/omega3.asp)

[71] International Fish Oils Standard (2006). "Consumer Report (on contaminants in fish oil)." (http://ifosprogram.com/IFOS/ConsumerReport.aspx)

[72] Harding A (2005). "Fish & Your Heart: Eating more of it is good for you – but there's a catch." (http://cholesterolmatters.msn.com/article.aspx?aid=20)

[73] Food & Water Watch (2007). "Smart Seafood Guide 2007." (http://www.foodandwaterwatch.org/fish)

[74] Kirschmann GJ & Kirschmann JD (1996). *Nutrition Almanac*, 4th Edition. New York, NY: McGraw-Hill.

[75] AHA (2010 October 6). "Fish, Levels of Mercury and Omega 3 Fatty Acids." (http://www.americanheart.org/presenter.jhtml?identifier=3013797)

[76] Kris-Etherton PM, Harris WS, Appel LJ (2002). "Fish consumption, Fish Oil, Omega 3 Fatty Acids, and Cardiovascular Disease." *Circulation* **106**(21): 2747-57.

[77] http://www.mltoku.com/products/umeboshi/healthbenefits.html

[78] Gray R (1990 June). *The Colon Health Handbook: New Health through Colon Rejuvenation*. Scarborough Yorkshire, United Kingdom: Emerald Publishing.

[79] Barrett M (2012 May 17). (http://www.naturalsociety.com/average-american-diet-infographic)

[80] David W (2011). *Wheat Belly: Lose the wheat, lose the weight, and find your path back to health*. New York, NY: Rodale, Inc.

[81] Hamilton-Miller JMT; Gibson GR; Bruck W (2003). "Some insights into the derivation and early uses of the word 'probiotic'." *British Journal of Nutrition* **90** (4): 845.

[82] Mindell E, Mundis H (2011). *Earl Mindell's New Vitamin Bible*, Revised & Updated. New York, NY: Grand Central Life & Style.

[83] U.S. FDA Press Release (2010 October 4). "FDA issues warnings to marketers of unapproved 'chelation' products." (www.fda.gov/NewsEvents/Newsroom/PressAnnouncements/ucm229320.htm)

[84] http://naturalhealthdossier.com/2012/06/doctor-accidentally-discovers-natural-chelation-therapy-in-vietnamese-soup-2/

[85] Geleijnse JM, et al. (2004). "Dietary intake of menaquinone is associated with a reduced risk of coronary heart disease: the Rotterdam Study." *J. Nutr.* **134** (11): 3100-5.

[86] Spronk HMH, et al. (2003). "Tissue-Specific Utilization of Menaquinone-4 Results in the Prevention of Arterial Calcification of Warfarin-Treated Rats." *J. of Vascular Research* **40** (6): 531-537.

[87] James AM, et al. (2005 June 3). "Interactions of mitochondria-targeted & untargeted ubiquinones with the mitochondrial respiratory chain & reactive oxygen species: Implication for the use of exogenous ubiquinones as therapies and experimental tools." *J. Biol. Chem* **280** (22): 21295-312.

[88] Sarich C (2013 July 1). (http://naturalsociety.com/11-foods-support-liver-cleanse-diet-toxins/)

[89] Guo Z, et al. (2011 November). "Influence of consumption of probiotics on the plasma lipid profile: a meta-analysis of randomized controlled trials." *Nutr. Metab. Cardiovasc. Dis.* **21**(11): 844-50.

[90] Gucciardi A (2012 May 29). (http://naturalsociety.com/Liver-cleansing-foods/)

[91] Nie L, et al. (2006 June). "Avenanthramide, a polyphenol from oats, inhibits vascular smooth muscle proliferation and enhances nitric oxide production." *Atherosclerosis* **186** (2): 260-6.

[92] Dunnick JK (2011 February 7). "Investigating the potential for toxicity from long-term use of the herbal products, Goldenseal & Milk Thistle." *Toxicol. Pathol.* **39** (2): 398-409.

[93] Mozaffarian D, et al. (2006 April 13). "Trans Fatty Acids and Cardiovascular Disease." *New England J. of Medicine* **354** (15): 1601-1613.

[94] National Dairy Council (2004 June 18). "*Comments on Docket No 2003N-0076 Food Labeling: Trans Fatty Acids on Nutritional Labeling (PDF).*" http://fda.gov/ohrms/dockets/.../June04/.../03N-0076-emc00228-01.pdf

[95] Food and nutrition board, institute of medicine of the national academies (2005). *Dietary Reference Intakes Energy, Carbohydrate, Fiber, Fat, Fatty Acids, Cholesterol, Protein, and Amino Acids (Macronutrients)*. National Academies Press. Pp. 423, 424, 447, 504.

[96] http://www.reorbit.com/news/health/2608879/trans-fats-from-ruminant-animals-may-be-beneficial

[97] Mayo Foundation for Medical Education and Research (MFMER). "Trans-fat: Avoid this cholesterol double whammy." (http://www.mayoclinic.com/health/trans-fat/CL00032)

[98] Labarthe D (2011). "Chapter 11: Adverse Blood Lipid Profile." *Epidemiology and prevention of cardiovascular disease: a global challenge* (2nd Ed.). Jones & Bartlett Publishers. Pp. 277, 290.

[99] Lewington S, et al. (2007 December). "Blood cholesterol and vascular mortality by age, sex, and blood pressure: a meta-analysis of individual data from 61 prospective studies with 55,000 vascular deaths." *Lancet* **370** (9602): 1829-39.

[100] Thijssen MA, Mensink RP (2005). "Fatty Acids and Atherosclerotic Risk." In von Eckardstein A. *Atherosclerosis: Diet and Drugs*. Springer Science + Business Media. Pp. 171-194.

[101] Giraldo EA (Author); Porter RS, Kaplan JL, et al. (editors) (2011). "Stroke." *The MERCK MANUAL of Diagnosis & Therapy*, 19th Ed. Whitehouse Station, NJ: Merck Sharp & Dohme Corp. Pp. 1643-55.

[102] Libby P (Author); Longo DL, Fauci AS, Kasper DL, Hauser SL, Jameson JL, Loscalzo J (editors) (2012). "The Pathogenesis, Prevention, & Treatment of Atherosclerosis." *Harrison's Principles of Internal Medicine*, 18th Edition. New York, NY: McGraw-Hill Co., Inc. Pp. 1983-92.

[103] Mitchell RS, et al. (2007). *Robbins Basic pathology: With Student CONSULT Online Access* (8th Ed.). Philadelphia, PA: Saunders. Page 345.

[104] Mayo Clinic (2008, March 27). "Normal Weight Obesity: An Emerging Risk Factor for Heart & Metabolic Problems." *Science Daily*. (http://www.sciencedaily.com/releases/2008/03/080327172025.htm)

[105] Cacciatore L, Cerio R, et al. (1991). "The therapeutic effect of L-carnitine in patients with exercise-induced stable angina: a controlled study." *Drugs Exp. Clin. Res* **17** (4): 225-235.

[106] Bartels GL, et al. (1994 July). "Effects of L-propionylcarnitine on ischemia-induced myocardial dysfunction in men with angina pectoris." *The American J. of Cardiology* **74**(2): 125-130.

[107] U. of Maryland Medical Center (http://www.umm.edu/altmed/articles/carnitine-1-000291.htm)

[108] Mohr D, et al. (1992 June). "Dietary supplementation with coenzyme Q10 results in increased levels of ubiquinol-10 within circulating lipoproteins and increased resistance of human low-density lipoprotein to the initiation of lipid peroxidation." *Biochem. Biophys. Acta* **1126**(3):247-54.

[109] Alleva R, et al. (1995 September). "The roles of coenzyme Q10 and vitamin E on the peroxidation of human low density lipoprotein subfractions." *Proc. Natl. Acad. Sci. U.S.A.* **92**(20): 9388-91.

[110] Konkle B (Author) & Weitz JI (Author); Longo Dl, Fauci AS, et al. (editors) (2012). "Bleeding & Thrombosis: Herbal supplements associated with increased bleeding; Antiplatelet, Anticoagulant & Fibrinolytic Drugs." *Harrison's Principles of Internal Medicine*, 18th Ed., New York, NY: McGraw-Hill Co., Inc. Pp. 457-464; & 998-1004.

[111] Turpie AGG (Author); Porter RS, Kaplan JL (editors) (2011). "Treatment & Prevention of

DVT." *The Merck Manual of Diagnosis & Therapy*, 19th Ed. Whitehouse Station, NJ: Merck Sharp & Dohme Corp. Pp.2228-31.

[112] Dept. of Nursing @ U. of Wisconsin Hospitals & Clinics Authority (2011 June 20). "Medications and Herbs Which Affect Bleeding." (http://www.uwhealth.org/healthfacts/B_EXTRANET_HEALTH_INFORMATION-FlexMember-Show_Public_HFFY-1126651115765.html).

[113] Levison ME (Author); Porter RS, Kaplan JL, et al. (editors) (2011). "Common effects of antibiotics on other drugs." *The Merck Manual of Diagnosis & Therapy*, 19th Ed. Whitehouse Station, NJ: Merck Sharp & Dohme Corp. P. 1183t.

[114] Suttie JW (1995). "The importance of menaquinones in human nutrition." *Annu. Rev. Nutr.* 15: 399-417.

[115] Havrda DE, et al. (2005). "Enhanced anti-thrombic effect of warfarin associated with low-dose alcohol consumption." *Pharmacotherapy* 25: 303-7.

[116] Tonelli J, Fleming JH, et al. (editors) (2011). "Cymbalta & Abnormal Bleeding of SSRIs & SNRIs; Celebrex & Risk of bleeding from NSAIDs List." *Physicians' Desk reference*, PDR 66th Ed., 2012. Montvale, NJ: PDR Network, LLC. Pp. 1602-1612, & 2723-2731.

[117] Shulman S (2006). "Herbal Drugs (phytomedicines) that can cause bleeding." (http://www.wfh.org/2/1/1_1_6_Drugs_list.htm) World Federation of Hemophilia (WFH).

[118] http://www.webmd.com/drugs/drug-6306-diazepam.aspx?drugid=6306&drugname=diazepam&source=1&pagenumber=6

[119] Schroder H, et al. (1990). "Helenalin and 11 alpha, 13-dihydrohelanin, two constituents from *Arnica Montana L.*, inhibit platelet function via thiol-dependent pathways." *Thromb. Res.* 57: 839-45.

[120] Murray L, Reed J, et al (editors) (2010). "Dietary Supplement Profiles; Herbal Medicine Profiles." *PDR for NonPrescription Drugs, Dietary Supplements, & Herbs*, PDR 32nd Ed., 2011. Montvale, NJ: PDR Network, LLC. Pp. 579-610.

[121] Guivernau M, et al. (1994). "Clinical & Experimental study on the long-term effect of dietary gamma-linolenic acid on plasma lipids, platelet aggregation, thromboxane formation, & prostacyclin production." *Prostaglandins Leukot. Essent. Fatty Acids* 51: 311-16.

[122] Fundukian LJ, et al. (editors) (2009). *The Gale Encyclopedia of Alternative Medicine*, 3rd Ed. Farmington Hills, MI: Gale Cengage Learning.

[123] Elvin-Lewis M (2001). "Should we be concerned about herbal remedies?" *J. of Ethnopharmacology* 75(2-3):141-164.

[124] Iwakami S, et al. (1992). "Platelet activating factor (PAF) antagonists contained in medicinal plants: lignans & sesquiterpenes." *Chem. Pharm. Bull* (Tokyo) 40: 1196-98.

[125] Hogaboam CM, Wallace JL (1991). Inhibition of platelet aggregation by capsaicin. An effect unrelated to actions on sensory afferent neurons." *Eur. J. Pharmacol.* 202: 129-131.

[126] Teng CM, Lee LG, et al. (1985). "Inhibition of platelet aggregation by apigenin from Apium graveolens." *Asia Pac. J. Pharmacol.* 3: 85.

[127] Yoona S-J, Yub M-A, et al. (2003). "The nontoxic mushroom *Auricularia auricular* contains a polysaccharide with anticoagulant activity mediated by antithrombin." *Thrombosis Research* **112** (3): 151-8.

[128] Chen SJ, et al. (1996). "Antiplatelet & calcium inhibitory properties of eugenol & sodium eugenol acetate." *Gen. Pharmacol.* 27: 629-33.

[129] Unger M, Frank A (2004). "Simultaneous determination of the inhibitory potency of herbal extracts on the activity of six major cytochrome P450 enzymes using liquid chromatography/mass spectrometry & automated online extraction." *Rapid Commun. Mass Spectrum* 18: 2273-81.

[130] Petroni A, et al. (1995 April 15). "Inhibition of platelet aggregation and eicosanoid production by phenolic components of olive oil." *Thrombosis Research* 78 (2): 151-160.

[131] Beauchamp GK, et al. (2005 September). "Phytochemistry: ibuprofen-like activity in extra-virgin olive oil." *Nature* 437 (7055): 45-6.

[132] Gadkari JV & Joshi VD (1991). "Effect of ingestion of raw garlic on serum cholesterol level,

clotting time, & fibrinolytic activity in normal subjects." *J. Postgrad Med.* 37: 128-131.

[133] Cupp MJ (1999). "Herbal remedies: Adverse effects & drug interactions." *American Family Physician* **59** (5): 1239-45.

[134] Gruenwald J, et al. (2007). *PDR for Herbal Medicines,* 4th Ed. Montvale, NJ: Thomson Healthcare Inc.

[135] Freedman JE, et al. (2001). "Select flavonoids and whole juice from purple grapes inhibit platelet function and enhance nitric oxide release." *Circulation* 103: 2792-8.

[136] Vitseva O, et al. (2005 October). "Grape seed & grape skin extracts inhibit platelet function and release oxygen intermediates." *J. Cardiovasc. Pharmacol.* **46**(4): 445-51.

[137] Shanmuganayagam D, et al. (2002 December). "Grape seed & grape skin extracts - elicit a greater antiplatelet effect when used in combination than when used individually in dogs & humans." *J. Nutr.* **132**(12): 3592-8.

[138] Bydlowski SP, et al. (1991). "An aqueous extract of guarana (*Paullinia cupana*) decreases platelet thromboxane synthesis." *Braz. J. Med. Biol. Res.* **24**(4): 421-4.

[139] Yu Z, Zhang G, Zhao H (1997). "Effects of Puerariae isoflavone on blood viscosity, thrombosis, and platelet function." *Zhong Yao Cai* 20: 468-9.

[140] Ge T, Sun Z, et al. (2005). "Cloning of thrombolytic enzyme (lumbrokinase) from earthworm & its' expression in the yeast." *Protein Expression and Purification* **42**(1): 20.

[141] Zou QZ, et al. (1989). "Effect of Motherwort on blood hyper-viscosity." *Am. J. Chin. Med.* **17**(1-2): 65-70.

[142] Chang YY, et al. (2008). "Cerebellar hemorrhage provoked by combined use of nattokinase and aspirin in a patient with cerebral micro-bleeds." *Intern Med.* **47**(5): 467-9.

[143] Mozaffarian D (2005). "Does alpha-linolenic acid intake reduce the risk of coronary heart disease? A review of the evidence." *Alternative Therapies in Health & Medicine* **11**(3): 24-30; quiz 31, 79.

[144] Matthaus B (2011 November). "Seed Oil Fatty Acids – SOFA Database Retrieval." (http://sofa.mri.bund.de/)

[145] Li Thomas SC (1999). "Sea buckthorn: New Crop opportunity." *Perspectives on new crops and new uses.* Alexandria, VA: ASHS Press. Pp. 335-7.

[146] von Schacky C (2003 March). "The role of omega-3 fatty acids in cardiovascular disease." *Curr. Atheroscler. Rep.* **5**(2): 139-45.

[147] Wang C, et al. (2006). "N-3 fatty acids from fish or fish-oil supplements, but not alpha-linolenic acid, benefit cardiovascular disease outcomes in primary- and secondary-prevention studies: a systematic review." *The American J. of Clin. Nutr.* **84**(1): 5-17.

[148] Brenna JT (2002 March). "Efficiency of conversion of alpha-linolenic acid to long chain n-3 fatty acids in man." *Curr. Opin. Clin. Nutr. Metab. Care* **5**(2): 127-132.

[149] Burdge GC & Calder PC (2005 September). "Conversion of alpha-linolenic acid to longer-chain polyunsaturated fatty acids in human adults." *Reprod. Nutr. Dev.* **45**(5): 581-597.

[150] Wang Y & Ma R (1990). "Effect of an extract of *paeonia latiflora* on the blood coagulative and fibrinolytic enzymes." *Zhong Xi Yi, Jie He Za Zhi* **10**(2): 101-2, 70.

[151] Putter M, et al. (1999). "Inhibition of smoking-induced platelet aggregation by aspirin & pycnogenol." *Thrombosis research* **95**(4): 155-61.

[152] Murphy KJ (2003 June). "Dietary flavanols and procyanidin oligomers from cocoa (*Theobroma cacao*) inhibit platelet function." *Am. J. Clin. Nutr.* **77**(6): 146-73.

[153] Wang S, et al. (1999). "The effect of pycnogenol on the microcirculation, platelet function, and ischemic myocardium in patients with coronary artery disease." *Eur. Bull Drug. Res.* 7: 19-25.

[154] Hubbard GP, et al. (2004). "Ingestion of quercitin inhibits platelet aggregation and essential components of the collagen-stimulated platelet activation pathway in humans." *J. Thromb. Haemost.* 2: 2138-45.

[155] Liu J, et al. (2006 December). "Structure-activity relationship for inhibition of 5 alpha-reductase by triterpenoids isolated from Ganoderma lucidum." *Biorg. Med. Chem.* **14**(24):8654-60.

[156] Olas B & Wachoxicz B (2005 August). "Resveratrol, a phenolic antioxidant with effects on blood platelet functions." *Platelets* **16**(5): 251-60.

[157] Stef G, et al. (2006 August). "Resveratrol inhibits aggregation of platelets from high-risk cardiac patients with aspirin resistance." *J. Cardiovasc. Pharmacol.* **48**(2): 1-5.

[158] Cheema P, et al. (2001). "Intraoperative hemorrhage associated with the use of extract of saw palmetto berry herb: a case report and review of the literature." *J. Intern Med.* 250: 167-9.

[159] Shah BH, et al. (1999). "Inhibitory effect of curcumin, a food spice from turmeric, on platelet-activating factor- and arachidonic acid-mediated platelet aggregation through the inhibition of thromboxane formation and Ca2+ Signaling." *Biochem. Pharmacol.* 58: 1167-72.

[160] Krivoy N, et al. (2001). "Effect of *salicis cortex* extract on human platelet aggregation." *Planta Med.* 67: 209-12.

[161] Hing Kwok Chu, Joe @ Complementary & Alternative U. of California (2013 September 21 – last updated). (http://alternativehealing.org/side_effect_of_some_herbs.htm)

[162] Cronin AJ, et al. (2002). "Aristolochic acid as a causative factor in a case of Chinese herbal neuropathy." *Nephrol. Dial. Transplant* 17: 524-5.

[163] Newman JH (Author); Porter RS, et al. (editors) (2011). "Drug, Herbal Preparation, & Food Interactions with Warfarin." *The Merck Manual of Diagnosis & Therapy*, 19th Edition. Whitehouse Station, NJ: Merck Sharp & Dohme Corp. Pp. 1917t, 1918t, 1919t.

[164] Suvarna R, et al. (2003). "Possible interaction between warfarin and cranberry juice." *Curr. Prob. Pharmacovigilance* 29: 8.

[165] Ziegler EE (2011 November). "Consumption of cow's milk as a cause of iron deficiency in infants and toddlers." *Nutr. Rev.* **69** Suppl 1: S37-42.

[166] Nutrient Data Laboratory, Agriculture Research Service, US Dept. of Agriculture (2010 May). "USDA Database for the Oxygen Radical Absorbance Capacity (ORAC) of Selected Foods, Release 2 – May 2010." (http://www.ars.gov/SP2UserFiles/Place/12354500/Data/ORAC/ORAC_R2.pdf)

[167] U.S. FDA, Center for Food Safety & Applied Nutrition (2008 June). "Guidance for industry, Food Labeling; Nutrient Content Claims; Definition for 'High Potency' and Definition for 'Antioxidant' for use in Nutrient Content Claims for Dietary Supplements and Conventional Foods." (http://www.fda.gov/OHRMS/DOCKETS/98fr/FDA-1995-N-0400-GDL.pdf)

[168] European Food Safety Authority (EFSA) Panel on Dietetic Products, Nutrition and Allergies (2010). "Scientific Opinion on the substantiation of health claims related to various food(s)/food constituents and protection of cells from premature aging, antioxidant activity, antioxidant content and antioxidant properties, and protection of DNA, proteins & lipids from oxidative damage pursuant to Article 13(1) of Regulation (EC) No 1924/20061." *EFSA Journal 2010* **8**(2): 1489.

[169] Renter E (2013 May 29). (http://naturalsociety.com/studies-apples-prevent-cancerous-tumors/)

[170] Garber L (2012 September 17). (http://naturalsociety.com/powerful-healing-properties-of-5-common-household-organic-spices/)

[171] Sarich C (2013 October 27). (http://naturalsociety.com/ginger-root-kills-ovarian-prostate-cancer-cells-better-chemo/)

[172] Renter E (2013 October 28). (http://naturalsociety.com/4-herbs-need-medicine-cabinet/)

[173] Sarich C (2013 July 13). (http://naturalsociety.com/cauliflower-treats-prevents-various-cancers-sulforaphanes/)

[174] Chiu CJ, et al. (2011). "Informing Food Choices & Health Outcomes by Use of the Dietary Glycemic Index." *Nutr. Rev.* **69**(4):231-42.

[175] Blakau B, et al. (1998 March). "High blood glucose concentration is a risk factor for mortality in middle-aged non-diabetic men. Twenty-year follow-up in the Whitehall Study, the Paris Prospective Study, & the Helsinki Policemen Study." *Diabetes Care* **21** (3): 360-7.

[176] Mendez J (2004 August-September). "The Euglycaemic Status and Infections." *Townsend Letter for Doctors and Families.*

[177] Atkinson F, et al. (2008 December). "International Tables of Glycemic Index & Glycemic Load Values: 2008." *Diabetes Care* **31** (12): 2281-2283.

[178] Glycemic Research Institute (2010). "Glycemic Index Defined." (http://www.glycemic.com/GlycemicIndex-LoadDefined.htm)

[179] http://nutritiondata.self.com/topics/glycemic-index

[180] Pawlak, et al. (2004). "Effects of dietary glycaemic index on adiposity, glucose homeostasis, & plasma lipids in animals." *Lancet* **28364** (9436): 778-85.

[181] Temelkova-Hurtschiev TS, et al. (2000 December). "Post-challenge plasma glucose and glycemic spikes are more strongly associated with atherosclerosis than fasting glucose or HbA1c level." *Diabetes Care* **23** (12): 1830-4.

[182] Gucciardi A (2012 November 28). (http://naturalsociety.com/study-high-fructose-corn-syrup-causing-diabetes-us-citizen-eats-55-lbs-per-year/)

[183] Renter E (2013 April 16). (http://naturalsociety.com/revealing-connection-sugar-and-cancer/)

[184] Barrett M (2012 March 8). (http://naturalsociety.com/common-cancer-causing-chemical-in-soda-exposed-by-scientists/)

[185] Abdullateef RA & Osman M (2012 January 1). "Studies on effects of pruning on vegetative traits *rebaudiana Bertoni* (Compositae)." *International J. of Biology* **4**(1): 146.

[186] Goyal SK, et al. (2010 February). "Stevia a bio-sweetener: a review." *Int. J. Food Sci. Nutr.* **61**(1): 1-10.

[187] Ulbright C, et al. (2010 April). "An evidence-based systematic review of stevia by the National Standard Research Collaboration." *Cardiovascular Hematol. Agents Med. Chem.* **8**(2): 113-27.

[188] Chatsudthipong V & Muanprasat C (2009 January). "Stevio-side & related compounds: therapeutic benefits beyond sweetness." *Pharmacolo. Ther.* **121**(1): 41-54.

[189] FDA.gov (2012 April 4 – last updated). "What refined Stevia preparations have been evaluated by FDA to be used as a sweetener." (www.fda.gov/AboutFDA/Transparency/Basics/ucm214865.htm)

[190] World Health Organization (2008 July 4). *Joint FAO/WHO Expert Committee on food additives, 69th meeting.*

[191] The American Journal of Clinical Nutrition (2002 January 1). "International table of glycemic index and glycemic load values." (http://ajcn.nutrition.org/content/76/1/5/T1.expansion.html)

[192] Marti N, et al. (2008 July). "An update on alternative sweeteners." *International Sugar J.* **110** (1315): 425-429.

[193] Ritter AV, et al. (2013 June). "Tooth-Surface-Specific Effects of Xylitol: Randomized Trial Results." *J. of Dental Research* **92**(6): 512-517.

[194] Azarpazhooh A, et al. (2011 November 9). "Xylitol for preventing acute otitis media in children up to 12 years of age." *Cochrane Database of Systemic Reviews* (11): CD007095.

[195] Wang YM & van Eys J (1981). "Nutritional Significance of fructose & sugar alcohols." *Annual Review of Nutrition* **1**: 437-75.

[196] Dunayer EK, et al. (2006 October). "Acute hepatic failure & coagulopathy associated with xylitol ingestion in eight dogs." *J. of the American Veterinary Medical Association* **229**(7): 1113-1117.

[197] Garber L (2012 September 17). (http://naturalsociety.com/is-diet-soda-bad-for-you-4-major-negative-impacts/)

[198] Renter E (2012 November 24). (http://naturalsociety.com/aspartame-cancer-link-exposed-increasing-cancer-risk/)

[199] Golay A, et al. (2000). "Similar weight loss with low-energy food combining or balanced diets." *Int. J. Obes. Relat. Metab. Disord.* **24**(4): 492-496.

[200] Diamond H & Diamond M (1985). *Fit for Life I*; & (1989) *Fit for Life II*. Diamond H (2003) *Fit for Life: Not Fat for Life*. Deerfield Beach, FL: Health Communications, Inc.

[201] Vasey C (2003 – English Translation from French 1999). *The Acid-Alkaline Diet: for Optimum Health*. Rochester, Vermont: Healing Arts Press.

[202] ScienceDaily.com (2011 August 8). "Buyer Beware: Herbal Products Missing Key Safety Information." (http://www.sciencedaily.com/releases/2011/08/110808202506.htm)

[203] U.S. FDA & Web MD Partnership (2012, April 20). (http://www.webmd.com/fda/fda-101-dietarysupplements) & (http://www.webmd.com/fda/avoiding-drug-interactions)

[204] Centers for Disease Control (CDC) & Prevention, National Center for Injury Prevention & Control (2012 February 1). "Web based Injury Reporting System (WISQARS)." (http://www.cdc.gov/injury/wisqars)

[205] 2010 Annual Report of the American Association of Poison Control Centers National Poison Data System (NPDS): 28th Annual Report. (http://www.aapcc.org/dnn/NPDSPoisonData/NPDSAnnualreports.aspx)

[206] Bengmark S, et al. (2001 Nov-Dec). "Use of pro, pre-, & synbiotics in the ICU – future options." Nutr. Hosp. 16(6): 239-56.

[207] Tursi A, et al. (2010 October). "Treatment of relapsing mild-to-moderate ulcerative colitis with the probiotic VSL H3 as an adjunctive to a standard pharmaceutical treatment: a double blind, randomized, placebo-controlled study." Am. J. Gastroenterol. 105 (10): 2218-27.

[208] Baldassarre ME, et al. (2010 March). "Lactobacillus GG improves recovery in infants with blood in the stools and presumptive allergic colitis compared with extensively hydrolyzed formula alone." J. Pediatr. 156(3): 397-401.

[209] Hayes GL, et al. (2011 Oct-Dec). "Nutritional Supplements in Critical Illness." AACN Adv. Crit. Care 22(4): 301-16; quiz 317-8.

[210] Krass P, et al. (2006). "Decreased gum bleeding and reduced gingivitis by the probiotic Lactobacillus reuteri." Swed. Dent. J. 30(2): 55-60.

[211] Aiba Y, et al. (1998 November). "Lactic acid-mediated suppression of Helicobacter pylori by the oral administration of Lactobacillus Salivarius as a probiotic in a gnotobiotic murine model." Am. J. Gastroenterol. 93(11): 2097-2101.

[212] Pang QF, et al. (2009 May 1). "Protective effects of a heme oxygenase-1 – secreting Lactococcus lactis on mucosal injury induced by hemorrhagic shock in rats." J. Surg. Res. 153(1): 39-45.

[213] Balamuruyan R, et al. (2010 Oct.). "Low levels of fecal lactobacilli in women with iron-deficiency anemia in south India." Br. J. Nutr. 104(7): 931-4.

[214] D'Arrigo T from American Gastroenterological Association (2010 April 24). "Probiotics: What they are & what they can do for you." (http://www.gastro.org/patient-center/diet-medications/probiotics)

[215] American Academy of Pediatrics Committee on Fetus and Newborn (2003 July). "AAPCFN: Controversies concerning vitamin K and the newborn." Pediatrics 112(1 Pt 1): 191-2.

[216] Didangelos A, et al. (2009 May). "Proteomics of acute coronary syndromes." Current atherosclerosis reports 11(3): 188-95.

[217] Sparrow CP & Olszewski J (1993 July). "Cellular oxidation of low density lipoprotein is caused by thiol production in media containing transition metal ions." J. of lipid research 34(7): 1219-28.

[218] Tsujioka T, et al. (2006 May). "The mechanisms of vitamin K2-induced apoptosis of myeloma cells." Haematologica. 91(5): 613-9.

[219] Habu D, et al. (2004 July 21). "Role of vitamin K2 in the development of hepatocellular carcinoma in women with viral cirrhosis of the liver." JAMA 292(3): 358-61.

[220] Harrington DJ, et al. (2008 April). "A study of the prevalence of vitamin K deficiency in patients with cancer referred to a hospital palliative care team and its association with abnormal haemostasis." J. Clin. Pathol. 61(4): 537-40.

[221] Salminem S, et al. (1998). "Functional food science & gastrointestinal physiology & function." Br. J. Nutr. 80(Suppl): S147-71.

[222] Sazawal S, et al. (2006 June). "Efficacy of probiotics in prevention of acute diarrhea: a meta-analysis of masked, randomized, placebo-controlled trials." Lancet Infect. Dis. 6(6): 374-82.

[223] http://www.nutraingredients.com/Regulation/EFSA-calls-for-characterisation-work-as-probiotic-resubmissions-loom

[224] Tsukamoto Y (2000). "Intake of fermented soybean (natto) increases circulating vitamin K2 (menaquinone-7) & gamma-carboxylated osteocalcin concentration in normal individuals." J. Bone Miner. Metab. 18(4): 216-22.

[225] Ansell J, et al. (2004). "The pharmacology and management of the vitamin K antagonists: the

Seventh ACCP Conference on Antithrombotic and Thrombolytic Therapy." *Chest* **126** (3 Suppl): 204S-233S.

[226] Booth SL, Centurelli MA (1999). "Vitamin K: a practical guide to the dietary management of patients on warfarin." *Nutr. Rev.* **57** (pt. 1): 288-296.

[227] Community Anticoagulation Therapy (CAT) Clinic @ Cedar Rapids Health Care Alliance (2006 Copyright).
(http://www.crhealthcarealliance.org/Portals/0/CRHA%20files/warfarin/My%20Guide%20to%2
0Warfarin%20therapy.pdf).

[228] Faloon W (2009 January). (http://www.lef.org/magazine/mag2009/jan2009_Vitamin-K-Protection-Against-Arterial-Calcification-Bone-Loss-Cancer-and-Aging/)

[229] Beulens JW, et al. (2008 July 19). "High dietary menaquinone intake is associated with reduced coronary calcification." *Atherosclerosis* **203**(2): 489-93.

[230] Schurgers LJ, et al. (2007 April 1). "Regression of warfarin-induced medial elastocalcinosis by high intake of vitamin K in rats." *Blood* **109**(7): 2823-31.

[231] Masterjohn C (2007 Spring). "On the trail of the Elusive X-Factor: Vitamin K2 Revealed." *Wise Traditions in Food, Farming, & the Healing Arts* (http://www.westonprice.org/fat-soluble-activators/x-factor-is-vitamin-K2).

[232] Cheung AM, et al. (2008). "Vitamin K Supplementation in Postmenopausal Women with osteopenia (ECKO Trial): A Randomized Controlled Trial." *PLoS Med.* **5** (10): e196.

[233] Tsuka (2004). "Studies on action of menaquinone-7 in regulation of bone metabolism and its preventative role of osteoporosis." *BioFactors* **22**(1-4): 5-19.

[234] Rasmussen SE, et al. (2006 March). "A safe strategy for addition of vitamins & minerals to foods." *European J. of Nutrition* **45**(3): 123-135

[235] Asakura H, et al. (2001). "Vitamin K administration to elderly patients with osteoporosis induces no hemostatic activation, even in those with suspected vitamin K deficiency." *Osteoporosis International* **12**(12): 996-1000.

[236] Elder SJ, et al. (2006 January). "Vitamin K contents of meat, dairy, & fast food in the U.S. diet." *J. Agric. Food Chem.* **54**(2): 463-7.

[237] Conly J, Stein K (1994). "Reduction of vitamin K2 concentrations in human liver associated with the use of broad-spectrum antimicrobials." *Clinical & investigative medicine* **17**(6): 531-539.

[238] Mullen BA, et al. (2002). "Ascorbic Acid Reduces Blood Pressure & Arterial Stiffness in Type 2 Diabetes." *Hypertension* **40** (6): 804-9.

[239] Khaw Kay-Tee, Bingham S, et al. (2001 March). "Relation between plasma ascorbic acid and mortality in men & women in EPIC-Norfolk prospective study: a prospective population study. European Prospective Investigation into Cancer & Nutrition." *Lancet* **357**(9257): 657-663.

[240] Rebouche CJ (1991). "Ascorbic acid & carnitine biosynthesis." *The American J. of Clin. Nutrition* **54** (6 Suppl): 1147S-1152S.

[241] Patrick L (2006). "Lead Toxity, Parts I & II." *Alternative Medicine Review* **11**(1): 2-22; & **11**(2): 114-27.

[242] Patrick L (2003 May). "Toxic Metals & Antioxidants." *Alternative Medicine Review* **8**(2): 106-128.

[243] U.S. Dept of Agriculture Research Service (2010). USDA National Nutrient Database for Standard Reference, Release 23. Nutrient Data Laboratory.
(http://www.ars.usda.gov/ba/bhnrc/ndl)

[244] Wilson JX (2005). "Regulation of vitamin C transport." *Annu. Rev. Nutr.* **25**: 105-125.

[245] Hemila H, et al. (2007). "Vitamin C for preventing & treating the common cold." *Cochrane database of systematic reviews* (3): CD000980.

[246] USDA SR-21 "Cilantro" (2012). (http://nutritiondata.self.com/facts/vegetables-and-vegetable-products/2414/2)

[247] Ebo DG, et al. (2006 April 16). "Coriander anaphylaxis in a spice grinder with undetected occupational allergy." *Acta Clinica Belgica* **61**(3): 152-156.

[248] Garber L (2012 September 25). (http://naturalsociety.com/7-best-foods-for-weight-loss-

274

overall-health/)

[249] Droge W & Holm E (1997). "Role of cysteine & glutathione in HIV infection and other disease associated with muscle wasting and immunological dysfunction." *The Fed. Of Amer. Soc. For Exp. Bio. (FASEB) J.* **11** (13): 1077-89.

[250] Dean O (2011 March). "N-Acetylcysteine in psychiatry. Current therapeutic evidence and potential mechanisms of action." *J. Psychiatry Neurosci.* **36**(2): 78-86.

[251] Droge W & Holm E (1997). "Role of cysteine and glutathione in HIV infection and other diseases associated with muscle wasting & immunological dysfunction." *The Fed. of Amer. Societies for Exp. Bio. (FASEB) J.* **11**(13):1077-89.

[252] Gondwe M, et al. (2008 Jan-Feb). "Effects of *Persea Americana Mill* (Lauraceae) ["Avocado"] ethanol leaf extract on blood glucose and kidney function in streptozocin-induced diabetic rats and on kidney cell lines of the proximal (LLCPK1) & distal tubules (MDBK)." *Methods Find Exp. Clin. Pharmacol.* **30**(1): 25-35.

[253] Renter E (2012 Sept. 29). (http://naturalsociety.com/how-to-increase-dopamine-levels-foods/)

[254] Patterson S (2012 Dec 6). (http://naturalsociety.com/worried-about-flouride-exposure-protect-yourself-selenium/)

[255] Garber L (2012 Dec 8). (http://naturalsociety.com/4-natural-liver-detox-foods/)

[256] Lau-Benjamin HS (2001). "Suppression of LDL oxidation by garlic." *J. Nutr.* **131** (3S): 958S-988S.

[257] Gucciardi A (2012 Nov 1). (http://naturalsociety.com/5-powerful-healing-properties-of-garlic/)

[258] Fassa P (2013 July 17). (http://naturalsociety.com/12-tips-extinguishing-disease-causing-Inflammation/)

[259] Barrett M (2012 April 24). (http://naturalsociety.com/benefits-of-ginger/)

[260] Chuengsamaen S, et al. (2012 Nov). "Curcumin Extract for Prevention of Type 2 Diabetes." *Diabetes Care* **35**: 2121-2127.

[261] Renter E (2013 Sept 15). (http://naturalsociety.com/turmeric-oral-health-gingivitis-mouth-cancer-more/)

[262] Dutton PL, et al. (2000). "4 coenzyme Q oxidation reduction reactions in mitochondrial electron transport." In Kagen VE & Quinn PJ. *Coenzyme Q: Molecular mechanisms in health and disease.* Boca Raton, FL: CRC Press pp. 65-82.

[263] Sandor PS, et al. (2005). "Efficacy of coenzyme Q10 in migraine prophylaxis: a randomized controlled trial." *Neurology* **64**(4): 713-5.

[264] Tracy MJ (2003). "Ch. 4: Coenzyme Q10 (ubiquinone, Ubidecarenone)." *Dietary Supplements: Toxicology and Clinical Pharmacology.* Humana Press pp. 53-85.

[265] Ghirlanda G, et al. (1993). "Evidence of plasma CoQ10-lowering effect by HMG-CoA reductase inhibitors: a double-blind, placebo-controlled study." *J. of clinical pharmacology* **33**(3): 226-9.

[266] Golumb BA, Evans MA (2008). "Statin adverse effects: a review of the literature and evidence for a mitochiondrial mechanism." *Am. J. Cardiovasc. Drugs* **8** (6): 373-418.

[267] Hathcock JN, Shao A (2006 Aug). "Risk assessment for coenzyme Q10." *Regul. Toxicol. Pharm.* **45**(3): 282-8.

[268] U.S. NIH: Medline Plus (2012 May 17 – last updated). "Vitamin D." (www.nlm.nih.gov/medlineplus/druginfo/natural/929.html)

[269] Sarich C (2013 October 20). (http://naturalsociety.com/8-foods-high-in-magnesium-mineral/)

[270] Shaw D, et al. (1997). "Traditional remedies and food supplements: a 5 year toxicology study (1991-1995)." *Drug Saf.* 17:342-56.

[271] Steinberg D (2007). *The Cholesterol Wars: The Cholesterol Skeptics vs the Preponderance of Evidence.* Boston, MA: Academic Press.

[272] Ravnskov U (2000). *The Cholesterol Myths: Exposing the Fallacy that Saturated Fat and Cholesterol Cause Heart Disease.* New Trends Publishing, Incorporated.

[273] D'Agostino RB, Sr., et al. (2008 Feb. 12). "General Cardiovascular Risk Profile for use in

primary care: The Framingham Heart Study." *Circulation* **117** (6): 757-63.

[274] AHA (2010 May 21 – last updated). "Frequently Asked Questions about Fats." (http://www.heart.org/HEARTORG/GettingHealthy/NutritionCenter/HealthyDietGoals/Frequentl y-Asked-Questions-About-Fats_UCM_306069_Article.jsp)

[275] Siro-Tarino PW, et al. (2010 March). "Meta-analysis of prospective cohort studies evaluating the association of saturated fat on cardiovascular disease." *The American J. of Clin. Nutrition* **91**(3): 535-46.

[276] Hu FB, Stampfer MJ (1999 November). "Nut consumption and risk of coronary heart disease: a review of epidemiological evidence." *Current Atherosclerosis Reports* **1**(3): 204-209.

[277] Mozaffarian D, et al; Katan MB, editor (2010 March). "Effects on Coronary Heart Disease of Increasing Polyunsaturated Fat in Place of Saturated Fat: A Systematic Review & Met-Analysis of Randomized Controlled Trials." *PLoS Medicine* **7**(3): 1-10.

[278] Sarich C (2013 November 19). (http://www.naturalsociety.com/essiac-tea-4-secret-ingredients-cured-thousands-cancer-patients/)

[279] Fallon S, Enig M (1996 May). "How Safe is SOY?" *Newlife* Pp. 37-39.

[280] Park YW (1991). "Relative buffering capacity of goat's milk, cow milk, soy-based infant formulas, & commercial non-prescription antacid drugs." *Journal of Dairy Science* **74** (10): 3326-3333.

[281] Duckett SK, et al. (1993). "Effects of time on feed on beef nutrient composition." *J. Anim. Sci.* **71**(8): 2079-88.

[282] Omega-3centre.com (2008 July 18). (http://www.omega-3centre.com/sources_long_chain.html)

[283] Duckett SK, et al. (2009 Sept). "Effects of winter stocker growth rate and finishing system on: III. Tissue proximate, fatty acid, vitamin & cholesterol content." *J. of Animal Sci.* **87**(9): 2961-70.

[284] Sheepandgoat.com (2005 Feb 15 – last updated). (http://www.sheep101info/labeledlamb.html).

[285] Donsbach K (1988). *Glandular Extracts*. Rosarito Beach, Baja CA: Wholistic Publishers.